BEST BREAST 2

BEST BREAST 2

The

ULTIMATE

*discriminating
woman's resource
for breast
augmentation*

John B. Tebbetts, MD
Terrye B. Tebbetts

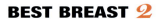

BEST BREAST 2

The Ultimate Discriminating Woman's Resource
for Breast Augmentation

Manufactured in China.

For information, please contact:

Brown Books Publishing Group

16200 North Dallas Parkway, Suite 170

Dallas, Texas 75248

www.brownbooks.com

972-381-0009

A New Era in Publishing™

ISBN-13: 978-1-933285-77-1

ISBN-10: 1-933285-77-X

LCCN 2007925310

1 2 3 4 5 6 7 8 9 10

If you are considering breast augmentation surgery,

If you are discriminating, and like to know the facts before making decisions,

If you believe in the value of common sense combined with knowledge,

If you want one resource that contains the most information about breast augmentation,

If you want to take full advantage of recent innovations that have redefined the patient and surgeon experience in breast augmentation, enabling most patients to be out to dinner the evening of surgery and return to full, normal activities in twenty-four hours,

If you want information based on experience from two of the world's experts in the field of breast augmentation—a surgeon and a woman who cares for augmentation patients every day, with a combined experience of over forty years,

If you decide to have breast augmentation and you'd like to get the BEST BREAST,

THIS BOOK IS FOR YOU!

TABLE OF CONTENTS

PREFACE

Where is the wisdom we have lost in knowledge? Where is the knowledge we have lost in information?

—*T.S. Eliot*

This book is for women considering breast augmentation.

In 2006, approximately 300,000 women in the United States had breast augmentation surgery. Worldwide, more than three million women have breast implants. The vast majority of these women are pleased with their results, but some are not. Why not? In many cases, prospective augmentation patients make poor decisions based on minimal information, impulse, and self-derived logic—then question the less-than-optimal results.

Your best chance for the best breast is the first operation. The questions you ask and the decisions you make *before* that first operation will largely determine the results. The more seriously you **pursue information and knowledge before making decisions**, the better the decisions and the better the chance of an optimal result.

Even in this age of exploding technology and information exchange, there was no single, comprehensive information resource for prospective breast augmentation patients—until now. This book is a comprehensive guide derived from forty-two years of combined experience treating augmentation patients, designing surgical techniques and implants, and, during the past seven years, redefining virtually every aspect of the patient and surgeon experience in breast augmentation. Information becomes knowledge when combined with a logical, common-sense, stepwise approach to making decisions that will help you in your quest for the best breast. This book provides information, knowledge, and common-sense tools to help you make the important decisions.

Decisions without knowledge are often flawed.
The more you know, the better decisions you'll make.
The better decisions you make, the more likely you'll have a good result . . . the best breast.

INTRODUCTION

"It's normal to want to feel normal. It's also normal to want to be the best you can be."

A NEW WORLD FOR BREAST AUGMENTATION PATIENTS

Out to Dinner the Evening of Surgery, Full Normal Activities within Twenty-four Hours

In just six years since the first edition of *The Best Breast*, the world of breast augmentation has changed more than it changed in the previous three decades. A new world of breast augmentation is now available for patients—a redefined patient experience that enables most patients to go out to dinner the evening of surgery and return to full, normal activities within twenty-four hours.

Routine 24-Hour Return to Normal Activities Following Breast Augmentation

Today, our patients routinely (with 96 percent predictability) return to full, normal activities within twenty-four hours following their breast augmentation,[1,2] raising their arms fully above their heads, lying on their breasts, driving their cars, lifting normal objects and small children, and immediately resuming their normal daily activities. *More than 80 percent of our augmentation patients are out to dinner the evening of surgery with no drain tubes, no narcotic pain medications, no bandages, no special bras, and no pain pumps.*

Many surgeons today consider this type of patient recovery and patient experience totally impossible, but patients can expect to see more and more surgeons delivering this level of care to patients as surgeons attend our educational venues and read and apply information from the peer-reviewed scientific articles we have published during the past decade[1-13] in the most respected journal in plastic surgery.

Every Major Area of Breast Augmentation Redefined for Patients and Surgeons

Beginning a decade ago, we set a goal to redefine every aspect of breast augmentation—to dramatically and conclusively change the patient and surgeon experience. That goal is now reality. Seven years of clinical research have produced patient education, surgical planning, implant selection, and surgical techniques that redefine the patient experience in breast augmentation:

- New patient choice, patient education, and informed consent systems provide you with more information and help you make more informed decisions than ever before.[9] You can make more informed choices based on more thorough, complete information.

- This is the first system in history that bases implant selection on your personal, individual tissue characteristics with the goal of reducing long-term risks, complications, and reoperations. The TEPID™ system[8] and the latest High Five™[12] system are completely unique, new systems that replace our previously published dimensional system and enable surgeons to tailor breast implant selection to individual patients' tissue characteristics, eliminating many previous unrealistic and unpredictable selection methods such as stuffing materials into bras or relying on pictures to define choices. Bra-stuffing and pictures never match your individual patient tissue characteristics and cannot optimally evaluate the two most critical factors in assessing optimal implant size—the width of your breast and the amount your tissues stretch.

- A new decision and operative planning system, the High Five™ system,[12] defines the five most critical decisions in augmentation and uses five simple measurements to allow surgeons and patients to base decisions on individual patient tissue characteristics. This new system enables surgeons to make more important decisions before you are asleep in the operating room, shortening the time you are under anesthesia, reducing the amounts of drugs that are administered, reducing your time to awaken and leave a surgery center, reducing nausea and vomiting, and speeding your overall recovery.

- New Dual-Plane[6] techniques no longer require patients to choose between placing the implant either under or over muscle; instead, they combine the two pocket locations. A dual-plane pocket for the implant combines a submuscular pocket above that transitions to a submammary pocket in the lower breast, enabling surgeons to maximize the benefits of both locations while minimizing the trade-offs of each previous pocket location.

- New 24-Hour Recovery[1,2] surgical techniques and instruments dramatically reduce bleeding and surgical trauma to your tissues during surgery, enabling an almost unbelievably rapid recovery with minimal pain for most patients. More than 80 percent of our patients are out to dinner the evening of surgery, and 96 percent return to full, normal activities within twenty-four hours.[2] These techniques can be applied through any of three different incision approaches that you choose, and the techniques are now being learned and applied by surgeons worldwide.

- The largest body of peer-reviewed and published scientific data in history about full-height, anatomically shaped implants (the Inamed-Allergan Style 468 full height, textured, anatomic saline implant and now in FDA studies, the Style 410 cohesive, form stable gel implant), which are now available in form-stable silicone gel and saline filled versions in a matrix of sizes and shapes. Peer-reviewed data published in the most respected professional journal in plastic surgery and further validated by our data in FDA studies of the new implants confirm information that we published in the first edition of *The Best Breast*:

  - Adequate implant fill in an anatomically shaped implant device may significantly reduce deflation rates and reoperation rates due to visible wrinkling and rippling.[3]

  - Malposition risks with a full-height anatomic implant are minimal (only three reoperations for malposition in over 1,600 cases [0.2 percent] in our published studies).[2,5,6] When these implants are used optimally by surgeons with optimal training, risks of malposition are lower than malposition risks for round implants in FDA PMA studies.[14,15]

  - When used with optimal patient tissue selection criteria and surgical techniques, textured anatomic implants have as low or a lower rate of visible wrinkling or rippling compared to round, smooth shell implants (0 percent in our 1,662 cases[2,5,6] using anatomic implants compared to 15.5 percent in averaged FDA study data of round implants).[14,15]

- Recently completed FDA clinical studies show the newest, most advanced technology likely to reach patients in the

United States is the form-stable cohesive gel, anatomic implant (Allergan Inamed Style 410). The impressive five-year results with this product in FDA clinical studies in the United States reinforce the extensive experience of surgeons in Europe and Asia with the Inamed Style 410 implant over the past thirteen years. Most impressively, and for the first time in the history of FDA studies of breast implants, the style 410 had a zero percent device failure rate at two years in all first-time augmentation patients enrolled in the FDA study.[16]

• An unprecedented opportunity for dramatically lower reoperation rates following breast augmentation can be realized by using processes that we have defined and published in the November 2006 issue of *Plastic and Reconstructive Surgery Journal*, the most respected professional journal in plastic surgery. For the first time in the history of FDA studies on breast implants in the United States, we were able to document a 0 percent reoperation rate at three-year follow-up in a series of fifty consecutive patients enrolled in an independently supervised and monitored FDA study of the Allergan/Inamed Style 410 form-stable, cohesive-silicone-gel implant.[13] The systems, processes, and implant devices that we defined in this publication offer surgeons worldwide an opportunity to apply these processes to dramatically lower reoperation rates compared to average 15 to 20 percent reoperation rates in previous FDA studies.[14,15,17]

These dramatic improvements in breast augmentation offer patients choices and opportunities that are unprecedented in the history of breast augmentation. Motivated surgeons worldwide are now offering patients the benefits of the processes, methods, and techniques that we have developed over the past decade.

In order to take advantage of these advancements, patients must be willing to become educated about all of the options and trade-offs in breast augmentation. Optimal decisions require knowledge. A surgeon can provide information and assist with decisions, but every patient must assume responsibility for her choices and requests. The more educated the patient, the better her choices and decisions and the better her chances of achieving the best breast.

The best breast is the natural female breast—until nature misses a beat or takes a toll, or a woman decides that it's not.

It's normal to want to feel normal. It's also normal to want to be the best that you can be.

WHAT IS NORMAL? WHAT IS BEST?

What is normal? If you asked a hundred women, you might get one hundred different answers. What is normal is personal to each individual—something that's most important to that person alone. Wanting to feel normal and be the best you can be are human traits that motivate and reward on a very personal level.

Every woman's breasts are special. Special in ways that may differ among women, but special in a personal way to each woman. Breasts change significantly during a woman's lifetime. During adolescence, the breasts usually enlarge. With pregnancy, the breasts enlarge, cycle during nursing, become smaller after pregnancy, and change in shape. Aging also changes the shape and position of a woman's breasts (Figure 1-1). A woman's breasts never match. Enlargement during puberty and pregnancy is not predictable, and the effects of pregnancy on the breast can vary widely. A woman's tissue characteristics and the size of her breasts affect changes in the appearance of her breasts as she ages.

Women for whom nature "took a toll" during pregnancy and nursing

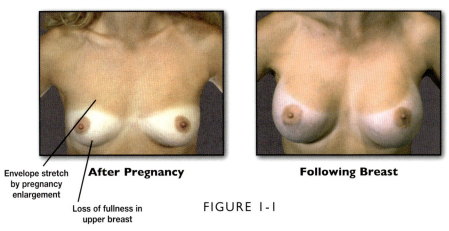

Envelope stretch
by pregnancy
enlargement

After Pregnancy

Loss of fullness in
upper breast

Following Breast

FIGURE 1-1

A woman may view her breasts differently at different times in her life, so the best breast at one time may not necessarily be the best breast at another time. In this book, we define the best breast for any woman as a personal decision, defined by that one woman's personal feelings, wishes, her tissues, and what her body will allow her to have (Figure 1-2). In this book, we will help you understand the choices available for breast augmentation, provide facts about those choices, and guide you in your decision-making process.

Women who, for personal reasons, would like to improve the appearance or shape
of their breasts

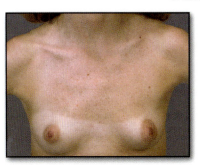

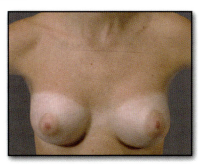

**Unsatisfactory Appearance to
Patient**

Following Breast Augmentation

FIGURE 1-2

Women for whom nature "missed a beat" during breast development

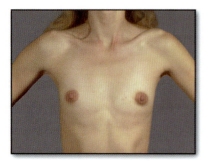 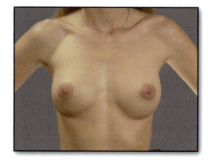

Inadequate Breast Development during Puberty   **Following Breast Augmentation**

FIGURE 1-3

The best breast is the natural female breast—until nature misses a beat or takes a toll, or a woman decides that it's not (Figures 1-1, 1-2, 1-3). The only totally natural breast is a totally natural breast. An augmented breast is not totally natural, and you should not expect it to be. If you want a totally natural breast, you should probably not have a breast augmentation. On the other hand, if the benefits outweigh the trade-offs, and the risks of breast augmentation are acceptable to you, augmentation provides options that can improve what you otherwise can't improve or restore what you otherwise can't restore.

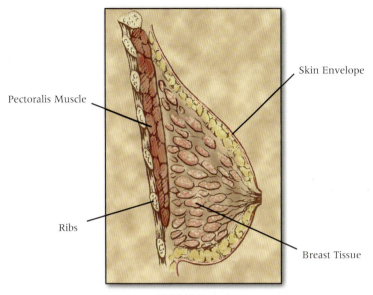

Pectoralis Muscle

Ribs

Skin Envelope

Breast Tissue

FIGURE 1-4

PRACTICAL ANATOMY OF THE BREAST

The basic components of the breast are

1) a **skin envelope**, and 2) **breast tissue** filler (parenchyma).

In simple terms, the breast consists of a skin envelope that surrounds and contains the breast tissue. The breast tissue lies on top of the pectoralis muscle. Beneath the muscle layer are the ribs that form the chest wall (Figure 1-4).

The skin envelope is the main support of the breast. Attachments are present between the back of the breast tissue and the front of the muscle, but these attachments don't contribute significant support to the breast. The larger the breast, with or without pregnancy and with or without an implant, the more gravity pulls downward on the breast tissue, stretching the lower skin envelope and allowing the breast to sag.

Following augmentation, the components of the breast are

1) the **skin envelope**, 2) the **breast tissue**, and 3) the **implant**.

WOMEN WHO CONSIDER AUGMENTATION

Three groups of women frequently consider breast augmentation:

ABNORMAL DEVELOPMENT DURING PUBERTY: WHEN NATURE MISSES A BEAT

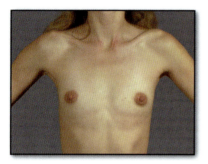

Before Augmentation

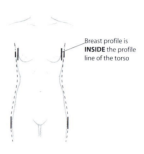

Breast profile is **INSIDE** the profile line of the torso

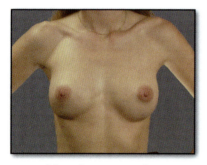

After Augmentation

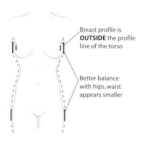

Breast profile is **OUTSIDE** the profile line of the torso

Better balance with hips, waist appears smaller

FIGURE 1-5

When breast development is inadequate during puberty, the breasts are disproportionately small compared to the rest of a woman's figure (Figure 1-5). Some women refer to this disproportion as a "bowling pin" figure, with the hips and lower body appearing wider than the narrower upper body. Buying clothing can be difficult. If it fits the bottom, it doesn't fit the top. Pushing up what you have is an option, provided you have enough to push up. Fillers are also an option, but a constant nuisance, and the balance provided by pushing up or fillers disappears when clothing is removed. Fillers and enhancers never feel like they belong to you. They never become a natural part of your body image.

Inadequate breast development during puberty produces breasts that don't appear normal.

The abnormal appearance can be a deformity or an imbalance with the rest of a woman's figure.

Before   **After**

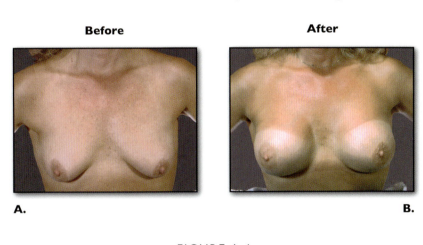

A.   **B.**

FIGURE 1-6

If the breasts develop abnormally during puberty, the shape of the breast can be abnormal (Figure 1-6) and can affect how a woman feels about herself. No woman has two breasts that are the same, but sometimes the normal amount of variation in breast shape and size is too much (significant asymmetry). Imagine the difficulty when you are trying to buy clothing and dressing to feel normal and how you might feel when clothing is removed.

The patient in Figure 1-6 illustrates an important point—that while routine breast augmentation enlarges and improves the breast, the procedure does not dramatically relocate the nipple-areola complexes. The down-pointing and outward-pointing configuration of this patient's nipples were not a major concern to her, and prior to her augmentation, she elected not to have the incisions and scars around her areolas that would be required to relocate them or risk sensory changes. By making these choices, the patient minimized possible trade-offs of nipple relocation while maximizing the benefits of breast augmentation. Each individual patient must make personal decisions about priorities and trade-offs before surgery.

CHANGES FOLLOWING PREGNANCY

Hundreds of women who consult us for breast augmentation following pregnancy have said, "I had no idea what pregnancy and nursing would do to my breasts. Not that it isn't worth it, I just had no idea. I loved it when they were full, but now they're saggy and almost gone!" The effects of pregnancy and nursing on the breast are variable but usually predictable. During pregnancy, tissue inside the breast enlarges and the skin envelope stretches. As the skin stretches, usually more in the lower breast, the larger, heavier breast is pulled downward by gravity, regardless of how much it is supported by a bra. During nursing, the breast cycles up and down, stretching the skin repeatedly. Following pregnancy and nursing, the tissue inside the breast (the breast parenchyma) usually decreases substantially in size, often to a size less than before the pregnancy, but the skin almost never shrinks back to its original size.

A stretched and enlarged skin envelope with less breast tissue to fill it is common following pregnancy.

The result is an empty upper breast and a sagging appearance in the lower breast.

More skin with less filler is typical following pregnancy and nursing. The stretched skin envelope with insufficient tissue to fill it produces predictable changes in breast appearance. The breast tissue filler predictably falls to the bottom of the envelope, leaving the upper breast appearing empty. Most women describe the empty upper breast and fuller lower breast as "saggy." Many women who consult us for augmentation following pregnancy ask for more fill in the upper breast to help restore a breast form closer to the breast they had before pregnancy.

WOMEN WHO WANT TO IMPROVE APPEARANCE OF THEIR BREASTS

The third group of women who seek augmentation usually want to improve the shape and/or size of their breasts for a variety of personal reasons. These are normal women who want to feel better, who want to be the best they can be. Some developed very unattractive breasts during puberty. Others have so much variation between the breasts that they have difficulty with clothing options. Still others want to improve the balance between the upper and lower portions of their body. Each woman's reasons are personal. Every woman has the right to want to optimize any aspect of her appearance.

THE IMPORTANCE OF REALISTIC EXPECTATIONS

Your expectations for augmentation must be realistic for you to be happy with the results.

The goal of augmentation is to improve the size and shape of your breasts. To the extent that the results meet your goals, you can have a more positive self-image, and these feelings may allow you to project a more open, positive image to others. But the only predictable change is larger breasts. This is an operation on the breasts, not on the brain. Positive psychological effects are common, but are not necessarily predictable. Certainly, your breast augmentation cannot be expected to have any predictable effect on other people. Some will notice, some may not—depending on your choices of clothing and breast exposure. Your love life may improve, but it may not. The breasts are only one of the many factors that affect the quality of one's love life! A better figure doesn't necessarily guarantee a model more modeling jobs or an actress more roles. The decision to have a breast augmentation should be based on realistic, personal objectives that you discuss with your surgeon.

Your surgeon can only work with what you bring—your tissues and your expectations.

The better you communicate with your surgeon, the more thoroughly your surgeon presents your options. The more expertly your surgeon executes your choices, the more rapid your recovery will be and the more likely you will have a result that pleases both of you.

THE IMPORTANCE OF INFORMATION AND KNOWLEDGE

A patient motivated us to write this book with the following challenge, "Knowing everything that twenty-nine years of experience has taught you, help me and other patients with the tough questions we all face. To make the best decisions about augmentation, what do I need to know, how do I go about learning it, and what is the logical sequence of making informed decisions? Walk me step-by-step through a thorough, logical approach to making good decisions about breast augmentation."

Based on our experience in treating thousands of breast augmentation patients over the past twenty-nine years, we are convinced that patients need more information to guide them through the research and decision-making process when considering this operation. You can't be helped by what you don't know. The more you know, both good and bad, the more realistically you can evaluate your options, the more equipped you are to deal with surgeons and the surgical experience, and the more likely you are to enjoy the benefits and minimize the risks and trade-offs of augmentation.

Knowledge is the basis of a logical approach to good decision-making.

Based on our experience with patients, we believe in a simple premise. The more you know, the better you can make informed decisions. The more thoroughly you research and understand your options, the better your decisions. The better your decisions, the more likely you are to achieve your goals with minimal risks and trade-offs. The better you communicate your desires and questions to your surgeon, the more likely you'll make good team decisions. Knowledge, common sense, and communication skills are important.

HOW THIS BOOK IS ORGANIZED AND FORMATTED

We have organized this book for flexibility. For the most complete information in the most logical sequence, read from beginning to end. If you want an overview without details, read the emphasized text in each chapter, and use the appropriate checklists. Refer back to specific chapters for more details. We have included removable cards in the back of the book that include the most critical information and checklists. References to peer-reviewed and published scientific articles that verify the statements in the book are included at the end of each chapter that includes references.

The formatting of emphasized text is continued in this edition based on the majority of feedback from readers of the first edition. A few readers felt the emphasized text was "shouting' at them or questioning their intelligence. That was not and is not our intention. Emphasized text is included to allow rapid scanning to acquire important content.

This edition contains more information compared to the first edition for two specific reasons: 1) More information is available today, especially scientifically published evidence that confirms information in the first edition, and 2) this book is intended to be the most comprehensive reference available for patients considering breast augmentation. Each patient can consider her individual information needs and use the book as she wishes. The book is designed to allow patients to focus on essentials, yet have the most definitive information and scientific references available in one volume. Based on our more than 30 years' experience, it is impossible for a patient to have too much information, because the quality of each patient's decisions depends on the knowledge base the patient develops. "Too much information" is something no patient feels she needs . . . until something occurs which makes her wish she had acquired the information before surgery.

WHAT WE ARE ABOUT- OUR BELIEFS AND BIASES

We believe that patients should be offered every option in breast augmentation. While offering options, surgeons are responsible for informing patients of the potential benefits, tradeoffs, and risks of each option. Every statement that we make in this book is backed by published scientific evidence and more than 30 years' clinical experience. Biases based on scientific evidence are the basis of our track record.

We believe that most patients are not provided optimal quality and quantity of information prior to having breast augmentation, and that some patients, despite the availability of quality information, do not commit adequate time and effort to become knowledgeable before making decisions about augmentation. Our commitment is to provide as much quality, science-based information as possible, and to assist every patient who wants to learn.

We believe that the best measures of the quality of breast augmentation surgery are 1) patient recovery, and 2) surgeon complication and reoperation rates documented in scientific publications or by the surgeon's record in FDA monitored studies. Rapid, 24-hour return to normal activities, is a criteria that surgeon's cannot easily manipulate for marketing purposes, provided patients insist on documentation of surgeon claims. The more tissue trauma and bleeding that a patient experiences during surgery, the longer the patient's recovery, and the greater the risk of complications following surgery. Rapid recovery correlates directly with fewer complications and less risk of reoperations as confirmed in our scientific studies listed at the end of this introduction. Surgeon complication and reoperation rates are critically important, but are of limited reliability unless they are confirmed by peer reviewed and published scientific studies.

Other measures of results, including before and after pictures, are far less reliable as long-term yardsticks of patient outcomes. Pictures are often carefully selected by surgeons, and without at least five views of each patient preoperatively and at intervals postoperatively, even the most expert surgeons cannot make valid judgments of aesthetic results. Most patients, despite education, make very superficial and often incorrect judgments when viewing pictures. This statement is not meant to offend; it is simply true.

We believe that a patient's highest priorities when considering various breast implant design options are 1) the scientific data and FDA data regarding the device shell failure rate (because device shell failure means a likely reoperation for the patient), and 2) each surgeon's specific experience (numbers of cases treated) with each type of implant the surgeon recommends or does not recommend. The more experience a surgeon has with every type of implant, the more qualified the surgeon is to comment positively or negatively on that type of implant.

In our practice, we follow very strict guidelines that have evolved from our more than 30 year clinical experience—guidelines that are confirmed by our peer reviewed and published studies to deliver a level of recovery and reoperation rates that are currently unmatched in published studies worldwide. We have specific criteria for declining to perform augmentation. Some of those criteria include patients who do not wish to follow our patient education requirements, patients who make requests that we feel we will be unable to deliver for any reason, patients who do not fit clinical criteria for our practice, and especially patients whose tissue qualities are such that a breast implant could cause negative and irreversible tissue changes after augmentation.

We would like for all patients to enjoy our practice, our personalities, and our care. Most do; some do not. Patients we decline to care for, despite the reasons, are usually not pleased, though a few have been very thankful. We are human; we are driven to deliver the best possible care for every patient, and we are far more concerned about documented quality of patient outcomes compared to any measure of popularity.

We love what we do, we are proud of our track record and encourage all patients to judge us and compare us to other surgeons based on track record, that is substantiated by scientific evidence and peer reviewed publications, not by unsubstantiated or unverified claims or marketing hype. Our goal is to deliver the best breast with the best recovery, and the best complication and reoperation rates, all documented by peer reviewed and published scientific studies.

VISUALIZING YOUR QUEST FOR THE BEST BREAST

Visualize your quest for the best breast as a staircase (Figure 1-7). Each chapter of this book represents one step on the staircase. The steps are divided into four main categories that approach augmentation in a logical sequence.

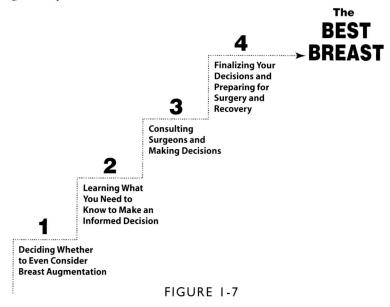

FIGURE 1-7

PART I

Deciding Whether Even to Consider Breast Augmentation

To decide whether you even want to consider augmentation, you will need some information. In Part 1, we will present some hard choices and hard facts. If they aren't acceptable, you don't need to waste your time and additional resources.

PART 2

Learning What You Need to Know to Make an Informed Decision

Most patients don't even know what they need to know to start considering augmentation. You need knowledge before you ever consult a surgeon. We think it's critical for you to build a base of knowledge so that you can make the most of the time and money you spend consulting surgeons. A little homework in preparation for your consultations is invaluable. You will learn how to ask the right questions, how to separate substance from hype, and how to evaluate the surgeons you consult.

PART 3

Consulting Surgeons and Making Decisions

In part 3, you will learn how to locate qualified surgeons with appropriate credentials, how to gather and assess information from surgeons, how to define your expectations before seeing the surgeon, and how to get the most out of your consultations.

PART 4

Finalizing Your Decisions and Preparing for Surgery and Recovery

Finally, we will put it all together. In part 4, we will help you with the final choices—picking the surgeon, the implant, the pocket location, the incision location, and the time to have your surgery. After the choices, you will learn how best to prepare for surgery physically, mentally, and financially; what to expect during recovery; and how to live with your new breasts in the future.

Our purpose is to help you climb the stairs and meet your goals for the BEST BREAST. If you are considering breast augmentation, we want you to know as much as we can possibly share with you, based on our experiences as a team who provides information and surgical care to breast augmentation patients. Our hope is that sharing our combined knowledge and experience will help you, logically, one step at a time.

Let's get started!

SUMMING UP:

- The best breast is the natural female breast—until nature misses a beat or takes a toll, or a woman decides that it's not.

- The basic components of the breast are
  1. a skin envelope and
  2. breast tissue filler (parenchyma).

- Following augmentation, the components of the breast are
  1. the skin envelope,
  2. the breast tissue, and
  3. the implant.

- Your expectations for augmentation must be realistic for you to be happy with the results.

- Your surgeon can only work with what you bring—your tissues and your expectations.

- The decisions that you and your surgeon make and the surgeon's knowledge and execution determine your result, your experience, the rate of your recovery, and your risks of reoperations in the future.

References

1. Tebbetts, J. B. Achieving a predictable 24-hour return to normal activities after breast augmentation, part I: Refining practices using motion and time study principles. *Plast. Reconstr. Surg.* 109: 273-290, 2002.

2. Tebbetts, J. B. Achieving a predictable 24-hour return to normal activities after breast augmentation, part II: Patient preparation, refined surgical techniques and instrumentation. *Plast. Reconstr. Surg.* 109: 293-305, 2002.

3. Tebbetts, J. B. What is adequate fill? Implications in breast implant surgery. *Plast. Reconstr. Surg.* 97(7), 1996.

4. Tebbetts, J. B. Use of anatomic breast implants: Ten essentials. *Aesthetic Surg. J.* 18: 377, 1996.

5. Tebbetts, J. B. Patient acceptance of adequately filled breast implants. *Plast. Reconstr. Surg.* 106(1): 139-147, 2000.

6. Tebbetts, J. B. Dual plane (DP) breast augmentation: Optimizing implant-soft tissue relationships in a wide range of breast types. *Plast. Reconstr. Surg.* 107: 1255, 2001.

7. Tebbetts, J. B. The greatest myths in breast augmentation. *Plast. Reconstr. Surg.* 107(7), 2001.

8. Tebbetts, J. B. A system for breast implant selection based on patient tissue characteristics and implant-soft tissue dynamics. *Plast. Reconstr. Surg.* 109(4): 1396-1409, 2002.

9. Tebbetts, J. B. An approach that integrates patient education and informed consent in breast augmentation. *Plast. Reconstr. Surg.* 110(3): 971-878, 2002.

10. Adams, W., Bengtson, B., Glicksman, C., et al. Decision and management algorithms to address patient and Food and Drug Administration concerns regarding breast augmentation and implants. *Plast. Reconstr. Surg.* 114(5): 1252-1257, 2004.

11. Tebbetts, J. B. Out points criteria for breast implant removal without replacement and criteria to minimize reoperations following breast augmentation. *Plast. Reconstr. Surg.* 114(5): 1258-1262, 2004.

12. Tebbetts, J. B., and Adams, W. P. Five critical decisions in breast augmentation using 5 measurements in 5 minutes: The high five system. *Plast. Reconstr. Surg.* 116(7): 2005-2016, 2006.

13. Tebbetts, J. B. Achieving a zero percent reoperation rate at 3 years in a 50 consecutive case augmentation mammaplasty PMA study. *Plast. Reconstr. Surg.* 118(6): 1453-1457, 1996.

14. U. S. Food and Drug Administration. General and Plastic Surgery Devices Panel Meeting Transcript. http://www.fda.gov/ohrms/dockets/ac/03/transcripts/3989T1.htm, accessed January 13, 2007.

15. U. S. Food and Drug Administration. General and Plastic Surgery Devices Panel Meeting Transcript. http://www.fda.gov/ohrms/dockets/ac/00/minutes/3596ml.pdf, accessed January 21, 2007.

16. Health Canada. Transcript of expert advisory panel meeting on silicon filled breast imlants. http://www.hc-sc.gc.ca/dhp-mps/mdim/activit/sci-consult/inpmlant-breastmammaire/breast_implants_intro_implants_mammaires_e.html. September 29-30, 2005. Accessed: November 26, 2006.

17. U. S. Food and Drug Administration. Product labeling data for Mentor and Allergan/Inamed core studies of conventional silicone gel implants. http://www.fda/gov/cdrh/breastimplants/labeling.html. Last accessed December 5, 2006. Updated November 17, 2006.

PART I

BREAST AUGMENTATION:
SHOULD YOU EVEN CONSIDER IT?

HOW CAN THIS BOOK
HELP ME?

"If there were one best answer to each question, all breast augmentation would be done the same."

If you are considering breast augmentation, you probably have a lot of questions, questions that need answers before you decide to have an augmentation. Most patients begin thinking about this procedure and, hopefully, soon realize that they have more questions than answers.

How much does it cost?
How big should I be?
What is the best place to put the incision?
What is the best type of implant?
How do I find a good surgeon?
How does that surgeon do the procedure?
How long will I be off work?
When can I return to normal activities and exercise?
How long until my breasts look natural?

Surely, there is one best answer to each of these questions.

YOU ARE AN INDIVIDUAL—DIFFERENT FROM OTHER WOMEN

In reality, the answer to each of these questions is the same, "It depends." If there were one best answer to each question, all breast augmentations would be done the same. You are an individual, different from every other woman. Your tissues are different, your breasts are different, and your desires and expectations are probably different. Ask yourself, "Do I want a rubber stamp, standard augmentation, or would I prefer that every aspect of my augmentation be tailored to my specific desires and my tissues?" If given a choice, do you buy the same size and style of dress that you think other women would buy or wear? Of course not, and it's not logical to think that the best choices in breast augmentation for your friend who had the procedure are necessarily the best choices for you.

If a surgeon does all breast augmentations the same, the surgeon is probably doing a lot of them wrong.

No two women are the same.
Their tissues are not the same.
The best breast for each woman is not the same.
How do you know what's best for you?
You begin by asking the right questions.

This book helps you ask the right questions based on knowledge.

HELPING YOU ASK THE RIGHT QUESTIONS

If someone you know has had an augmentation, have you seen the result? Do you like it? Even if you do, are your tissues exactly the same as her tissues before she had the operation? If not, your result won't be the same either

A common practice by surgeons, implant manufacturers, and Internet Web sites is to show pictures and imply (even with disclaimers) that you can look at pictures and choose what type or size implant might be best for you. If you see pictures in a magazine of breasts that you like, can you take the pictures to a surgeon (like you would take pictures of a hairstyle to your hairstylist) and expect to get the breast that is pictured? Not if you or the surgeon are very sophisticated. Can you manipulate images on a Web site or a surgeon's office computer and reliably predict how your tissues might respond to a certain type or size of breast implant? Can you make good choices based on pictures? The answer is no, but you should understand why it is impossible to logically compare what you'd like to have to any picture, whether it's in a magazine or on the Internet.

Is the woman pictured your age? Did her breasts start out looking like your breasts? Are your pregnancy histories similar? Is the picture taken to enhance the look of the breasts? Has the picture been retouched? Most importantly, you can't stretch the skin in a picture, and skin stretch is one of the two most important factors that determine optimal implant size to avoid tissue damage while optimizing the aesthetic result. You can't accurately judge the width of the breast in the picture, and breast width is another critical factor in choosing an optimal implant that is compatible with your tissues. If a surgeon asks you to bring a picture and casually assures you that you will get that breast or if the surgeon asks you to stuff trial implants or bags into a bra the size you would like to be, beware! If you see pictures on the Internet, and anyone implies that you can even remotely make decisions based on pictures, beware! Using pictures to help understand what you like is logical, but you should thoroughly understand all the factors that make you different from the woman in the picture and understand and accept what your individual tissues will allow you to have. The same is true for trial implants or bags of fluid in a bra. The bra is not your tissue. It doesn't respond to the presence of an implant in the same way that your tissues will respond. A bra never stretches in response to an implant like your tissue stretches. A bra doesn't predictably age and stretch more with time as your tissues will age and stretch. Did your surgeon discuss all of these issues with you? More importantly, did your surgeon discuss how your choices now may affect your breasts in the future as you get older? How do you know what you need to know? How do you go about researching all of the important information? How do you ask the right questions in the right order?

How can this book help? By asking some basic questions and providing information to help you answer the questions in a logical sequence. **As you read and review this chapter, ask yourself: Are these the**

logical questions I should be asking? Are the topics presented in an order that seems logical and helpful to me? If these questions and topics sound reasonable to you, you will find this book useful. Let's look at an overview of the questions we will ask and the information we will cover, and you can determine how the information can best help you.

ASKING THE RIGHT QUESTIONS IN THE RIGHT ORDER

This book helps you ask the right questions in a logical order. Each chapter adds **information** that builds your **knowledge**.

What does augmentation really do?

Is augmentation medically safe? Do I understand the medical evidence?

What are basic questions I should ask before proceeding?

Am I just being vain?

Can I correct the problem any other way?

Am I willing to do my homework and make this my own decision?

Am I willing to realistically accept the trade-offs and risks?

Can I handle the costs financially?

How can I locate qualified surgeons?

How do I prepare for my visit with a surgeon?

How do I "interview" a surgeon?

How do I judge a good result and a bad one when I see it?

How do I define what I want, and how do I reconcile my desires with reality?

How do I "grade" the surgeons I consult?

How do I finalize my decisions and prepare for surgery?

How might my choices and decisions affect my recovery, how do I make choices to make my recovery as easy and rapid as possible, and how do I care for my breasts later?

How might my decisions affect my risks of additional reoperations or problems in the future?

If you want the best breast, you need to know the answers to each of these questions. This book will help you with the answers.

WHAT DOES AUGMENTATION REALLY DO?

Breast augmentation enhances what you already have and what you already are.

Breast augmentation works with your tissues and your wishes to improve what you have.

It fills the skin envelope of your breast (what you already have) to enlarge and improve the shape of your breast and usually helps you feel better about you (what you already are). Now that we know what it does, where do we start? You will need a lot of information, but the information is more useful if you learn it in a logical, stepwise process.

HOW CAN THIS BOOK HELP ME?

By now, you should a have definite feel for how this book can help you. If the questions sound logical, the topics sound intriguing, and the order of our information sounds logical, **you'll find this book helpful**.

STEP 1:

DOES IT MAKE SENSE TO EVEN THINK ABOUT IT?

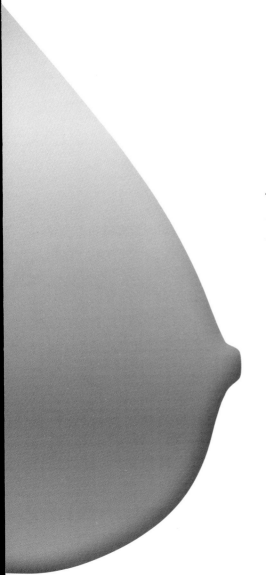

"One good way to start thinking about breast augmentation is to ask yourself some very basic important questions."

One good way to start thinking about breast augmentation is to ask yourself some very basic, important questions. Is the procedure medically safe? Are there specific issues in my medical history that I should consider before proceeding? Am I just being vain? Can I achieve the changes I want any other way? If the answers to this first series of questions are positive, then it's time to ask yourself some "Am I? Can I?" types of questions. Am I willing to do my homework and make my own decisions? Am I willing to realistically accept the trade-offs and risks? Can I handle the costs or the financial burden? Am I willing to use common sense when making my decisions? Am I willing to remove my implants if necessary? Answering these questions is the first step. If you can't take the first step successfully, you probably shouldn't try to climb the stairs.

IS IT SAFE? THE MEDICAL EVIDENCE

To judge whether something is safe medically, you need to know a little about medical science. Medicine is not an exact science. The answers to most medical questions are rarely black and white. Instead, most answers are usually shades of gray. Good decisions in medicine are based on 1) weighing evidence scientifically (does the data prove the hypothesis in a scientific study?) and 2) clinical experience (the sum of a physician's experience treating patients). Part science and part art, plastic surgery relies on scientific evidence and experience.

No procedure in plastic surgery is perfect. Perfection isn't an option—improvement is the only option.

What is "best" and what is "right" are always shades of gray. Don't expect many black and white answers.

No procedure is without trade-offs and risks (the grays).

Whether something is reasonable depends on whether the potential benefits outweigh the potential trade-offs and risks. Whether something is safe is relative. The best decisions are based on scientific evidence and your comfort level with the trade-offs and risks.

CURRENT SCIENTIFIC STUDIES AND EVIDENCE

Somewhere, someone can always tell you a personal horror story about almost any experience in life, even having a baby. Does that stop us from having babies? No. We weigh the pros and cons and make a personal decision. Most potential gains involve some risks. For most "pros," some "cons" usually exist. Breast augmentation is no exception.

Sound medical decisions are usually based on scientifically tested and proven evidence that is reinforced by substantial clinical experience treating patients (on-the-job training). What is "scientifically tested and proven" evidence? First, a well-designed scientific study is performed (tough to do), and then the evidence is reviewed by professional peers (other plastic surgery experts in the field). If the study is scientifically sound after review, it is usually published in well-respected medical journals. That process takes time. When you hear, read, or see something in the media about breast implants or augmentation, it may or may not be true, especially when a technique or device is new. The questions to ask are, How long has it been tested? Do we really know yet? It takes time to treat and follow enough patients to know if something is good. Good scientific studies that answer the important questions are very time consuming. Compiling meaningful clinical experience takes years. When we try to answer the following important questions, our answers are based on the best scientific evidence available and on twenty-four years of clinical experience treating and following breast augmentation patients.

THE MOST COMPELLING ANSWERS TO DATE . . .

To date, one of the most conclusive, compelling, and reassuring sources of information is the report of the National Science Panel appointed by U.S. District Judge Sam Pointer, the presiding judge over the class action breast implant litigation. This panel was appointed by Judge Pointer to evaluate all existing scientific evidence and determine whether silicone gel breast implants cause any type of autoimmune diseases, connective tissue diseases, or immune-system dysfunctions. Four disciplines were represented on the panel by world-recognized experts in each discipline: immunology, epidemiology, toxicology, and rheumatology. What were their conclusions?

Immunology—"The main conclusion that can be drawn from existing studies is that women with silicone breast implants do not display a silicone-induced systemic abnormality in the types or functions of cells of the immune system."

Epidemiology—"No association was evident between breast implants and any of the individual connective tissue diseases, all definite connective tissue diseases combined, or the other autoimmune/rheumatic conditions."

Toxicology—"In conclusion, the preponderance of evidence from animal studies indicates little probability the silicone exposure induces or exacerbates systemic disease in humans."

Rheumatology—"Furthermore, many of the rheumatologic complaints reported are common in the general population as presenting complaints in physician's offices. No distinctive features relating to silicone breast implants could be identified."

This panel of unbiased experts unequivocally concluded that breast implants do not cause any of these diseases.

Their findings point out one of the greatest hoaxes ever perpetrated on American women by the FDA and plaintiff lawyers—banning a device that does not cause disease, depriving American women of their rights to valid information and valid choices with regard to breast implants, and making plaintiff lawyers wealthier in the process!

Do breast implants cause breast cancer? NO

Appendix 2 summarizes pertinent medical studies that have been published in respected, peer-reviewed medical journals with regard to breast implants and breast cancer. Each of these studies reaches a similar conclusion: breast implants do not cause breast cancer. Approximately 10 to 11 percent of women in the United States, with or without breast implants, will develop breast cancer during their lifetimes. The best scientific studies compared similar large groups of women with and without breast implants and found that the occurrence of breast cancer was not significantly different in women with implants compared to women without implants.

Do breast implants cause autoimmune disease? NO

Autoimmune diseases are conditions that cause the body's own immune system to malfunction and result in certain symptoms, conditions, or groups of symptoms and conditions that have been categorized as diseases. Examples of autoimmune conditions include scleroderma, rheumatoid arthritis, lupus, and fibromyalgia. One of the most respected organizations in the world that deals with these diseases is the American College of Rheumatology. The following statement was issued by the American College of Rheumatology regarding breast implants and the risk of autoimmune diseases:

American College of Rheumatology Statement on Silicone Breast Implants
Approved by Board of Directors on Oct. 22, 1995

The American College of Rheumatology recognizes that many women who have received silicone breast implants have musculoskeletal complaints that are also very common in the general population. Many rheumatologists have examined women with implants who have scleroderma, lupus, fibromyalgia, or other well-defined disorders. The problem has been to determine whether any cause-and-effect relationship exists between silicone implants and the musculoskeletal symptoms. Previous data were solely based on anecdotal evidence. In 1994, the American College of Rheumatology stated the importance and great need for scientific analysis of this question.

Two large studies now have been completed. The first was conducted on all women in a single county in Minnesota who received implants between 1964 and 1991. At a mean follow-up of 7.8 years, there was no association between breast implants and connective tissue or rheumatic disease (NEJM 330:1697-702, 1994). The second study was a follow-up of the Nurses Health Study. Among this very large cohort, after 14 years of follow-up, no evidence existed for an association between silicone breast implants and connective tissue diseases (NEJM 332:1666-70, 1995).

The American College of Rheumatology believes that these studies provide compelling evidence that silicone implants expose patients to no demonstrable additional risk for connective tissue or rheumatic disease. Anecdotal evidence should no longer be used to support this relationship in the courts or by the FDA. Clinicians, scientists, academicians, and editors who have been harassed by plaintiffs' attorneys for their involvement in scientific research efforts related to silicone implant deserve the continued support of their institutions and professional societies.

In future cases involving rheumatic diseases possibly associated with an environmental agent, we call upon the FDA and other regulatory agencies to allow professional societies, such as the American College of Rheumatology, to foster appropriate and scientifically developed epidemiological studies. Anecdotal reports, while of importance to call attention to a potential problem, should not be utilized to formulate decisions and regulations.

The American College of Rheumatology is the most respected, professional organization of rheumatologists. It includes practicing physicians, research scientists and health professionals who are dedicated to healing, preventing disability, and eventually curing the more than 100 types of arthritis and related disabling and sometimes fatal disorders of the joints, muscles and bones.

Appendix 3 summarizes pertinent medical studies about autoimmune disease that have been published in respected, peer-reviewed medical journals.

A certain percentage of women, based on hereditary or environmental factors, will develop autoimmune diseases during their lifetimes. Logically, some women who have breast implants will develop autoimmune diseases. This does not mean that the breast implants caused the autoimmune disease.

What We Currently Tell Patients about Autoimmune Disease

If you have a family history of autoimmune disease, you should understand that although you may be genetically destined to develop the disease at some point, there may be factors that could stress your autoimmune system and possibly cause you to develop the disease sooner (though we have no scientific proof of that risk). Emotional stress or physical stress of any kind, even having a surgical procedure, might theoretically stress your system excessively. At the very least, if you have a family history of autoimmune disease, we want you to consult a board certified rheumatologist or immunologist and get a written opinion regarding the safety of your having breast augmentation. Before having an augmentation, you should ask yourself: If I know that I might be prone to develop an autoimmune disease because of heredity or other factors and a breast augmentation might cause me to develop it sooner, is it worth it to me to have a breast augmentation?

Internet references

If you want to dig deeper into scientific studies and additional information, check out the Internet references.

FDA Information and Position Statement re: Breast Implants:

www.fda.gov/cdrh/breastimplants

The American Society for Aesthetic Plastic Surgery:

www.surgery.org

American Society of Plastic and Reconstructive Surgeons:

www.plasticsurgery.org

24-hour recovery website:

www.24hrrecovery.com

The book Web site:

www.thebestbreast.com

Institute of Medicine, National Academy of Sciences Report and Book

In 1999, the Institute of Medicine of the National Academy of Sciences organized a committee of thirteen respected medical specialists from a wide variety of medical specialties to serve on a committee and review all current research and evidence regarding the safety of silicone breast implants. The committee's findings are presented in detail in the book *Safety of Silicone Breast Implants*, edited by Stuart Bondurant, Virginia Ernster, and Roger Herdman; Committee on the Safety of Silicone Breast Implants, Institute of Medicine, published by The National Academies Press, Washington, D.C., in 2000. This book contains the most comprehensive information available in a single source currently available regarding the safety of silicone breast implants and is available from The Academies Press, Washington, D.C. Web site at **www.nap.edu/catalog/9602.html**.

According to the American Society of Plastic Surgeons, the committee's report "emphatically showed there to be no health problems associated with silicone breast implants." The report also stated that there is no evidence that silicone breast implants contribute to an increase in autoimmune (connective-tissue) diseases.

The committee could find no proof or significant evidence of a "novel" systemic disease caused by the presence of silicone implants. In addition, evidence from the study suggests that various systemic complaints or conditions are no more common in women with breast implants than in women without them.

Do breast implants cause any other known diseases?

NO

At this time, there is no credible, scientific evidence that breast implants cause any type of disease, regardless of the type of breast implant.

This does not mean that there could not be a disease or diseases of which we are unaware that are affected by breast implants. It simply means that, currently, no such disease has been documented scientifically.

For over thirty years, breast implants have been used in the United States in over two million women. Complications from breast implant surgery certainly occur in a small percentage of patients, and these complications can produce significant problems if they are not treated promptly and correctly. Later in this book, we will address the specific risks of complications so that you can determine whether those risks are reasonable.

If breast implants don't cause any of these diseases, why all the lawsuits? Why do I hear about all these breast implant disasters?

When humans get diseases, it's human nature to ask, Why me? What caused this? The physical and emotional stress of disease causes most people to lose their feeling of being "normal" and frightens them. Regardless of the disease, most of us instinctively want to blame it on something. When potential financial gain is added to the equation, regardless of the disease or condition, a plaintiff lawyer feeding frenzy is predictable. "Would you like some money? We can probably get some for you!" Whether from a plaintiff lawyer or a con man (not a totally incidental comparison), these words can be hard to resist. Our judicial system has been called an example to the world—good in some ways, for sure, but not so good in other ways.

In medical cases in this country, there is no requirement that evidence introduced in the courtroom must be based on quality, scientific evidence. Any lawyer can hire any "expert" whose testimony becomes evidence, whether or not the expert's opinion has been tested in peer-reviewed, published scientific studies. Needless to say, there are plenty of "experts" who, in exchange for money, will testify to almost any-thing regarding a medical situation. Fortunately, recent federal court decisions have emphasized the importance of basing judgement on scientific data, an encouraging sign for the future. Until that happens, remember: The facts in a case don't necessarily need to be scientifically "right" or justifiable to get an award. The plaintiff lawyer only needs to convince a jury. How many juries would you want making your medical decisions for you?

Companies that are sued face a dilemma that is great for the plaintiff lawyer and not so great for the company. Fighting the suit with a trial is often more expensive than settling the suit by paying a monetary settlement (some have called it legalized bribery), so the company makes a business decision to settle. Legalized extortion? Certainly sounds like it to us. Judgements that are not based on scientific evidence ultimately cost all of us. The company pays. The company does not have as much money left for research and development of better products. The company is forced to raise the price of its product (breast implants). A higher priced, less state-of-the-art product is the result.

How good is that for you?

Are all lawsuits bogus and without merit? Certainly not. Plastic surgeons aren't perfect. We make mistakes. If a surgeon makes mistakes that are below the standard of usual and customary medical practices, then the surgeon should be held accountable for malpractice. There should not be a double standard. If we want tort reform to reduce frivolous cases without merit, surgeons must perform to an acceptable level and be held responsible for our actions when we do not. We also must be willing to police ourselves by holding our colleagues accountable to an acceptable standard of care.

Team decisions and accountability

During my career, I have been asked to review a large number of breast implant cases in which "disasters" occurred. What was to blame? The implant? Almost never! In almost every case, problems were directly related to bad team decisions by the patient and the surgeon. What do we mean by "team" decisions? The team consists of you and your surgeon. Both of you are responsible for decisions you should make jointly. Let me tell you about a case that illustrates the point.

Julie (a fictitious name but a real patient) came to see us after having an augmentation and after four reoperations for excessive breast firmness due to capsular contracture, each time placing larger and larger implants. Her surgeon (she let the same surgeon reoperate four times and had never sought a second opinion until now) continued to honor her wishes to try to achieve softer breasts and get larger implants! Bad team decisions. Her breasts were like rocks, and only thin skin, stretched from excessively large implants, covered her implants. We told Julie, "Enough is enough. More operations will only mean more potential complications, costs, risks, and possible permanent deformity. The best option is to remove the implants. You are one of a very small percentage of patients who persistently form tight capsules around your implants. We can't change your body's response, and we can't continue to surgically assault your tissues."

Julie's response? "No way. Not a chance. No way I'm giving up my implants. I know I can find someone who'll operate on me again!" True, no doubt. Also true: bad decision by Julie. When the inevitable complications occur, who is the last person Julie will blame? Julie. You guessed it! She will almost never blame herself. Instead, the surgeon and the implant will get the blame. The surgeon probably deserves some blame; the implant does not. The last surgeon who operates on Julie will get most of the blame, but it's Julie and the first surgeon who made the bad team decisions.

Most surgeons want to please their patients. Most patients want to keep their implants at any cost. Under certain circumstances, this combination can present problems. Going in, you should be aware of both good and bad results. You should know, if bad happens, what will be done. You and your surgeon should also set limits up front that define: If bad happens, when do we stop? When do we remove implants? Plan up front for the worst-case scenario, commit to limits prior to surgery, and disasters will be almost nonexistent. Problems are rare, but if you beat a dead horse, you get a beaten, dead horse. You are responsible for your decisions. A qualified surgeon will help inform you so that you can make good decisions, but remember, the decision is still yours. Do your research, think past dinner, and make your decisions carefully.

Disaster = Device (implant) alone? Almost never.

Disaster = Device + poor surgeon judgment + poor patient judgment
BAD TEAM DECISIONS

Is augmentation medically safe? Yes, provided you use good judgement and make good decisions. But if for any reason, you are not comfortable and convinced after considering the medical evidence, don't have an augmentation.

WHAT IN MY MEDICAL HISTORY SHOULD I CONSIDER?

Few hard rules exist that specify who should or should not have an augmentation based on medical history alone. Here, too, there are more grays than blacks or whites. Each case is different, and each surgeon approaches these issues differently. Here's what we tell our patients.

Recognizing that augmentation is a totally elective procedure (it's not medically necessary), if you have any of the following, we advise careful consideration about augmentation:

1. **A strong family history of breast cancer**

Mother with breast cancer—you probably should reconsider.

Mother and grandmother with breast cancer—forget it. You definitely shouldn't have augmentation.

Any breast implant can interfere with mammograms to some degree. Mammograms are not 100 percent accurate even without a breast implant. From 5 to 15 percent of breast cancers do not show up on a mammogram. The techniques used to do the mammogram and the experience of the person interpreting the mammogram also affect accuracy. But if you know that you have a significantly increased risk of breast cancer due to a strong family history, a breast augmentation just doesn't make good sense.

2. A personal history of autoimmune disease such as scleroderma, rheumatoid arthritis, lupus, or fibromyalgia

Even though breast implants have been shown **NOT** to cause these diseases, any stress (a surgical procedure, for example) could possibly affect the course of the disease. Why take a chance?

Interestingly, we have seen patients in consultation who had autoimmune diseases and brought written statements from their immunologists stating that the immunologist did not think that having an augmentation would affect their disease. A real chance for a bad decision? Do we know absolutely that just having an elective operation might not make the disease worse? If the disease did get worse, even if the implant didn't cause it, guess who and what would get the blame? We didn't do the augmentation.

3. HIV

Since HIV is also a disease that affects the immune system, the same logic applies for HIV that applies for other autoimmune diseases.

Any avoidable event that could possibly stress the immune system, especially when it is not medically necessary, probably isn't a good idea.

Add to that the increased risk of transmission to all of the medical personnel involved for a procedure that is not medically necessary. Make good sense? No.

Having said no, I would hasten to add that exceptions exist for every generalization in medicine. Our medical knowledge and, hopefully, our control of this dreaded disease are improving. If this disease is controlled, if we can prove that augmentation wouldn't make the disease worse, and if we have better measures to protect the patient and personnel, a patient's quality-of-life issues deserve careful consideration.

4.   Any other medical disease or condition

If you are not totally healthy or if you have ever had any other disease or condition diagnosed by your family physician or internist, you should consult that physician about the advisability of having an augmentation. We require a written letter from the physician confirming their opinion that your having an augmentation is reasonable, safe, and will not interfere with the management of your other conditions.

AM I JUST BEING VAIN?

Do you like feeling normal? For whatever personal reasons, do you feel that your breasts are less than normal or optimal? Do your breasts make dressing difficult? Do you have difficulty shopping for clothing? Do you like feeling that you are the best you can be, given what you have to work with and what you can't do for yourself? If you answer yes to these questions, you are very normal. If being vain is a desire to feel normal and wanting to be the best you can be, so be it. But it's not. Fact is, almost all of us do things that someone else might consider vain—personal things that are our own business that we do only for ourselves (and don't need to explain to anyone else)—things that make us feel better about ourselves. The key is doing those things responsibly.

Earlier, we discussed three large groups of women who consider augmentation:

1. The **"I never developed much to begin with"** group

2. The **"I lost everything I had after my baby"** group, and

3. The **"I want to improve for personal reasons"** group.

All perfectly normal women with perfectly normal, personal reasons to consider augmentation? Maybe, maybe not. There are always weird exceptions in any large group of people. Weird situations make the sensational stories you see in the media. The vast majority of all women we see who are considering augmentation are perfectly normal and approach this decision responsibly.

CAN I CHANGE ANY OTHER WAY?

Devices—and Their Vices

Aren't "wonder" bras wonderful? Compared to what? If you have got something the bra can push where you want it to go, usually up and in, then they are more wonderful than without them. But what if you don't have much to push somewhere? If you have enough to push, and you are happy with that, why have an augmentation? "Wonder" bras are cheaper and involve fewer trade-offs and risks. But if you don't have anything much to push and you want something to push, how can you get it?

Fillers and enhancers simply fill and enhance. From washcloths to tissues, from balloons to commercially available breast enhancers, every imaginable material has probably been tucked into a bra at one time or another. The good news? Any of them can fill and enhance provided they stay put. The bad news? They don't always stay put, and even if they do, they can be a huge nuisance. They are hot, itch, move around, and move out of place. The worst news about fillers and enhancers? As one of my patients told me, "They are slightly less than special when I undress, especially in front of or with the help of my lover."

A true patient story . . .

> Another patient was a tall, lithe, beautiful executive who happened to have a lovely figure except that she had virtually no breast tissue. She had considered all options and decided that the most state-of-the-art, shaped "enhancers" that fit inside her bra were the best answer. Everything went well until she was informed that she had been honored with her company's highest achievement award and that the award would be presented at a black tie gala that required a new black dress. Unfortunately, the perfect dress was strapless. Undaunted and resourceful, this patient decided to solve her problem with a large amount of electrical tape. Preparations for the evening were something akin to wiring the Pentagon. After applying several rolls of electrical tape, everything was perfectly in place. Enhanced didn't even begin to describe the result!
>
> As this beautiful but somewhat nervous executive stood accepting her award and anticipating her speech, she began perspiring heavily. The instant she stepped to the microphone to address her audience, something "enhanced" started to move. One sentence into the speech, something started sliding. With a deft grab of the

award plaque, she clutched it to her chest and stopped the downward sliding enhancer with one hand while she turned the page of her speech with the other. One minute later, the unthinkable—the other side started shifting to the side and sliding down! In one motion, she not so deftly swept the other elbow downward and up to get things hitched back up, then hugged the plaque to her chest with both arms. The next sentence became the last line of the speech as she unconsciously backed away from the microphone and hastily exited the stage: "I'm so honored and happy with this award that I may not let it go all night."

What about the water bra? As another patient told us, "Just imagine, if you're caught out in the desert, you have a built-in canteen! Wonder if it sloshes?" Another device, same problems. It's a thing.

External devices aren't as good as something that you don't have to think about, something that you incorporate unconsciously into your body image, then forget that it's there: Something that to many women seems more normal.

The Muscle Myth

Ever hear this? "If you just work out enough and build up your pec (pectoralis major) muscles, you can enlarge your breasts." Muscle is not breast tissue, and no matter how much you exercise it, you can't make it look like or act like breast tissue.

To make a pectoralis muscle enlarge significantly, you have to do serious, regular, bodybuilding exercises. Assuming you have the time and motivation, what you get is a bigger, thicker pectoralis muscle. Since most normal women don't have big, thick pectoralis muscles, you don't notice the muscle when you look at the breasts of most normal women. It's under there, but you don't see it. When you see a breast sitting on top of a big, thick pectoralis, you will almost always notice it because it doesn't look like something you normally see. The bigger muscle almost never blends naturally with the lines of the breast, so instead of seeing larger breasts, what you see is larger pectoralis with still small breasts on top of it. Bottom line?

You can't predictably make the breast appear larger (and you definitely can't make the breast appear natural) by exercising or building up the pectoralis muscle—or by any other exercises.

Other Magic Remedies?

Whenever you are dealing with an area of the body that affects one's sense of well-being and relates to sex, you will see every imaginable solution (and some you can't imagine) to any perceived problem relating to that area. Somehow, there seems to always be a definite, surefire cure for what ails you. The breast is no exception.

Drugs, herbs, lotions, massage, suction devices: you name it, and it has been touted as a predictable way to enlarge women's breasts.

We are not aware of a single one that really works and predictably enlarges the breast enough to satisfy a majority of patients and surgeons.

The only thing that predictably gets larger is the bank account of whoever sells it. Worse, some remedies, especially drugs, have effects or side effects that can be harmful if used improperly. Good examples are some types of hormones—steroids, estrogens, testosterone. Used properly for specific conditions under qualified medical supervision, each of these drugs works wonderfully for specific conditions. **Used to enlarge the breasts? No. Purely and simply, no.**

Maybe there is a better way predictably to enlarge the breasts other than augmentation, but we don't know a better, safer, and more predictable method. Assuming you are convinced that you can't do it on your own, you will logically need some help, but *help* is the key word. Part of the job is yours. Part of the responsibility is yours. All of the costs are yours. How much you are willing and able to do and the quality of the decisions you make will have a lot to do with the result now and in the future.

WHAT OTHER PEOPLE THINK AND SAY . . .

In deciding whether to consider breast augmentation, you will probably hear a lot of different opinions. Listen carefully, consider the content and source of the opinions, and filter out what you consider useful information. **Asking the following questions can be enlightening and helpful:**

> **Am I capable of making my own, personal decisions?**
>
> **Why would someone else want to make a decision for me or influence my decision?**
> Is my personal business their business?
>
> **Has this person had a breast augmentation?**
> If not, how does he or she know?

Did this person have a good result?

If so, why? How much does she know? Is she like me? What can I learn from her? What do I want to learn from her?

Did this person have a bad result?

Why? Did she do her homework? Did she and her surgeon(s) make good team decisions? If she had a problem, was it because of the implant? Is there any reason to expect that I would have the same problem? How much does she know? Is she like me? What can I learn from her? What do I want to learn from her?

Is this opinion based on facts and knowledge, or is it based on fluff?

The Media and Breast Augmentation

Breast augmentation is a popular topic. The media is interested in breast augmentation because you, their customers, are interested in breast augmentation. You will hear about whatever the media thinks you want to hear about—good or bad—as long as the media thinks the topic will make a good story and that you will read, watch, or listen. Negative stories are more common than positive stories. In the media, if it bleeds, it leads (to quote a news anchor patient). What percentage of stories on the evening news are "good news" stories? I can't prove it, but I'd bet that over 90% of media stories about augmentation are problem based. How productive is time spent hearing about problems? Why not spend the time offering **knowledge-based solutions** to avoid the problems at the outset?

What percentage of media stories focuses on problems? What you need are solutions!

Which is more productive: hearing about problems and negatives or learning about solutions to avoid problems?

What you don't need is sensationalism. What you do need is substance! Sensationalism can help you become the next sensational story. Substance helps you avoid becoming the next headline.

Are magazines, television, and radio a good source of information? Sometimes yes, sometimes no. It's your job to listen carefully, filter fact from fluff, consider the sources and the content, and then use good information appropriately. **At the end of any time spent watching, reading, or listening to media presentations, ask yourself:**

What did I learn that added to my knowledge?

What did I learn that will help me make better decisions?
Write down a list! I bet it will be a short one!

When you see information about augmentation in magazines or on TV, consider the following:

Media information is only as good as the sources.
If you don't know the sources, don't bet on the accuracy of the content.

If it's not stimulating, exciting, or new, you are not likely to hear about it.
How often have you seen stories about plastic surgery that focus on common sense and decision-making skills?

How many important, long-term personal decisions do you base on something stimulating and new?
If a lot, how did the decisions work out long term?

To make good decisions about plastic surgery, you need far more information than you can find in magazines or on television.

How often does the media take responsibility for the decisions that result from its information?

What most patients hope for and get is a routine, excellent result after an augmentation! How often do you hear this story in the media?

Balance is important, but sometimes the routine isn't exciting, stimulating, or "new" enough to be reported.

Are confrontation and controversy more important than basic information about augmentation?

What percentage of your time is best spent on basic information versus controversy and confrontation?

What can the media never tell you? Just how good your surgeon is at planning and performing your augmentation! And that has a lot to do with your recovery and result.

Use media information responsibly, but don't neglect your homework!

And, most important . . .

You can't educate yourself with sound bites.

You need information and a willingness to use it!

Breast augmentation is a complex topic. You need a lot of information to develop a broad perspective that helps you make good decisions. Most media articles and stories address one or two aspects of augmentation. Print space and television time don't allow adequate coverage of all the important issues. You will get pieces of information that are important to the pie; you just never get the whole pie. You see steps on the stairs, but you never see the whole staircase.

What does this say about our culture?

Why would a woman want to put some foreign object in her body just to have larger breasts? If I've heard this question once, I've heard it a hundred times. My answer? It depends on your assumptions. If you assume that the only reason that women have breast augmentations is to have a large chest (and many people make that assumption) and be noticed, then perhaps it says that our culture notices large breasts. After all, breasts have been a visual, sexual symbol since the beginning of civilization.

To generalize that most women want augmentation to have a large, noticeable chest is tenuous, if not patently absurd!

I wouldn't want to try to sell that concept to most women I know!

Another assumption is that women are intelligent individuals who are capable of making personal decisions based on valid information and their right to choose.

Most of our patients fall into this category!

There's a lot of ax-grinding with respect to augmentation. You have folks who want to sell stories and television time. Their axe is to always tell you about the new, the wonderful, or the controversial. You have unhappy patients whose axe is, unfortunately, a bad result or experience that they are just sure you will have, too (regardless of whether your decisions are the same as theirs). You have surgeons who make their living doing augmentations (we are in this category), so their axe is to tell you how good augmentation is! The only person you rarely get ax-grinding from is the happy patient who would have an augmentation again, in an instant, but doesn't feel compelled to discuss it with anyone!

How many "good-news," "I-am-thrilled-with-the-improvement," "I-would-do-it-again-in-an-instant" stories have you seen, heard, or read?

If you think it's because they are rare, just ask around!

THE "AM I" AND "CAN I" QUESTIONS

If you can't answer **YES** to every question that follows, you might consider stopping on this first step of the stairs.

Am I willing to do my homework and make this my own decision?

What homework? The more you learn and understand about breast augmentation, the more likely you are to make the right decisions that ultimately determine your result. The homework isn't heavy, and some women hardly do it at all. Some women also aren't happy with the results. Even if they are, some women don't really know whether they have a good result or not. If you care and you want to know, our goal is to help give you the tools.

Your homework consists of reading this book and every piece of informational material that you accumulate from surgeons and other sources.

Make a list of issues and questions.
Get answers before making decisions.

If the answers don't make sense, seek more information and other answers. Organize your questions, and ask them over and over to different surgeons until you are satisfied. Follow the steps outlined in this book, and you will be far better prepared and informed than most prospective augmentation patients who don't do their homework. Most of all, you will be more comfortable making decisions that can affect your result, and the decisions will be better ones.

Who else would make your decisions for you? I hope that the answer is no one. I hope that those close to you will be supportive and respect your intelligence, privacy, and decisions. What about everyone else? What will they think? Who cares? It doesn't matter, and it isn't their business. But for the sake of discussion, let's assume someone else feels they could (or should) make decisions for you. What about a boyfriend, husband, or significant other? Should they be interested? You bet. Interested in you (if they really care), and if they are normal, in your breasts as well. Should they become informed, provide input, and ask questions? Yes, great! But make decisions for you? That's something else. **Whenever a patient mentions the demands made by a significant other with respect to augmentation, we have two ready replies:**

1. We hope the statistics never apply to you, but the divorce rate is 50 percent in the United States, so you have a coin-toss chance that the person who enjoys your breasts with you now won't be the same person enjoying them with you in the future. If you are doing it for someone else and not specifically for yourself, how do you plan to deal with the next significant other wanting something different? Another operation?

Make your own decisions for yourself and only for yourself. If you are happy with the results, you can credit yourself.

If not, you know whom to blame.

2. Have you ever seen the person who wants to make your decision for you change his or her mind about anything? What do you do when that person has a change of heart after placing the order? This isn't McDonalds! We are not talking about fast food, a little more mustard or cut the onions. It isn't even Neiman Marcus. We are not talking about a gown that can be altered or replaced with another gown. We are talking about making changes to your body that you will live with forever.

Think long term. Don't make decisions that you are likely to want or need to change.

Nothing gets better when you need to change things later.

Am I Willing to Realistically Accept the Risks and Trade-offs?

Later, we will go into a lot more detail about specific risks and trade-offs. For now, let's just assume (because it's true) that every augmentation involves trade-offs and risks. No matter who does it, no matter how well it's done, no matter what technique, incision location, pocket location or implant, there are trade-offs and risks. The only question is whether you learn what they are, consider them, and, hopefully, avoid them, or whether you never know. Never knowing can be nice, but only if you are the luckiest person in the world, a person who magically, with minimal thought and preparation, gets the best result by a surgeon, whom you located fortuitously, who never has complications using an implant that is perfect and lasts forever, and who can control every aspect of your body's healing processes. Fairy tale. Never happens.

You need to know details about risks and trade-offs before you can decide whether you are willing to accept them. We'll supply the details later. **For now, just ask yourself:**

> **Do I fully understand that this is not magic?**
> It is surgery that involves factors that neither I nor any surgeon can fully control.
>
> **Do I understand that nothing material, even a breast implant, lasts forever?**
>
> **Do I accept that any surgery is serious and that I will live with the results forever?**
>
> **Do I understand that perfection is not an option, only an improvement?**
>
> **Can I accept that although risks are very low, bad things can happen?**

If you can't answer YES to all of these questions, breast augmentation may not be the best thing for you.

STOP ON THE FIRST STAIR STEP.

Can I Handle the Costs?

For a first-time augmentation (primary), costs can vary a lot, and we'll go into more detail later. For now, assume that you will spend between $5,000 and $10,000 for an augmentation by a board-certified surgeon. Less than $4,000, you are most likely getting a "bargain" that may not be a bargain later. More than $8,000, you are likely paying more than you need to pay to get a top-quality augmentation with a state-of-the-art implant. Like everything else, these costs will increase in the future.

When it comes to price, think value. If ever value is important, it's when you are hiring someone to operate on you!

Can I afford it? Not can I somehow get the money to get the implants, but can I really afford it? If not, don't do it until you can afford it.

In our experience, patients who plan carefully and save for their augmentations are often happier than patients who stretch beyond their means to borrow money or spend money they don't have, and then later have difficulty paying it back. A financial burden can detract from fully enjoying the result. Financing options that we discuss later are available, but financing is a reasonable option only when the payments fit your income and your budget.

If someone else pays for the augmentation, the question, "Can you afford it?" takes on an entirely new meaning and raises other issues. Under the correct circumstances, wonderful (a gift from your husband). Under other circumstances, not so wonderful. How good will it feel if later someone informs you that they own a piece of you? Is it worth it to afford it?

Am I Willing to Use Common Sense? Can I Think Past Dinner?

These questions are certainly not meant to insult or demean. Neither question, however, should be taken lightly. The anticipation prior to augmentation and the positive effects after surgery are powerful and can affect even highly intelligent, accomplished, reasonable people. Once you decide to have implants, you want them now, and you want to keep them forever.

Throughout your quest for the best breast, common sense is invaluable.

The more you use it, the easier and better your decisions.

If you don't feel confident that you have common sense and that you can use it no matter how appealing something becomes, be careful. Many patients and, regrettably, some surgeons focus on the here and now. Think past dinner? Dinner is here and now, tonight. Think at least five years ahead.

Thinking past dinner means recognizing that what you do now you will live with for the rest of your life.

Choose for now and for when you are sixty or older.

We will tell you how later. If you use common sense and think past dinner, you will make better decisions. Can you do it? If the answer is yes, take a step upward.

Am I Willing to Remove an Implant if Necessary?

Once you get the implants, if you are like 99 percent of patients, you will want to keep them, no matter what. Our advice to patients is that implants are wonderful for the overwhelming majority of patients. If for any reason they are not, especially if there's any hint that they could affect your health or well-being in the future, remove them. We both need to make that commitment before doing your augmentation. What makes implant removal necessary? Very rare incidences of infection and multiple recurrences of capsular contracture are reasons that I recommend implant removal to patients. More about that later.

Before having an augmentation, if you can't commit to removing your implants if it becomes necessary, I would recommend you don't have an augmentation.

Many surgeons don't discuss this specific issue during consultations, but it's better to address the issue *before* surgery than to first hear about it *after* surgery.

So, does it make sense to even think about augmentation?

I hope that you have a better feeling for the answer to this question by now. If it makes sense to continue to think about it, the next step on the stairs is learning what you need to know and how to go about it.

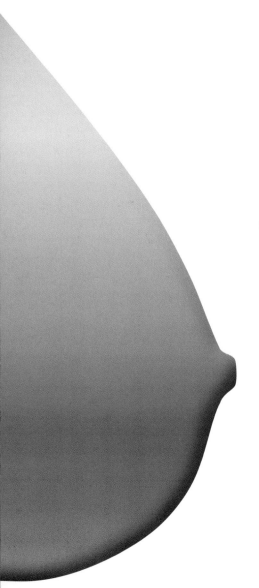

FIRST THINGS FIRST:

WHAT YOU NEED TO KNOW AND HOW TO GO ABOUT FINDING IT

"If you want to make the best decisions for your future, you will consider at least ten topics . . . before you think about the only three decisions that a less-informed patient considers."

Before we go into detail about the many different options and choices in breast augmentation, let's start by making a **shopping list of what you need to know**. Then we will give you a guide for learning what you will need to know. Armed with your shopping list and your guide, you can better explore each step in detail. Before you climb the stairs, we will give you a look at the entire staircase.

You need to know the answers to more than three questions.

When considering augmentation, many women focus only on three basic questions:

1. What cup size am I going to be? (What size implant?)

2. Where will the incision be?

3. Will my implant be over the muscle or under the muscle? Or maybe the newest option, dual plane (more about dual plane later), partly over and partly under muscle to maximize benefits and minimize trade-offs of the other pocket locations?

Why these three questions? For many patients, these are the only issues they ever hear from friends, other patients, and the media. Believe it or not, many patients only hear about the first two. They don't ask. They often don't know *what* to ask. Regrettably, some surgeons don't volunteer information about *choices* and *options*. Some surgeons are not committed to patient education. If you don't know, if you don't care to ask, and if your surgeon doesn't help as much as possible, the result can be less-than-optimal decisions.

WEAK TEAM PREPARATION can lead to BAD TEAM DECISIONS.

We want good team decisions. Good team decisions begin with you.

If you aren't armed with knowledge, one member of the team is weak—you. Without the basics, why bother researching surgeons? You won't be able to distinguish fact from fluff. If you can't evaluate a surgeon, you will likely not select the best surgeon for you. Then another member of the team is weak—the surgeon. Two weak team members increase the chances of weak or bad team decisions.

If you want to make the best decisions for your future, you will consider at least ten topics . . . before you think about the only three decisions that a less-informed patient considers.

Let's start with a shopping list of 10 topics you need to research before you contact a surgeon:

What You Need to Know Before Consulting a Surgeon

1. What do you want, and what will your body allow you to have?

2. Implant types and options: shape, smooth or textured shell, type of filler material.

3. Possible complications, risks, and trade-offs.

4. Implant pocket location: Over muscle (retromammary) or partially under muscle (partial retropectoral) or the newest option, dual plane (a combination of over and under muscle) to maximize benefits and minimize trade-offs compared to the other two locations.

5. Incision-location options.

6. Implant size.

7. Options and trade-offs: Sorting them out.

8. Complications and trade-offs: things you and the surgeon can't control.

9. Recovery: ask about it up front because what you hear can tell you a lot.

10. How to organize your information to use it effectively.

Learn about these topics before you call a surgeon's office.

HOW TO GO ABOUT IT

In this chapter, we give you an overall outline of what you need to know to make good team decisions. In the chapters that follow in Part II of the book, we will explore the details of every topic on this list to let you look at the stairs thoroughly before you start climbing. Having armed you with knowledge, in Part III, we will move to the next logical step—contacting and consulting surgeons and making decisions. Finally, in Part IV, you will finalize decisions and prepare for surgery and recovery. Our reason for this sequence is: It's best to know what you need to know, learn it, then apply what you know to surgeon selection and the decision-making process.

The "How to Go About It" List

1. List what you need to know (the ten topics).

2. Research each topic.

3. Armed with knowledge, prepare for surgeon consultations.

4. Consult surgeons and evaluate what they tell you (using what you have learned). Ask in detail about your recovery (drains, bandages, special bras, time to resume full, normal activities) because it will tell you a lot about how much bleeding or tissue trauma you are likely to have during your surgery.

5. Choose your surgeon.

6. Select from your options and discuss the trade-offs with your surgeon (team decisions).

7. Think about the choices you have made and the trade-offs you have accepted. Be sure you are comfortable.

8. If you have any questions or if anything is not clear, talk with your surgeon again. The time to clarify every detail is before, not after, your surgery.

9. Have your surgery and follow your surgeon's instructions for recovery.

10. Enjoy!

Now that we understand the process, let's begin learning what we need to know!

PART II

ARMING YOURSELF WITH INFORMATION:
LEARNING WHAT YOU NEED TO KNOW TO MAKE AN INFORMED DECISION

RECONCILING DESIRES WITH REALITY:

WHAT DO I WANT AND WHAT WILL MY BODY ALLOW ME TO HAVE?

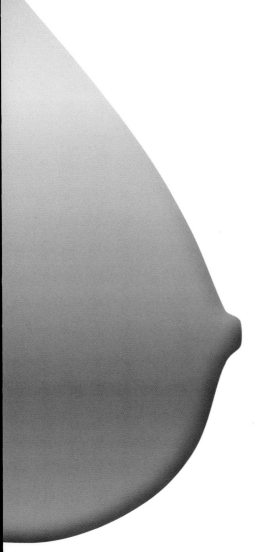

"If you and your surgeon don't recognize and acknowledge what your body tissues will allow you to have now and for the future, one or both of you may pay a penalty you don't want to pay."

One of the first and most important steps on the staircase is understanding the importance of reconciling desires with reality—reconciling your *wishes* with your *tissues*. What you want with what your body will allow you to have. It's much easier to find a surgeon who will tell you he can produce what you want than to find a surgeon who knows and will tell you how what you want is likely to affect you now and in the future. The choices you make now may decisively influence your risks of having problems and reoperations in the future.

It is critically important that you understand not only what you want but also how what you want is likely to affect you and your breasts in the future. Wishes are fine, but good wishes come true only when you and your surgeon reconcile your wishes with what your tissues will realistically allow you to have.

WHY DEFINE WHAT YOU WANT, AND HOW DEFINITIVE SHOULD YOU BE?

Let's start by assuming that you would like to have breasts that are beautiful or, at the least, better than they are now. But what is a "beautiful" breast? What is "better than they are now?" You probably have some feelings about the answers to these questions, but the feelings may be general and not well defined. That's okay for starters. In fact, that's probably a good start. Think first in generalizations, then focus and define your desires more clearly as you learn more. You don't like what you have now, but how do you make a surgeon understand what you want?

The more clearly you define your expectations and the better you communicate your specific desires to your surgeon, the more likely you will achieve your goals.

ONCE YOU HAVE DEFINED IT, IS IT ACHIEVABLE?
AT WHAT PRICE?

Assume we have defined our goals and expectations in detail. Great! We know what we want, but getting it can be another matter. Reality sets in. Is it achievable? What are the costs? Will circumstances allow me to get what I want? These questions always require answers.

Let's assume you would like to have beautiful, full C cup or small D cup breasts with a naturally sloping upper breast (they look like breasts, not volleyballs), a nice hang to the lower breast without sagging, and nipples that point slightly upward that will maintain that look as you grow older. But, you are forty years old, have never had children, have virtually no breast tissue (your chest is absolutely flat); you are a workout fanatic with almost no body fat; and you hate wearing bras. Can you get what you want? Will your body allow you to have what you want? Is it doable with current implant options and surgical techniques? No way, no how, not gonna happen. Your body is not going to allow you to have what you want, and if you push it, your body and you will pay the price! If you get implants large enough to produce the D cup you want, your tissues will change due to the weight, your already thin tissues will sag and thin more, and you are likely to see edges of the implant and see visible rippling as the implant pulls on the thin overlying tissues! Over time, excessively large implants or very highly projecting implants can cause your breast tissue to shrink away (atrophy) and can cause deformities of your ribs and chest wall beneath the implant.

In breast augmentation, one of the most difficult steps on the staircase is reconciling what you want with what your body will allow you to have.

To make the right choices, you will need to understand more about your tissues.

Unfortunately, few surgeons and even fewer patients spend enough time with this step before doing an augmentation. A skilled, experienced surgeon can deliver almost anything you can dream up. With today's surgical techniques and implant options, you can create almost any size breast. What can be unfortunate is the price you may pay, now or later.

You come with only one set of tissues, you can't change those tissues for the better, and you can't replace those tissues.

If you choose options that exceed what your tissues can tolerate, sooner or later you are likely to pay with visible edges, loss of breast tissue, visible rippling, or other uncorrectable deformities.

Many patients never know before their augmentation what price they may pay years later if they don't recognize and respect what their tissues will allow them to have.

A classic example? Too large an implant with thin overlying tissues, excess tissue stretch, excess tissue thinning, shrinkage of your breast tissue, further aging and thinning of tissues, visible implant edges, and visible rippling from implants pulling on thin overlying tissues. Maybe even operations to try to correct rippling or visible edges that usually can't be corrected because no surgeon can change the qualities of tissues that have been compromised by excessively large implants.

Another classic example? An excessively highly projecting implant that is trying to force tight tissues to create a more projecting breast. The price over time is loss of breast tissue (atrophy) and possible rib and chest wall deformities, both uncorrectable deformities.

Unless you like problems, more surgeries, more costs, and more disappointments, you don't want to ignore what your tissues will allow you to have.

Is there any excuse for not knowing and not respecting your tissues? Maybe not good excuses, but there may be some mitigating circumstances. Some surgeons, especially early in their careers, have not followed enough patients long enough to fully appreciate what happens to tissues over time and how implant options can affect the equation. Happy augmentation patients often do not return for long-term, follow-up appointments, so the surgeon can't learn from what the surgeon doesn't see. The last thing that many younger patients want to think about is getting older (to be honest, even I don't like thinking about it, and I am older). But you will get older. Your tissues will change and not for the better (visualize your grandmother's breasts). How your implant affects those tissues can change over time. If you **make good team decisions now**, you have a much better chance of having nice grandmother breasts in the future.

A concept and a mission . . . to avoid penalties in the future

One of the missions of this book is to raise the level of awareness of this important concept:

If you and your surgeon don't recognize and acknowledge what your body tissues will allow you to have now and for the future and try to match your implant choice to your tissue characteristics, one or both of you may pay a penalty you don't want to pay.

Any team decision that ignores this concept is a bad team decision. You can make it be a bad decision by asking for the wrong thing(s). Your surgeon can present or encourage choices that make a bad team decision. Or your surgeon can, with perfectly good intentions, try to deliver what you ordered without helping you understand the implications of your choices. Any one or combination of these can result in bad team decisions that penalize you and your surgeon in the future.

WHERE DO WE START? WITH WHAT YOU DON'T LIKE OR WITH WHAT YOU WANT?

Both, actually. Start with what you don't like; then list what you want. To help, here's a list of steps:

Defining what you don't like and what you want—a list

1. List the things you dislike about your breasts.

2. List how those dislikes affect your feeling of being normal or how those dislikes affect your lifestyle.

3. List the basics of what you would like to have based on what you know now.

4. Read the rest of this chapter to help you understand what your body may allow you to have.

5. Refine your list of what you'd like to have based on your new knowledge.

6. Look at your list carefully, and ask yourself if you are willing to live with your choices long term.

7. Finalize your list of "wants" that you will discuss with surgeons you visit.

8. Don't let window shopping (looking at pictures in magazines and surgeon's "brag books") fool you about reality and the future. Think about your own tissues.

LISTING YOUR DISLIKES

Make this easy. Pick simple things like these that we have heard from patients:

My breasts are too small for my figure.

I wish the top of me matched the bottom.

I look like a bowling pin.

I can't fill up any bra.

I wish I could wear a T-shirt or blouse without a bra.

I'm tired of buying things to fit the bottom, then having to spend more money altering or filling the top.

Cleavage is not a word in my vocabulary.

If I could take what's on my butt and put it in my breasts, I'd be deadly.

Every bathing suit I buy must contain helpful devices.

I'm sick of males asking me why I just don't wear trunks instead of that girlish bathing suit.

If I'm not careful, I'll trip on them.

Hold a pencil underneath? Hell, I could hold a barbell!

My upper breasts look like ski slopes! No, they look worse than a ski slope.

I wish I had what I had before I was pregnant.

I liked what I had when I was pregnant (or nursing) a lot better than what I have now.

I'm sure there are more, but you get the idea.

LISTING WHAT YOU WANT BASED ON WHAT YOU KNOW NOW

These are examples listed according to how often we hear them from patients:

Fuller upper breasts

More cleavage

X cup breast (Choose the cup size.)

Perkier breasts

Not huge, but proportionate to my figure

More fullness at the sides to balance my hips

A better shape to my breasts

Fix my weird nipples

Baywatch breasts—big and round

Now that we know what we don't like and what we would like to have, let's learn more about the implications of our wants.

HOW NOT TO DEFINE YOUR EXPECTATIONS

Although some methods of defining breast size are popular, they are not as accurate as we might like to believe. First, let's consider how not to define your desired breast.

Cup size—especially cup size alone

Cup size is not even a consistent fashion measurement, let alone a medical term that can accurately and consistently define breast size.

But it's probably the most common yardstick women use. Any woman who has ever shopped for bras knows that a B is not a B is not a B. Although the labels say the same size, when you put them on, some fit and some don't. For the same woman, some B cup bras fit better than her usual C cup and vice a versa. Some B cup bras fit better than other B cup bras. Check your own bra drawer! How many cup sizes do you have?

We frequently hear from patients, I'm sorta a B cup and I want to be a full C cup. Our response is simple. Tell me what a sorta B or a full C cup is! Can you go buy me a bra that is labeled sorta B or full C? If you can't define it and you can't buy a bra labeled it, how do you expect a surgeon to create it? And if a surgeon tells you he can create it, what should that tell you about the surgeon?

Cup size is extremely variable and inconsistent from one brand of bra to another.

If cup size is inconsistent and you know it from buying your own bras, why would you want to rely on cup size to specify what you want?

You can't define it because it isn't a consistent measurement from manufacturer to manufacturer, as much as they'd like you to think it is. If a surgeon guarantees you a cup size, that should tell you something about the surgeon. How can you deliver something that isn't consistently definable? What about the surgeon who doesn't even know that bra cup size is not consistent or definable?

How do we use cup size? We have no objection to using cup size as a general guideline, provided you recognize it is only a *general guide* that can't be ordered or delivered, and your surgeon doesn't talk to you about cup size *only* when defining your desired outcome.

We always ask our patients the following questions: What cup size were you before you were pregnant? Largest during pregnancy? What cup size after pregnancy and nursing if you nursed? What are you now? What would you like to be? If cup size is not a consistent measurement, why do we ask? The answers to these questions give us a clearer understanding of how our patient sees her breasts. During our exam, measurements will precisely define the size of the patient's skin envelope.

Knowing what a patient thinks she is (by asking the questions) and knowing what she really is (from our measurements) helps us better understand the patient's perspective and her wishes.

But we NEVER define the desired result by cup size alone.

Many women don't buy bras to fit their breasts . . . a personal revelation from Dr. Tebbetts

During my first several years in plastic surgery, I was baffled by the array of bra types and sizes that patients applied to breasts that all looked very similar and that measured similar in size on exam. One of the more enlightening milestones of my plastic surgery career was the day I realized that women don't buy bras to fit their breasts. Most women buy bras to push their breast tissue where they think it looks best. Women don't necessarily buy bras that fit their breasts. They buy bras that the breast will fill. What do I mean?

The width of a breast (from side-to-side, Figure 4-1) increases with increasing cup size. But I was amazed that women who had measurements indicating a D cup width were often telling me they were a B cup. What they really meant was that they were wearing a B cup bra. Then one day I asked a patient to please put her bra on as I observed. The B cup bra did not fit the fold beneath the breast. The breast was wide, more like a D cup width. The bra she had picked was much narrower than the width of the breast. When the patient put it on, she leaned forward and tucked the outside part of the wider breast inward to fill the cup of the smaller and narrower B cup bra. A light went on! Then I understood! She picked the smaller B cup bra because the amount of breast tissue that she had would fill it! When she pushed the outside portion of the breast inward into the bra, it not only filled the bra but bulged at the top of the breast and toward the middle. More cleavage! From that day on, I have been able to put bra cup size in perspective and rely more on measurements to document the size of breasts.

Breast Width and Cup Size

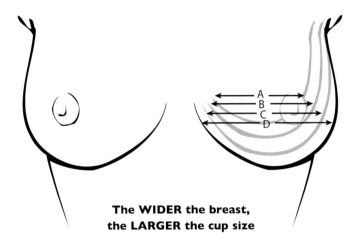

**The WIDER the breast,
the LARGER the cup size**

FIGURE 4-1

Women buy a bra that they can fill.

*Women buy bras to push breast tissue where they want
it to go to create a specific appearance.*

Women don't necessarily buy bras that fit their breasts!

Implant size in ccs

One measurement of the size of a breast implant is the volume (amount of filler) in the implant measured in cubic centimeters (ccs). Do you know how much a cc is? How much is 300 ccs? How many ccs are your breasts right now? How many ccs are in a B cup? How many ccs in a C cup? If you are thinking about trying to define what you want in terms of ccs, you should know the answers to all these questions. Fact is, some of these questions don't have an answer, at least not one correct answer. The answer to some of the questions is "It depends."

Join a conversation with a group of women discussing their breast implants, and you might hear, "I have 300 cc implants, and I'm a C cup." Another woman responds, "How can that be? I have 300 cc implants, and I'm a D cup." They could both be correct. The message? A certain implant size in ccs does not guarantee a certain cup size. Why?

When teaching courses to surgeons, I have frequently asked the question, how many ccs does it take to produce a C cup breast? Invariably, one or more surgeons will respond with a specific number of ccs that will predictably produce a certain cup size breast, usually a less experienced surgeon. Also invariably, another surgeon will answer correctly by pointing out the following:

An augmented breast consists of the skin envelope plus the implant plus whatever breast tissue the woman had before the augmentation.

Expressed as a formula for surgeons: Augmentation Result = Envelope + Parenchyma (breast tissue) + Implant

Now you can answer the question of how, if both women described above had 300 cc implants, one could have a C cup breast and the other a D cup breast. The woman who ended up having a D cup breast after augmentation had more breast tissue before her augmentation compared to the woman who ended up with a C cup breast.

A certain number of ccs in an implant does not make a certain cup size breast.

Be sure you understand this concept, and then ask yourself if your surgeon understands it, based on what the surgeon tells you.

The final size of the breast depends on the amount of breast tissue the woman had prior to surgery plus the size of the implant that was placed in the breast.

So a woman who has more breast tissue to begin with needs fewer ccs in an implant (smaller) to get to a C cup breast compared to another woman who had less breast tissue to begin with, and will need a larger implant to get to a C cup breast. If this concept is confusing, read it again until it makes sense.

Now you know why a certain size implant (in ccs) does not make a specific cup size breast!

The cup size an implant will make depends on how much breast tissue the woman had before her augmentation.

Now that we know how not to define our desired breast size, how do we define it? At this stage, it's fine for you to specify what you want with the simple "want list" you made. Don't worry too much about specifics until you understand more about how breast size affects your tissues. Later, you and your surgeon can make more realistic estimates of what is achievable (and the trade-offs) by thinking about your specific tissues. Do you have enough skin to create what you want? Do you have too much skin that will require more than what you want to fill it optimally? And a whole series of additional questions that will help answer the question, Will your tissues allow you to have what you want? To what degree? And for how long?

Do you have what it takes (your tissues) to get what you want? And what do you have when you get it (the long-term result)?

How Much Is Enough?

How much breast is enough? In the first edition of this book, we stated that breast size should be in proportion to body size or body shape. While that may be an ideal concept, it is not totally correct or realistic.

The amount of implant volume and the optimal size of the breast are defined only by the amount of skin available in that breast—the width of the breast envelope and the stretch of the breast envelope. The smaller and narrower the breast and breast envelope, the less fill or volume will fit into that envelope without causing tissue damage that can produce the uncorrectable deformities we just mentioned. While we might like to produce large, wide breasts to better balance large, wide hips, the amount of skin and breast fill that you come with may limit how much a surgeon can safely put in your breast without causing permanent damage.

Remember these important principles (we will go over them more later):

- The wider a woman's breast before augmentation and the more the skin stretches (and we will measure both), the more volume is required to fill the patient's envelope to get an optimal result.

- If we don't put enough fill (implant size) in the breast, allowing for skin stretch, you won't have enough fill in the upper breast, and the upper breast will appear empty.

- If we put too much fill to match the width and stretch of your breast, you will have too much fill in the upper breast with excess upper bulging and a *Baywatch* looking breast. (Some women like this look, and we can produce it, but excess fill always comes with a price later—increased risk of sagging, excess tissue thinning, visible implant edges, and visible rippling from the implant pulling on thin overlying tissues.)

From a practical, common-sense perspective, a woman's breasts are "designed" to enlarge an amount that approximates the amount of enlargement that usually occurs with pregnancy. For most women, the breast usually enlarges an average of one to one and one-half cup sizes during pregnancy. Of course, the larger the breast before pregnancy, the greater the degree of enlargement during pregnancy. The larger the breast during pregnancy, the more the skin stretches to accommodate the enlarged breast tissue. After pregnancy, the breast tissue shrinks and falls to the bottom of the larger, stretched skin envelope. The result is a more sagging breast that is emptier in the upper breast. Extreme enlargement with pregnancy usually results in a very sagging breast with thin skin and visible stretch marks.

If you have been pregnant and can remember the degree of fullness of your breasts at nine months (not necessarily the maximum fullness when your milk came in), the nine month amount of fill is approximately what is required to achieve an optimal amount of safe fill in your breast.

Similar changes occur following breast augmentation, and is the amount that the High Five™ measuring system recommends. The larger the implant, the larger the resulting breast. The larger the implant, the more the breast skin stretches and thins and the more the breast will ultimately sag as a woman ages, losing upper fill.

An augmented breast may not sag quite as much as an unaugmented breast of the same size, but the larger the implant, the more the breast will sag in the future as you age.

If a surgeon tells you that an augmented breast won't sag or that excessively large implants (usually over 350 cc) can't possibly cause the problems listed previously, locate another surgeon who understands tissue dynamics.

The Funnel Analogy

What is ideal fill for each woman's skin envelope? If a woman has had previous pregnancies, her skin envelope is already stretched. Envision a funnel and pitcher pouring liquid into a breast envelope (Figure 4-2, A). If the envelope has already been stretched, the fluid will initially fill the lower breast. As more fluid is added, at some point, the breast appears full and natural with a natural appearing upper breast slope (Figure 4-2, B). If more fluid is added, the upper breast begins to bulge outwardly as the skin envelope is overfilled.

What Is Ideal Fill?

If you want a natural appearing breast, there is a correct amount of fill that is both the *least* and the *most* for an optimal result.

Less fill leaves you an
empty upper breast.

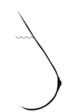

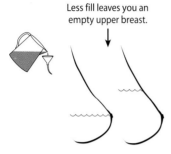

A. INADEQUATE FILL

B. IDEAL FILL
**Similar to maximal enlargement
with pregnancy**

Excess fill produces an unnatural excessively bulging upper breast.

C. EXCESSIVE FILL

Excessive Risks	May Require	Consequences	
	Breast lift (mastopexy)	More scars, Sensory loss, Costs, Risks	
Tissue thinning	No correction	Visible implant edges Visible rippling or wrinkling	Uncorrectable deformities
More Sagging, thinning	Another breast lift with higher risks and poorer results	Possible wound healing problems, even implants exposure requiring removal Possible disfigurement	Uncorrectable deformities
Shrinkage of existing breast tissue	Not correctable	Visible implant edges Feel shell of implant Impact on nursing	Uncorrectable deformities

FIGURE 4-2

Exactly the same principles apply to breast augmentation. To achieve an optimal aesthetic result, enough filler must be added (the size of the implant) to adequately fill the envelope (Figure 4-2, B). If a woman wants a very bulging upper breast, more filler (a larger implant) is required. But the larger the implant, the more the stretch, the more the breast will sag in the future, and the greater the risk of tissue thinning with stretch, which allows the implant edges to become visible and visible rippling or wrinkling resulting from the implants pulling on the thin overlying tissues. Visible implant edges and traction rippling are often uncorrectable by surgery.

How much is enough? If the best long-term result is the goal, the answer is to fill the existing envelope to ideal fill and a natural breast contour (Figure 4-2, B). Any overfill past this point virtually guarantees that the breast will sag more in the future, increasing risks of implant edge visibility and traction rippling, causing possible shrinkage (atrophy) of existing breast tissue, decreasing the quality of the result (Figure 4-2, C), and increasing risks of reoperations. For women who have never been pregnant, the surgeon must estimate a normal amount of stretch that would occur with pregnancy, given each woman's breast tissue characteristics.

Women who are very flat chested often ask surgeons to produce a breast that projects much more off their chest wall compared to what they have. Implants that have significantly more back to front thickness (projection) push the skin forward more and create more projection. These "high projection" and "extra high-projection" implants have become more and more popular recently for patients wanting a more projecting breast. Unfortunately, high-projection implants can cause significant and uncorrectable long-term tissue damage. The tighter a patient's skin and the more projecting (or large) the implant, the more pressure the implant exerts on the patient's breast tissue (parenchyma). This pressure, over time, causes the breast tissue to shrink or atrophy, decreasing soft-tissue coverage over the implant and possibly impairing a patient's ability to nurse or impairing sensation. Excessive implant projection and pressure can even cause rib-cage deformities. Highly projecting implants are sometimes needed in breast reconstruction, but are rarely indicated in primary breast augmentation.

A key concept is that a properly chosen breast implant does not force tissues to where they have never been or were never intended to go. An optimum implant either optimally fills the space present or stretches tissues no further than they are likely to stretch with a pregnancy.

When you choose an implant that is too large for your skin to support, the implant can cause tissue changes (listed in Figure 4-2, C) that cannot be reversed and that can result in unsatisfactory consequences and additional surgery. Remember that your choice of breast size has long-term consequences.

WHAT DO YOU HAVE NOW?

A surgeon can work only with the tissues that you bring to the surgeon.

Look at your breasts in the mirror. Do they look exactly like any other woman's breasts that you have ever seen? No. Do they match side to side? Never. And they will never exactly match following an augmentation! Do they look the same now as they looked five years ago? Probably not, if you look closely. No two women have exactly the same breast appearance because every woman's tissues and combination of tissues are different. The two breasts never match exactly because the tissues are never exactly the same in both breasts.

No woman has two breasts that are the same, and no surgeon can create two breasts that are exactly the same.

Your breasts don't look the same as they did five years ago because your tissues are five years older, and the characteristics of those tissues have changed. They will continue to change throughout your lifetime. I wish we could tell you they change for the better, but tissue quality predictably declines with aging.

Will what you have (your tissues) allow you to get what you want (your result)?

Since a surgeon can only work with what you bring, whether you can get what you want depends on what you bring the surgeon—your individual tissues—to work with. Will your tissues allow you to get what you want? Do you have the optimal amount and type of skin to accept the implant that will create the breast you are ordering? If your tissues will accept the implant, how will your choices affect your breasts in the future? These are complex questions that don't necessarily have a single correct answer. Begin by memorizing two inescapable truths, then tell every woman you know who is considering augmentation (and every surgeon you see who doesn't already know) the following:

The bigger the breast, the worse it will look over time— augmented or not! Think about the woman you knew at a younger age with large breasts. How do they look now?

Aging in the Excessively Augmented

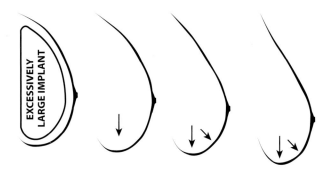

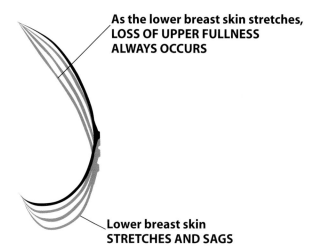

**As the lower breast skin stretches,
LOSS OF UPPER FULLNESS
ALWAYS OCCURS**

**Lower breast skin
STRETCHES AND SAGS**

The larger the implant, the more your tissue will stretch.

The more your tissues stretch, the more the breast will sag.

**Risks of visible rippling, visible edges, feeling the implant,
and reoperations increase.**

FIGURE 4-3

Your tissues won't get better as you age; they will get worse! Think about your grandmother's breasts or any woman's breasts after age sixty.

We aren't dealing with magic here. A little logic and common sense goes a long way. The bigger the breast you request (all other factors being equal), the bigger and heavier the implant and the more that implant will stretch your tissues over time (Figure 4-3). Stretched breast skin sags and thins. All this happens as you and your tissues are getting older and more stretchy on their own. You can't do anything about what you come with (genetics are inescapable) or how your breast envelope ages (aging is inescapable, too), but you certainly can affect how the implant may affect your tissues in the future by avoiding excessively large implants.

The bigger the breast you request, the worse it will look over time. Guaranteed.

Continue to remind yourself: The bigger the implant I request, the worse it will look over time, and the greater my risk of reoperations and uncorrectable deformities.

Not only will it look worse, the bigger the implant you get now, the more likely you may pay in the future for additional operations and additional costs. You may, for example, require a breast lift (mastopexy) with additional scars, more risk of loss of sensation, and additional costs sooner if you select implants large enough to accelerate sagging. More about that later. For now, just recognize and acknowledge that:

For the best long-term result, you might want to balance what you want with what your tissues will allow you to have. Your surgeon should help you understand the characteristics of your individual tissues and which options are realistic for you.

For the best long-term result, you might want to balance what you want with what your tissues can support over time. Ask you surgeon specifically how the implants you select will affect your individual tissues over time, and take notes. This will make your surgeon aware that you are concerned about this and want the best result for the longest time with the least risk of reoperations and uncorrectable deformities.

The real truth is that different patients' tissues react differently to the same implant over time. No surgeon can tell you exactly how your tissues will age, how soon you will sag, or when you may need a breast lift. But you should remember this: if a surgeon doesn't bring up the subject of your tissue characteristics and how your choice of implant might affect your long-term result, stop and think. Just what are the chances that you will get the best long-term result from that surgeon?

TWO GOLDEN RULES FOR GOOD RESULTS—SHORT TERM AND LONG TERM

For an optimal result, the surgeon must adequately fill the existing breast envelope.

Any fill more than that required for an optimal, aesthetic result will detract from the long-term result.

These principles will make more sense by applying them to two patient examples:

1. Sharon, a fictitious name but real patient, (patient number 1, Figure 4-4) had a C cup breast before pregnancy and enlarged to DD during pregnancy. After pregnancy, her envelope remained stretched (as usually occurs), but her breast tissue shrank and fell to the bottom of the envelope. She now has what appears to her a sagging breast, empty in the top and fuller and saggy at the bottom. Her breasts won't look good unless the stretched envelope is adequately filled. Imagine a funnel in the top of the breast. If we poured in liquid, the bottom of the breast would fill first. Pour more into the funnel, and the middle will fill next. The top fills last. At some point, with the patient sitting, the breast would look optimal with adequate but not excessive upper fill. At that exact point, the amount of filler that we added to the breast is precisely the amount required to produce an optimal result. Exactly the same thing happens with breast implants. Too small, and you won't fill the top. Too large and the top will bulge, and the breast will sag more rapidly.

    The size of implant that will be required to fill a larger, stretched envelope will be greater than the size required to fill a smaller, less-stretched envelope.

2. Consider a different patient we will call Janet (patient number 2, Figure 4-5). Younger, no children, with an A cup breast. The skin is tight, has never been stretched by pregnancy, and there is very little breast tissue (parenchyma). Janet's envelope is totally different than Sharon's envelope. It is tight, with less room for an implant. The larger the implant placed, the more the skin will push against the lower implant, and the more the upper breast will bulge. The bulging will decrease over time

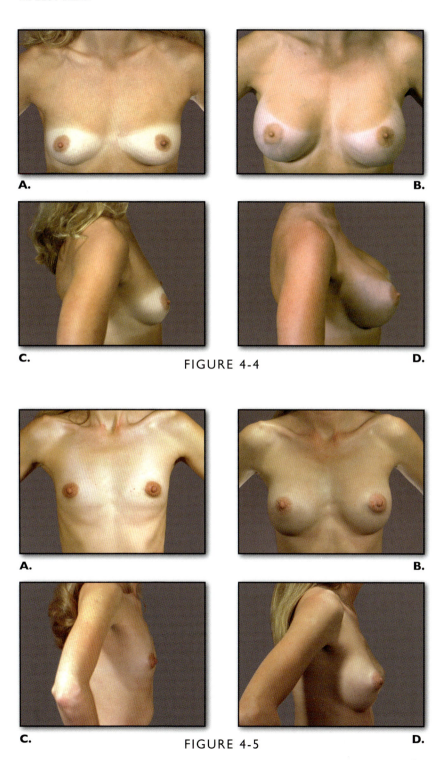

A.

B.

C.

FIGURE 4-4

D.

A.

B.

C.

FIGURE 4-5

D.

as the skin of the lower breast stretches, but if the implant is too large for the amount of stretch that can occur, the breast will have permanent, excessive upper bulging. If the implant is too large for the patient's skin characteristics, the lower breast skin will stretch excessively and the breast will appear saggy or have a "bottomed out" appearance—both are bad. The implant that will produce an optimal long-term result for Janet will be smaller than the ideal implant for Sharon. Janet has smaller breasts to begin with and skin that has never been stretched. To apply the principles, use enough implant to fill the envelope, allowing for stretch, but not so much implant that excessive stretch and sagging will occur with time.

The smaller and tighter (unstretched by pregnancies) the envelope, the less implant the envelope can accept and give an aesthetically optimal result and a good long-term result without problems.

No surgeon can totally predict what a patient's tissues will do over time, but every surgeon and patient should consider these issues when making implant choices. Even if Sharon and Janet were the same height with the same torso proportions and both wanted the same, optimal result, the implant required to produce that result would be different in the two patients. Why? Because their tissues are different.

No implant will produce the same result in two different patients.

Just because your best friend had a round, smooth, saline-filled, 300 cc implant that produced a certain result, rest assured that the same implant will not produce the same result in your breast because your tissues are different.

ARE YOU WILLING TO LIVE WITH WHAT YOU HAVE ORDERED?

Now, we get to balance what you want with the trade-offs of what you are willing to live with. What if you are Janet and you want *Baywatch* breasts? For those who were never treated to this prime example of video artistry, a *Baywatch* breast is very large, very round, and very bulging at the top, even without clothing. With your tight skin, can you get very large, round, bulging implants? You bet! If you can afford them and you can describe them, you can find a surgeon who will fill your order—guaranteed. I mean you are guaranteed to be able find a surgeon who will fill the order, but the surgeon would have to be brain dead to guarantee the work.

Assume that now you have got them—the *Baywatch* breasts. Awesome! You love them, your significant other loves them, and most men must love them because they can't look in your eyes when they talk to you. You got'em—now what have you got? What will predictably happen to the extremely large breasts over time?

This really isn't a tough question; just think about what always happens to large breasts. The skin can't adequately support the weight of the breast tissue over time, so the breast sags. It's a little different with implants: they usually don't sag quite as much over time as an unaugmented breast the same size, but they nevertheless sag. The weight of the implant stretches and thins the skin. The thinner the skin, the more the breast sags. The weight of the implant pulls on the skin enough to create visible ripples around the edges of the breasts or in the upper part of the breast. Whatever breast tissue you may have had before augmentation may shrink significantly. If you need a reoperation for sagging or rippling, now what does the surgeon have to work with? Thinner, stretched skin. Poorer quality tissues. Less breast tissue to cover your implants. Tissues that have been compromised or damaged by excessively large implants, tissue changes that can never be corrected. Operating on thinner or poorer quality tissues often brings poorer results and more potential problems. You ordered them. Now you have them. What have you got?

Does this mean that no woman should have larger breast implants? Not necessarily. Sometimes, larger implants are required to adequately fill a woman's existing breast envelope. Some women simply want to have larger breasts and implants, and they certainly have the right to have what they want. But they also should understand what will likely happen over time.

What's important is, regardless of personal choices and choices dictated by your tissue characteristics, you should be informed and aware of the potential long-term implications of those choices before surgery.

It's your job to see that this happens.

REALISM AND THE PERFECT BREAST

Regardless of how much homework you do, how well informed you become, and which choices you make, another inescapable truth is:

Perfection is not an option. Surgeons can only produce improvement.

We hope that you will view the improvement as perfection compared to what you had before, but perfection doesn't exist in plastic surgery. Your breasts won't exactly match, you likely won't get every single thing you want, and even if you select a perfectionist surgeon, I guarantee you the surgeon won't be able to achieve perfection. Your tissues aren't perfect. Time isn't kind to tissues, and neither you nor your surgeon can stop the clock.

Go in with your eyes wide open. Do everything you can right, but be realistic about your expectations. Pin your surgeon down with questions that help you be realistic. Hopefully, your surgeon will do all this automatically, but ultimately, it's your job to pick the surgeon who best meets these goals.

WHAT A BREAST AUGMENTATION DOES AND DOES NOT DO

A breast augmentation predictably does only one thing—enlarges your breasts. To avoid misconceptions, you should understand each of the following things that breast augmentation does not do predictably:

- In every woman, one breast is larger than the other. Breasts never match, and no surgeon can make breasts match. Putting a larger implant into the smaller breast will not make the breasts match and may create shape differences that are more apparent than a size difference.

- Breasts are never located at exactly the same level on the torso. One breast is always higher than the other, and one nipple is higher than the other. Breast augmentation does not move the breasts around on the torso and does not routinely relocate the nipple-areola, so these discrepancies will remain after a breast augmentation.

- Breast augmentation cannot predictably compensate for how you stand, for chest wall deformities you may have, or for spinal curvature deformities you may have. Breast augmentation only enlarges the breasts.

- In the gap between your breasts, only skin and a thin fat layer cover the underlying sternum. If you and your surgeon choose to move the edges of your implants into this area to narrow your cleavage, you are choosing to put your implants under inadequate tissue coverage. Over time, you are likely to experience visible implant edges and visible traction rippling that are largely uncorrectable.

- Regardless of the thickness of tissues overlying her implant, every augmentation patient should be aware that at some point in her life, she may be able to feel portions of her breast implant.

- A breast augmentation never produces a "natural" breast, because no natural breast contains a breast implant. The degree of naturalness of any type of implant is highly subjective and varies among patients and surgeons.

- Breast augmentation cannot make your breasts look like any picture or like any other person's breasts. Even though pictures might appear similar, vast differences can exist between the tissues in those pictures. Only tissue measurements tell the true story.

THE PLEASURES AND PERILS OF WINDOW SHOPPING FOR BREASTS

Although I'm risking putting myself in a position I might not want to be in (and I should know better by now), I have observed that most women like to shop! If you needed a new dress, chances are you would shop for it. If you were ordering a dress, you would want to see a picture before placing the order. Deep down, you know that shopping for a dress isn't the same as shopping for a breast, but instinctively, you are likely to apply some of the same principles. As an informed consumer, you would like to know what's available. You would really like to know what your breasts are going to look like before you proceed with your augmentation. Pictures and images are common ways to address these issues. Three commonly used media are magazine pictures, pictures from a surgeon's before-and-after ("brag") book, and pictures on a computer imager.

Before looking at pictures, *remember these principles.*

Three of the most important aspects of a woman's breast that determine breast size and the amount of implant required for optimal fill are the following:

1. BREAST WIDTH—the width of the breast prior to augmentation

2. SKIN STRETCH—how much the skin stretches prior to augmentation

3. AMOUNT OF BREAST TISSUE BEFORE AUGMENTATION

It is categorically impossible to accurately determine breast width, skin stretch, or amount of existing breast width, skin stretch, or amount of existing breast tissue from any picture.

Any decisions you make based on looking at pictures are inherently flawed and not based on your individual tissue characteristics.

Magazine Pictures

The only picture that truly represents breast characteristics is one totally without clothing, standing or lying down.

Most pictures in magazines don't meet these criteria. If nude, the model is almost always posed in a position that best complements her positives. Often the positioning interferes with (or contributes to) the appearance of the breast. At any rate, it doesn't allow an objective appraisal. If the model is wearing any clothing that touches the breasts (much less pushes the breasts to make them or the clothing look more appealing), you can't make objective judgements about the breast.

If you see breasts that you like, it's fine to take the pictures with you when you visit a surgeon. Pictures may help a surgeon understand what you like, and pictures may help you judge the surgeon:

If a surgeon looks at a picture and says, "Sure, we can make that breast! No problem!"
RUN THE OTHER WAY!

There could be a real problem if your tissues don't match the tissues of the person in the picture, and they never do. Either the surgeon may not know, or the surgeon may not care. Exception: The picture is a picture of a woman standing, nude, with tissues exactly the same as yours. Does she exist?

On the other hand, if the surgeon replies, "Let's look at your tissues and compare you as best we can to the person in the picture,"
BETTER!

Problem, still, is that the surgeon can't evaluate the tissues of the woman in the picture.

If the surgeon replies, "I'll use the pictures to help me understand what you'd like, and then I'll try to help you understand our best options and trade-offs, given your tissues,"
GREAT!

Surgeon "Before-and-After" Brag Books

We will cover this subject later when we discuss surgeon consultations. Some basic rules that we will mention again are:

If you can find a patient in the book who looks almost exactly like you BEFORE her augmentation, it's possible that you MIGHT be able to look SOMEWHAT like her result AFTER your operation.

Unfortunately, you can't accurately know the width of the breast and the degree of skin stretch of the skin in the picture, and these two measurements are the most critical in determining optimal fill for your breast.

If you can't find someone who looks like you before her surgery, it's still fun to look.

The best lessons you can learn from any before-and-after book are:

If the surgeon doesn't have pictures to show you, consult other surgeons.

If every result looks good, consult other surgeons.

If the book does not contain a wide variety of breasts with some results better than others, consult other surgeons.

A surgeon's habits are reflected in the quality of the pictures as well as the quality of the results. Look at the quality of the pictures! Are they standardized? Good quality? Is the background consistent in all the pictures?

If the surgeon or his personnel can't fully explain any question you ask about the pictures, consult other surgeons.

Computer Imagers and Images

Again, we will cover this topic more later, but keep in mind for now that anyone, even a technician, can produce changes on a computer that no surgeon can produce with living tissue.

If the surgeon uses the imager to help you understand some points, fine.

If a technician or the surgeon uses the imager to sell you something that doesn't make sense or to sell you other non-breast-related operations, BEWARE.

If the surgeon morphs (changes the appearance of) your breasts on the computer and prints you a simulated before-and-after picture, don't look at it too much, and try not to fix the image in your mind. Your result definitely won't match the image exactly.

We are all human. Once we have seen a simulated result, we tend to expect that result, even if the computer screen is covered with disclaimers informing us that this is only a simulation.

The computer can be a wonderful tool when used as a constructive tool to discuss options with you or provide you useful information. We use it a lot. When it's used primarily as a marketing tool to sell you an operation, you are likely not getting all that's best for you. To date, no one can precisely represent your tissue characteristics on a computer.

When it comes to images, shop all you want, but don't buy. Use pictures constructively, but base your buying on information and an evaluation of your tissues.

Internet- or Computer-Based "Modeling" Gimmicks

Almost every patient would like to know how their breasts might look following augmentation, with different sizes or types of implants. This natural human tendency makes patients easy prey for marketing gimmicks, such as computer- or Internet-based programs that show a model or mannequin and allow a patient to select implant sizes or types and see changes occur in the breasts. Virtually all of these marketing gimmicks are accompanied by long, detailed disclaimers stating that the images do not reflect actual results. Although the disclaimers may (and I emphasize "may") protect the marketers legally, prospective patients who use these gimmicks may make poor decisions if they don't carefully read all disclaimers. Despite any disclaimers, when most patients see an image based on a theoretical implant type and size that has nothing to do with their own personal tissue characteristics, the patient forms opinions. These opinions are often severely flawed, and in the best-case scenario, a very knowledgeable surgeon will need to spend considerable time reeducating the patient to reconcile the patient's desires with tissue realities. Worst-case scenario, a surgeon simply attempts to produce what the images showed without consideration of the patient's tissues (avoiding the additional time necessary to alternatively reeducate the patient). In the worst case scenario, problems may occur later as the result of poor decisions. Either surgeon scenario is not a good one for the patient (more time spent undoing bad ideas or ignoring tissue priorities or agreeing with poor decisions and suffering consequences later). Patients should recognize these types of marketing hype that may have little to no relationship to reality and avoid them.

AND NOW . . .

Now that you have a feel for reconciling your desires with reality, let's move on to the next step—implants.

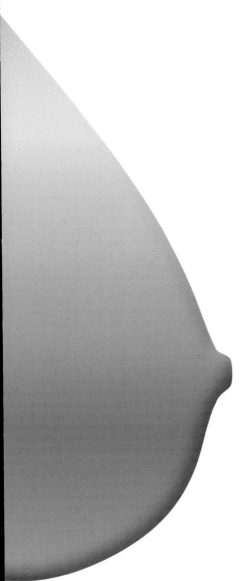

BREAST IMPLANTS:

THE DEVICES AND THE CHOICES

*"The implant you choose is the implant
you'll live with—understand the trade-
offs of different implants, and choose
carefully."*

Implant choices? There are many: round shape, anatomic shape, underfilled, adequately filled, overfilled, smooth outer shell, textured outer shell, saline filled, silicone gel filled, or filled with alternative fillers. Each of these choices is currently available somewhere, and each is a valid choice in certain situations. Each has benefits and trade-offs. How do you choose? Start by learning about the alternatives! This chapter contains a lot of information—maybe more than you think you would like to know! But the alternative—not knowing—could cost you significantly in the future. The only way to make the best decisions is to fully understand the many issues regarding implants.

You can't know too much about implants—the issues and the choices.

Not knowing now could cost you significantly in the future—in quality of results and in complications and need for additional surgery.

The future price of poor decisions from lack of knowledge is too high for any patient to pay.

BREAST IMPLANTS ARE DEVICES . . .

A breast implant is a device. Can you name any device that's perfect? Can you name any device that lasts forever? Can you name any sophisticated device that never requires maintenance? Probably not. So let's start out with three basic truths:

Breast implants are not perfect.

Breast implants don't last forever.

Breast implants may require some maintenance.

If you believe these three statements, you have taken a big step. If you accept that something's not perfect, you can begin learning about its imperfections and whether you are willing to accept them. If you accept that something won't last forever, you can begin to understand the factors that affect its longevity and make choices that help prolong its life. You can also decide whether you are willing to have maintenance if it becomes necessary.

If you can't accept the imperfections of implants or if you are unwilling to have maintenance, don't have a breast augmentation.

IMPLANTS: WHAT DO I NEED TO KNOW?

This chapter is organized to meet the information needs of two different groups of women. If you want basic information about the currently available alternatives and don't want to spend more time understanding all of the issues about implants, read the first half of the chapter. If you want more detailed information that focuses on the important issues that affect implant longevity and the trade-offs between naturalness and longevity, read the entire chapter. Many of the most important issues about breast implants are not addressed in any other written information for the public. Although some of these issues may seem too detailed, dry, or boring, they affect your long-term result, risk of reoperations in your future, and risks of complications and problems

As a potential patient, you will almost certainly learn about what is "the latest," what is "new," and what is supposedly "best." What you may not learn is that the first two of these (the latest and new) do not necessarily correlate with the last (what's best). Before we discuss current implant alternatives, we will offer you some interesting and potentially valuable background information.

Regardless of how much you may want to know, you can benefit from knowing a few facts about the history of breast implants, why many "new" designs that receive a lot of marketing hype and press coverage seem to disappear, and patterns of marketing behavior that have become common in the breast implant industry. The following are three "lessons" that may provide valuable insight.

LESSON I

When is "new" really new, and when are old products resurrected and recycled?

In the technology age, we all want what is "newest" and often equate what is "newest" to what may really be best. When it comes to breast implants, there are some important lessons here. Breast implant manufacturers recognize patients' desire for "newer" implants, and if the manufacturers really don't have anything that is truly "new" or really better, historically they have **reinvented old designs, and recycled old implant designs** under the guise of "new products."

The most recent example of this recurring trend occurred in 2000–2001 when Mentor Corporation began heavily marketing their "new" round, high profile implants (implants that have more front-to-back or forward projection compared to lower profile implants). The novelty and effective marketing resulted in patients' and surgeons' believing the hype, when in reality there is absolutely nothing new about high profile implants. This type of implant has been available since the 1970s—over three decades!—yet many younger surgeons (and some not so young) as well as many patients who didn't know the history fell prey to the marketing. What patients were told was that they could achieve a more "projecting" breast, and in some instances, they could. What many may not have been told is that high profile implants were largely discarded by some surgeons in the late 1970s (except for a few specific types of breasts) because they had all of the following potential trade-offs and potentially could cause all of the following tissue compromises:

- Pressure on overlying breast tissue, causing shrinkage or atrophy of existing breast tissue.

- For any given volume, more of that volume is placed in the lower breast, the area already most prone to stretching.

- Because the round, high profile implant has a narrower base (for a given volume) compared to lower profile implants, it will produce less upper breast fill (shorter vertical height).

- All current round, high profile implants collapse vertically when filled to a manufacturers' recommended fill (varying amounts depending on patient tissue characteristics), further decreasing upper breast fill.

- To achieve adequate upper fill, a larger volume implant is required, adding more weight, more stretch, and all of the potential compromises of excessive stretch: tissue thinning, visible implant edges, traction rippling, etc.

- For any given volume, the base width of the implant is less compared to lower profile implants. That means that for a given volume, the implant won't fill the breast side-to-side as much compared to lower profile implants, leaving a wider gap between the breasts.

- There are other potential compromises, but you get the point . . .

Here is a product that had limited applications three decades ago and, although useful for a very few specific breast deformities, has considerable potential compromises. Nevertheless, it was reintroduced as a "new" product and continues to be used by some surgeons.

When one company recycles old designs that are successful in the marketplace (patients and surgeons either don't know history and implant-soft tissue dynamics or don't care and buy the products), other companies often follow. When Mentor enjoyed success with the resurrected and recycled round, high profile design, Inamed/Allergan (formerly McGhan Medical) rapidly followed and reintroduced similar designs.

Since reality rarely changes, and the compromises listed above still apply, our prediction is that enthusiasm for round, high profile implants will decline as surgeons and patients experience potentially increased tissue compromises such as shrinkage (atrophy) of breast tissue (parenchyma) and excessive stretching, thinning, and sagging of the lower breast skin envelope.

The **important messages for patients** from the "new" high profile implant story:

1. **High profile implants do not necessarily produce more projection in the patient's breast.**

Remember that a higher-profile implant compresses the breast tissue more. What is gained by the few millimeters of additional projection of the implant is often lost by the compression and shrinkage (atrophy) of the overlying breast tissue over time.

2. **Don't rush to something "new" until you know the history.**

   Products that are really "new" and better will have stood the test of time and are supported by valid scientific data, not just marketing hype.

3. **Don't request something "new" until you and your surgeon have discussed potential long-term consequences.**

4. **Don't select something "new" if your surgeon can't (or won't) provide you in-depth explanations of how that product may interact with your tissues over time.**

LESSON 2

How "old and bad" can suddenly become "new and okay": The resurrection of old silicone-gel implant designs

Interestingly, the basic design of the old-style round, noncohesive silicone-gel-filled implants that were banned by the FDA in 1992 have suddenly become available again to patients in the United States in November of 2006. How can this be?

A large body of scientific evidence has shown that the old silicone gel implants do not cause many of the diseases or conditions that they were accused of causing. Nevertheless, the same data also show that this design of implant had a relatively high shell failure rate and that when the shells failed, the non-cohesive silicone gel in some instances escaped from the surrounding capsule and caused local complications in the breast or adjacent tissues. In addition, compared to saline-filled implants, the recently FDA-approved old-style silicone-gel implants also have a very high capsular contracture rate of 13.2 percent in the Allergan study and 8.1 percent in the Mentor study. So, why would the FDA allow the product back on the market? Is the round, non-cohesive silicone-gel implant that may reenter the market significantly different from the 1992 or earlier product that was banned? Go figure.

The facts are that the round, non-form-stable, silicone-gel-filled implants that have again become available in 2007 are not substantially different compared to the products that were banned in 1992 and not really very different compared to similar products from the 1970s—three decades ago! Although today's round, non-cohesive gel implants incorporate a barrier to "gel bleed" (minuscule amounts of silicone molecules escaping through the shell), and the shells may be somewhat more durable, the gel is essentially unchanged from previously, and the implants remain underfilled, allowing shell collapse and/or folding that could compromise shell life. So, why are they back?

Table 5-1 compares data on saline- and silicone-gel-filled-implants from FDA PMA studies to peer-reviewed data that the author has published in *Plastic and Reconstructive Surgery*. Scientific references to this data are listed after the table.

Compiled December 5, 2006, by John B. Tebbetts, M.D. Revised February 8, 2007.

TABLE 5-I

	Mentor Saline PMA (all saline)[6]	Allergan Saline PMA[6]	Tebbetts Saline Style 468 Studies[1-4]	Mentor Gel PMA[7]	Allergan Gel PMA[7]	Tebbetts Form Stable Gel Style 410 PMA series[5]
Date	Jan 2004	Nov 2004	Dec 2002	Nov 2006	Nov 2006	Dec 2006
Patients	1264	901	1662	551	455	50 consec-utive
Followup (years)	3 years (5 and 7 year FUs were 5% and 50%)	5 years (81% FU at 5 yrs)	up to 7 years, 83% FU	3 years 88% followup	4 years 82% followup	3 years 94% followup
	SPS study See ref #6	A95 Study See ref #6	*See refs #1-4	See ref #7	See ref #7	See ref #5
Complications & Reoperations (%)						
	At 3 yrs	At 5 yrs	Up to 7 yrs	At 3 yrs	At 3 yrs	At 3 yrs
Reoperations all causes %	13 20.2@ 7yrs[6]	26 30@7yrs	3	15.4	23.5	0
Capsular Contracture 3-4	9 10.1@ 7yrs[6]	11@5yrs 16 @7yrs	0.7	8.1	13.2	0

TABLE 5-2

	Mentor Saline PMA (all saline)[6]	Allergan Saline PMA[6]	Tebbetts Saline Style 468 Studies[1-4]	Mentor Gel PMA[7]	Allergan Gel PMA[7]	Tebbetts Form Stable Gel Style 410 PMA series[5]
Rupture, Leakage, Deflation	10.4@ 7yrs[6]	7@5yrs 10@7yrs	0.8%	0.5% (MRI Cohort)	2.7% (MRI Cohort)	0
Implant removal without replacement	14.2@ 7yrs[6]	15@7yrs	0.3%	2.3%	2.3%	0
Implant removal replacement any reason (size change, etc)	8%	12%	0.2%	2.8%	7.5%	0
Implant malposition	2.2%	9%	0.1%	NR	4.1%	0
Breast pain	5%	17%	0	1.7%	8.2%	0
Visible Wrinkling	21%	14%	0	NR	<1%	0
Asymmetry	7%	12%	0 reops	NR	3.2%	0 reops
Nipple Paresthesia	5%	10% (skin)	NR	2.2%		NR
Implant palpability/ visibility	2%	12%	0 visible	NR	<1%	0
Loss nipple sensation	10%	10%	0	NR	NR	0
Hematoma	2%	2%	0.2%	2.6%	1.6%	0
Seroma	NR	3%	0.1%	NR	1.3%	0

	Mentor Saline PMA	Allergan Saline PMA	Tebbetts Saline Studies	Mentor Gel PMA	Allergan Gel PMA	Tebbetts Style 410 PMA
Infection	2%	1%	0.3%	1.4%	<1%	0
Delayed wound healing	NR	1%	0	NR	<1%	0
Implant extrusion	NR	NR	0	NR	<1%	0
Tissue/skin necrosis	NR	NR	0			
Sagging/Ptosis	2% 3yr	28/901= 3.1%	0.1%	2.3%	1.4%	0
Scarring Complications		7%	0	6.7%	3.7%	0
"Nipple Complications" (gel studies only)	-	-	-	10.4%	7.9%	0

	Mentor Saline PMA	Allergan Saline PMA	Tebbetts Saline Studies	Mentor Gel PMA	Allergan Gel PMA	Tebbetts Style 410 PMA
Reasons for Reops (%)	* Reported as "% Types Additional Surgical Treatment at **3** yrs"	* Reported as "% Types Additional Surgical Treatment at **5** yrs	% reops in 1664 pts. up to **7** year followup	**3 years** % of 109 reoperations	**4 years** % of 135 reoperations	**3 years** % reops
Deflation/ Rupture (Suspected rupture in gels)	24% (calculated), NR	18% of 293 reops	0.8%	1/109= 0.91%	6.135= 2.2%	0
Removal with replacement (size or shape change)	32%	34 15% "Pt choice of 293 reops)	0.2%	16/109= 14.6%	7/135= 5.1%	0
Capsular contracture	22%	19%	0.7%	40/109= 36.7%	39/135= 28.8%	0
Scar/Wound Revision	19%	9%	0	NR	NR	0

	Mentor Saline PMA (all saline)[6]	Allergan Saline PMA[6]	Tebbetts Saline Style 468 Studies[1-4]	Mentor Gel PMA[7]	Allergan Gel PMA[7]	Tebbetts Form Stable Gel Style 410 PMA series[5]
Implant malposition/reposition implant	8%	5%	0.2%	2/109= 1.8%	21/135= 15.5%	0
Saline adjustment	8%	11%	0	NA	NA	0
Mastopexy/Ptosis	6%	6%	0	4/109= 3.6%	19/135= 14.0%	0
Implant removal without replacement	3%	2%	0.3%	NR	NR	0
Biopsy/Cyst removal	2%	5%	0	6/109= 5.5%	12/135= 8.8%	0
Nipple related	<1%	<1%	0	NR	1/135= 0.74%	0
Hematoma/ Seroma	See above	See above	See above	12/109= 11.0%	9/135= 6.6%	

Mentor 5-and 7-year saline follow-up were 5% and 50% respectively, so the 3-year data are more reliable.

1. Tebbetts, J. B. Patient acceptance of adequately filled breast implants. *Plast. Reconstr. Surg.* 106(1): 139-147, 2001.

2. Tebbetts, J. B. Dual plane (DP) breast augmentation: Optimizing implant-soft tissue relationships in a wide range of breast types. *Plast. Reconstr. Surg.* 107: 1255, 2001.

3. Tebbetts, J. B. Achieving a predictable 24-hour return to normal activities after breast augmentation, part I: Refining practices using motion and time study principles. *Plast. Reconstr. Surg.*109: 273-290, 2002.

4. Tebbetts, J. B. Achieving a predictable 24-hour return to normal activities after breast augmentation, part I: Refining practices using motion and time study principles. *Plast. Reconstr. Surg.* 109: 293-305, 2002.

5. Tebbetts, J. B. Achieving a zero percent reoperation rate at 3 years in a 50-consecutive case augmentation mammaplasty PMA Study. *Plast. Reconstr. Surg.* 118(6): 1453-1457, 2006.

6. U. S. Food and Drug Administration. Product labeling data for Mentor and Allergan/ core studies of saline-filled implants. http://www.fda.gov/cdrh/breastimplants/labeling. html. Accessed January 1, 2007; FDA web site updated November 17, 2006.

7. U. S. Food and Drug Administration. Product labeling data for Mentor and Allergan/Inamed core studies of saline-filled implants. http://www.fda.gov/cdrh/ breastimplants/labeling.html. Accessed December 5, 2006; FDA web site updated November 17, 2006.

IMPORTANT FACTS ABOUT THE SILICONE GEL IMPLANTS APPROVED BY THE FDA IN NOVEMBER OF 2006

The categories of silicone-gel-filled implants approved by the FDA on November 17, 2006, are smooth shell, round, silicone gel implants that ARE NOT FORM STABLE. (They collapse when tilted upright due to the amount of filler the manufacturer places in the shell.) Shell collapse and folding have been shown to be significant factors that shorten the life of an implant shell. While Mentor markets these products as containing "Memory Gel™", in fact the implant gel does not have "memory" and does not return to its original shape when deformed. Although all silicone gel is "cohesive" to some degree, none of the gels approved in 2006 is adequately cohesive to be "form stable," meaning that it maintains its shape or regains its shape following deformation.

When considering the round, smooth, non-form stable implants approved in 2006, patients should be aware of the high reoperation rates associated with these products, of the high capsular contracture rates associated with these products, and that the reported shell failure rates are early reports at a maximum of four years. Table 5-1 summarizes key data from the Allergan and Mentor FDA studies of these products and compares the rates to similar rates for saline implants. Although the FDA has not approved form-stable silicone-gel products, data on the Allergan Style 410 form-stable cohesive-gel implant reported to the Canadian equivalent of the FDA by Allergan in 2006 is included for comparison.

The data in this table is all data from FDA or Health Canada supervised and monitored studies. This data strongly suggests that compared to either saline or conventional silicone gel implants, the Allergan Style 410 form-stable, cohesive-gel anatomic implant has a lower shell failure rate and a dramatically lower capsular contracture rate. The 410 also virtually eliminates wrinkling problems associated with saline implants in these studies.

The excessively high reoperation rates in all of these studies is unquestionably related more to surgeon issues than to implant issues. The most common causes of reoperation in all of these studies include implant size or style change, capsular contracture, bleeding or fluid collection, and implant malposition. Each of these causes relates directly to patient and surgeon decisions in implant selection and to surgeons' techniques and accuracy in the operating room. During the past decade, studies that Dr. Tebbetts has published[1-4] have demonstrated that these reoperation rates can be dramatically reduced to approximately 3% by using specific tissue measurements and proved processes for surgical planning and surgical techniques.[5,6] In the most recent PMA study for the Style 410 form-stable, cohesive-gel implant, Dr. Tebbetts published a series of fifty consecutive augmentation patients who had a 0 percent reoperation rate at three years follow-up.[7] This is the first peer reviewed and published report of a zero percent reoperation rate at 3 years for a consecutive patient series by a single surgeon in any FDA PMA study of breast augmentation.

The FDA almost certainly recognizes the errors made in 1992 when banning a product in response to a media frenzy, at least partially for the wrong reasons. The alternative, saline filled implants, although offering a different set of trade-offs, aren't perfect either, with deflation and reoperation rates in clinical studies submitted to the FDA that fall short of wonderful (more about that later). Saline-filled implants are perceived by many patients and surgeons to feel less natural compared to the old silicone-gel implants, and there is a definite demand for "naturalness," even at the expense of shell durability.

Is there another alternative? Yes, cohesive, form-stable silicone-gel implants, with the most form-stable design under PMA studies for the FDA being the Allergan Style 410 anatomic cohesive-gel implant. The obvious question is why have the old round, non-cohesive, silicone-gel implants become available again before the newer, anatomic, cohesive, form-stable gel designs? The basic answer is that Inamed (now Allergan) management made a conscious decision to attempt to get FDA approval for the older design and instituted the studies on the older designs prior to initiating clinical PMA studies for the newer design. Why would they do that? Their answer might be that the FDA mandated studying the older implants first, but if so, where is the logic in that mandate? A skeptic might also consider that the potential market for the older type gel implant is potentially much larger than for newer designs because the newer implant designs place more demands on surgeons, and many surgeons may not want to adopt new designs that are more demanding.

Regardless, patients should be aware that the round, non-form-stable silicone-gel implants that were approved by the FDA on November 17, 2007, are not substantially different compared to three-decade-old round, non-cohesive gel implants. Even if clinical data to the FDA appear encouraging initially, the longer term failure rates of the shells of these implants will not be known definitively for at least a decade. They may feel more natural compared to saline or newer design cohesive gels (although no objective data exists to support this theory), but the difference is minimal in most patients, and there may be a substantial trade-off when long-term durability is compromised for perceived and unproved "naturalness."

LESSON 3

Why do "wonderful, new" designs suddenly disappear?

History can teach important lessons. Consider for a moment the history of three "wonderful, new" types of implants that were introduced in the United States during the past decade: The Misti Gold implant, the Trilucent™ peanut-oil- or soybean-oil-filled-implant, and the PIP pre-filled saline implant. Each of these implants was heavily marketed prior to introduction, each had limited clinical use prior to introduction, and the media and the public rushed to embrace (albeit transiently) the new products. Each has either disappeared completely or is currently severely compromised in the marketplace. Why?

- **When new products are introduced without adequate prior research and clinical use, they often have problems that are unrecognized.**

    The Misti Gold implant contained a filler that caused body fluids to enter the shell of the implant, making the implant grow larger with time in some patients. The almost wild enthusiasm for the Trilucent™ implant because it was "transparent" on mammography was quickly tempered when the British equivalent of the FDA raised concerns that breakdown products of the soybean oil filler might be carcinogenic (cause cancer). Both the Trilucent and prefilled saline PIP implants began to experience unusually high shell failure rates, requiring patients to undergo repeated reoperations for replacement of deflated implants.

- **When manufacturers, patients and surgeons prioritize "naturalness" above durability, compromises may occur (especially higher shell failure rates necessitating more reoperations for implant replacement).**

We won't say "we told you so," but "we told you so!" In the first edition of *The Best Breast,* and in scientific publications, we have repeatedly emphasized the potential role of adequate implant fill in reducing implant shell collapse or folding and the rate of implant shell failures. When patients and surgeons prioritize "soft" more than "durable," especially when there is scientific evidence that proves the difference is insignificant to a majority of patients studied,[1] manufacturers will continue to offer patients underfilled implants that according to marketing hype, "feel softer and more natural." If patients are fully aware of the possible compromises and trade-offs, they are certainly entitled to select a more natural feeling implant at the expense of durability, but they should be fully informed and sign informed consent documents verifying their understanding and acceptance of potential trade-offs.

Both the Trilucent™ and the prefilled PIP saline implant were touted as being more "natural feeling" in the breast compared to other implants, but this naturalness was because both were underfilled to make them feel softer. In both cases, the underfilled implants experienced a higher than expected shell failure rate, causing implant deflations and necessitating additional reoperations with additional risks and costs to patients.

The final messages from the lessons?

"New" is not necessarily better. The clinical track record of a new product is critical to determining just how good it really is.

When you rush to purchase something "new" in a breast implant, be sure that you know what you are getting and what trade-offs you may be purchasing!

Now let's focus on current implant choices.

THE BASIC CHOICES

Figure 5-1 outlines the basic choices in breast implants available in the world in 2006. In the United States, implant filler choices were limited to saline in early 2003. FDA studies on the older type silicone gel (not cohesive, not form stable) have been completed, and the older, conventional type gel implants were approved by the FDA November 17, 2006. FDA studies of the newer, cohesive, form-stable silicone-gel anatomic implants manufactured by Allergan (Style 410) are in progress, and the FDA may approve these devices in 2007.

A round implant is round. An anatomic implant is shaped. Which looks more like a breast?

You can get a good result with either a round implant or an anatomic implant. Which is better for you? It depends on your answers to the following questions: Write down your answers, then continue reading.

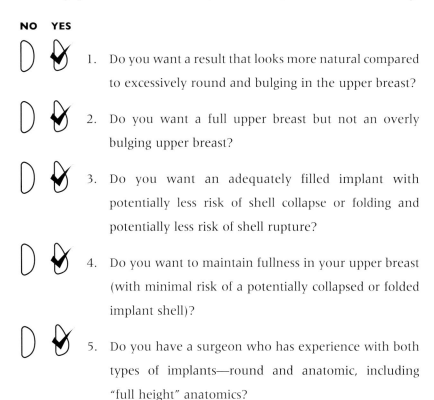

NO   YES

1.   Do you want a result that looks more natural compared to excessively round and bulging in the upper breast?

2.   Do you want a full upper breast but not an overly bulging upper breast?

3.   Do you want an adequately filled implant with potentially less risk of shell collapse or folding and potentially less risk of shell rupture?

4.   Do you want to maintain fullness in your upper breast (with minimal risk of a potentially collapsed or folded implant shell)?

5.   Do you have a surgeon who has experience with both types of implants—round and anatomic, including "full height" anatomics?

If your answer to all of the questions is "yes," you will likely want to consider an anatomic implant that is form stable and does not experience upper shell collapse when tilted upright.

Breast Implant Alternatives

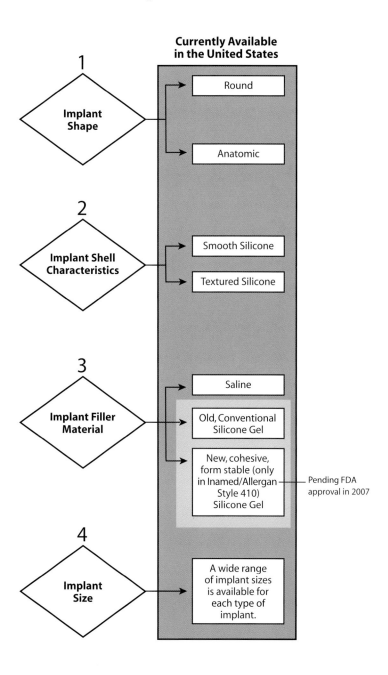

FIGURE 5-1

Basic implant shapes

Figure 5-2, A shows a side view of a round implant on the left and an Allergan Style 410, form-stable, anatomic implant on the right. Figure 5-2, B shows the implants tilted more vertically more closely simulate their orientation in the breast.

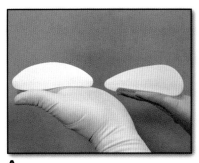 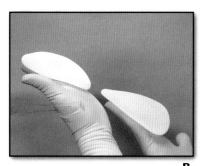

A. **B.**

FIGURE 5-2

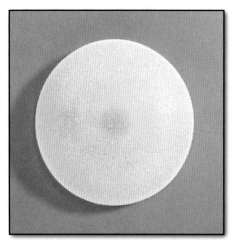

FIGURE 5-3

Round Implants

Round implants are designed on a round base (Figure 5-3), and *when adequately filled to minimize upper-shell collapse with the implant upright,* create a more round appearance in the breast, a more globular appearance with a more bulging upper breast. Is it possible to create a natural appearance using a round implant? Yes, and Figure 5-4 B is an example of a round implant creating a natural-looking breast—but there's a catch. What is it?

If an augmentation result looks natural (with a gradually sloping, full upper breast) and contains a ROUND implant, chances are overwhelming that the round implant is UNDERFILLED and the SHELL IS EITHER COLLAPSED OR FOLDED.

If the round implant were adequately filled to prevent upper shell collapse and folding, the upper breast would bulge more and/or the breast would appear more globular (Figures 5-4 B, 5-5 B)—in virtually every instance. To achieve a natural slope in the upper breast with a round implant, the upper portion of the round implant **must collapse downward** in the pocket (Figures 5-4 A, C). If the upper implant shell collapses, the implant shortens vertically and the shell collapses downward, reducing the bulging in the upper breast. One major problem is that the shell is collapsed or folded. The second major problem may be loss of upper fill in the breast when the upper shell collapses. Do you know what is likely to happen to a folded shell? It may wear out sooner. This phenomenon of upper shell collapse in a round implant explains what you might hear from some surgeons: "Round implants become anatomic in the pocket." No, round implants do not become anatomic. Round implants collapse because most are not filled adequately to prevent shell collapses, even if the surgeon fills the round implant within the manufacturer's recommended fill range.

ROUND Implants—What Happens Over

1–3 months after augmentation

1–5 years after augmentation

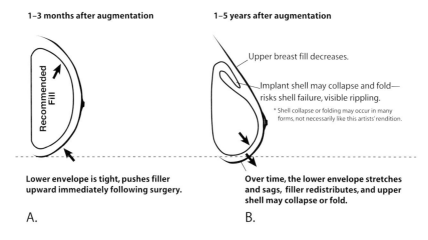

Recommended Fill

Upper breast fill decreases.

Implant shell may collapse and fold—risks shell failure, visible rippling.

* Shell collapse or folding may occur in many forms, not necessarily like this artists' rendition.

Lower envelope is tight, pushes filler upward immediately following surgery.

Over time, the lower envelope stretches and sags, filler redistributes, and upper shell may collapse or fold.

A.

B.

What happens when the skin envelope releases?
The shell **collapses** and **folds**—risking **shell failure, visible rippling** and **more reoperations.**

If Round Implant is OVERFILLED Past Manufacturer's Recommendations

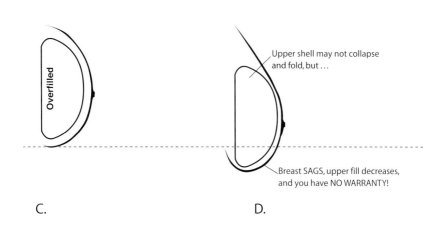

Overfilled

Upper shell may not collapse and fold, but …

Breast SAGS, upper fill decreases, and you have NO WARRANTY!

C.

D.

The patient CAN'T WIN—
Fill to recommendations—preserve warranty, but SHELL MAY COLLAPSE OR FOLD
Overfill to protect shell = MAY VOID WARRANTY

FIGURE 5-4

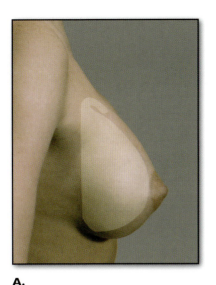

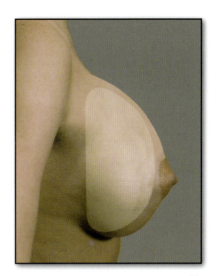

A.

**The upper shell is collapsed
and folded.**

B.

**If overfilled to protect the
shell, a round implant produces
more upper bulging.**

FIGURE 5-5

Round Implants: The Catch-22

To produce a natural appearing breast with a round implant, a surgeon
must underfill the round implant (if the implant is filled with saline),
or select an underfilled implant (if the implant is prefilled or silicone
filled) according to the tilt test. (We know already that we can't trust
manufacturer's recommendations alone to determine adequate fill.) If
the surgeon fills the round implant to manufacturer's recommendations, the implant shell may fold and collapse (Figures 5-4). The breast
may look natural, but the shell is likely collapsed or folded. If the
surgeon overfills past recommendations to prevent shell folding (Figure
5-4 C), the surgeon may void the implant warranty. When our patients
request a round implant or when we think a round implant may be
better (usually in a multiple reoperation case where it's difficult to
control an anatomic implant), the patient must sign a permit indicating
only one of the following choices:

The Catch-22 with ROUND IMPLANTS—

Solved by McGhan 468 and 410 Anatomic Implants With Adequate Fill.

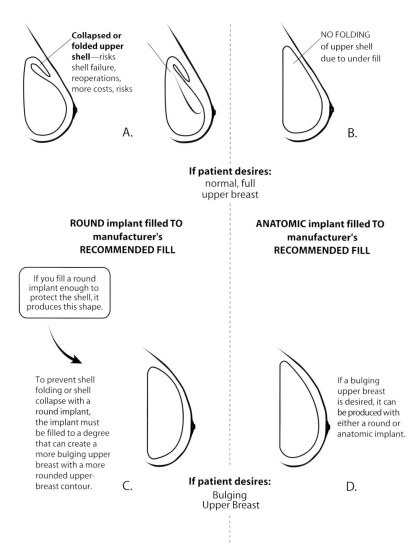

ROUND IMPLANTS

ANATOMIC IMPLANTS

Collapsed or folded upper shell—risks shell failure, reoperations, more costs, risks

A.

NO FOLDING of upper shell due to under fill

B.

If patient desires:
normal, full upper breast

ROUND implant filled TO manufacturer's RECOMMENDED FILL

ANATOMIC implant filled TO manufacturer's RECOMMENDED FILL

If you fill a round implant enough to protect the shell, it produces this shape.

To prevent shell folding or shell collapse with a round implant, the implant must be filled to a degree that can create a more bulging upper breast with a more rounded upper-breast contour.

C.

If a bulging upper breast is desired, it can be produced with either a round or anatomic implant.

D.

If patient desires:
Bulging Upper Breast

ROUND implant filled PAST manufacturer's recommended fill— MAY VOID WARRANTY

Or

ANATOMIC implant filled to manufacturer's recommended fill— WARRANTY INTACT

FIGURE 5-6

1. I want Dr. Tebbetts to fill my round implant to the manufac-
    turer's recommendations. I understand that this amount of fill
    may not prevent shell folding, and I accept that shell folding
    may cause my implant to wear out sooner.

OR

2. I want Dr. Tebbetts to fill my round implant to more than the
    manufacturer's recommendations until Dr. Tebbetts feels that
    the implant passes the tilt test and contains adequate filler
    to minimize risks of shell folding and shell collapse in the
    upper implant. I understand and accept that filling above the
    manufacturer's recommended fill may void the manufacturer's
    warranty, and I am responsible for all costs of implant replace-
    ment whenever it becomes necessary.

**With today's round implants, you must choose a rippled,
folded shell or give up the manufacturer's warranty if
you overfill the implant!**

**With current round implants from any manufacturer,
you can have only one of the two choices listed above,
not both. Neither is perfect, so . . . you choose.**

If you request that your surgeon overfill your round implants, be
sure to specify that you want the implants filled adequately to pass
the tilt test. Many surgeons intuitively overfill past manufacturers'
recommendations, but the amount of overfill is still inadequate for the
implant to pass the tilt test. Later in this chapter, we will explain the
tilt test in detail.

When overfilling past manufacturers' recommendations to protect the implant shell from folding, continue adding filler until the implant passes the tilt test.

Some surgeons fill round implants a fixed amount over manufacturers' recommendations. Others fill a fixed percentage above manufacturers' recommendations. Neither is as foolproof as filling the implant to pass the tilt test.

The larger a round implant, the more fill above manufacturers' recommendations is required to prevent shell folding.

In contrast, it is unnecessary to overfill Allergan anatomic, form stable implants past manufacturers' recommendations because at manufacturers' recommendations, Allergan Style 468 saline or Style 410 cohesive, form stable gel anatomic implants for augmentation pass the tilt test!

The fill volumes for Allergan anatomic implants were defined higher by the designer (Dr. Tebbetts) and the manufacturer (Allergan) to pass the tilt test. Round implants were not!

The upper shell of round implants may not collapse and fold immediately after surgery (see Figure 5-4 A) because the tight skin envelope pushes back against the lower implant. However, over the first six months following surgery, the lower breast envelope stretches, allowing the filler to redistribute into the lower implant (see Figure 5-4 B). As the filler redistributes into the lower portion of an underfilled round implant, the upper shell collapses and folds, risking premature shell failure.

When round implants are overfilled to protect the shell (see Figure 5-4 C), the upper shell may not collapse and fold, but the upper breast is likely to bulge excessively, and with current round implants, overfill technically voids the manufacturer's warranty (see Figure 5-6 D). Both Mentor Corporation and Allergan Corporation currently inform their sales representatives, who in turn inform surgeons, that both companies will warranty overfilled implants. At the time of this writing, and despite our concern written four years ago in the first edition of *The Best Breast*, no manufacturer currently specifies in their written warranties that they will warranty an implant that is filled past their recommended range.

Figure 5-6 depicts a patient's alternatives. If a patient desires a normal but full upper breast, the patient can select either a round implant filled to manufacturers' recommendations and accept risks of shell folding (Figure 5-6, A), or the patient can select a more form-stable implant that is less likely to experience shell folding. If a patient desires a more unnatural, globular, round, bulging upper breast, the patient can choose a larger or overfilled round implant (Figure 5-6, C) or choose a larger, form-stable anatomic implant that is less prone to upper shell collapse or folding.

To summarize, it is definitely possible to achieve natural appearing results with round implants, but to do so requires patient and surgeon to accept a more underfilled product, potentially more shell folding, and potentially less fill in the upper pole of the breast. To avoid these potential compromises, in 1993 we began working on alternative anatomic implant designs that could be adequately filled to reduce risks of upper implant shell collapse.

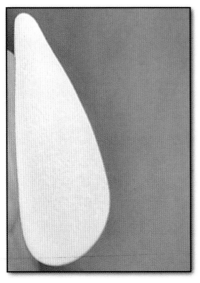 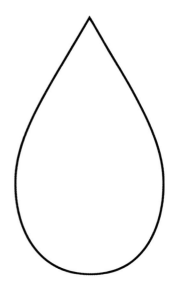

A. **B.**

FIGURE 5-7

Anatomic Implants

Anatomically shaped implants are shaped more like a natural breast (Figure 5-7 A). Some surgeons refer to anatomic implants as "teardrop-shaped" implants. Either the surgeon hasn't looked closely at a teardrop (Figure 5-7 B), or the surgeon hasn't looked closely at an anatomically shaped implant (see Figure 5-7 A). They don't look the same to me; do they to you? Fifteen years ago, I became very interested in full height anatomic implants after finding that I could not adequately fill round implants to protect the shell and simultaneously create a result that looked like a breast with optimal upper-breast fill.

> **With an anatomically shaped implant, it is possible to adequately fill the implant to prevent shell collapse and folding AND simultaneously produce an optimal aesthetic result.**

I was frustrated that I could never achieve OPTIMAL SHELL PROTECTION AND OPTIMAL AESTHETICS with any round implant.

The message? For most first-time augmentation patients, based on our twenty-six year experience, full height, adequately filled anatomic implants seem *safer* (less risk of shell folding and early rupture) and *more effective* (a more natural result with a full but not excessively bulging, upper breast). Since the first edition of *The Best Breast* published in 1999, we have published the largest amount of clinical data on anatomic implants in history, and this data supports our belief that shell failure rates are lower for adequately filled saline implants compared to underfilled implants.[1-7]

The first anatomic implants that I experienced were silicone gel filled and covered with polyurethane foam. Tissues attached to the polyurethane foam and held the implant in proper position. They produced excellent aesthetic results and dramatically reduced risks of capsular contracture—excessive tightening of the lining around a breast implant that makes the breast excessively firm. Capsular contracture will be discussed in more detail later. But polyurethane-covered, silicone gel implants were not perfect. (Remember, no implant is perfect.) The implants were underfilled and were designed on a round base with excessively tapered upper edges. Because the shells were thin and underfilled (which we didn't know back then), some of the shells failed, and the implants ruptured earlier than we liked. (Any time is too early for us.) We thought we could do better, so we began redesigning anatomic implants. We didn't try to redesign round implants, because if we filled any round implant enough to protect the shell, it was impossible to get the best possible aesthetic result.

Our design and clinical experience with anatomic implants began prior to 1993 working with McGhan Medical Corporation, then Inamed, and now Allergan Corporation, and resulted in the design of the Style 410 cohesive, form-stable, silicone-gel-filled anatomic implants and later the Style 468 full-height saline-filled implant. Hundreds of thousands of both types of implants have been in use around the world since 1994, and to date, the track record of these implants has been impressive.

What changes did we make with the new anatomic designs? We simply addressed the problems with the older designs. Instead of building the implant on a round base (since breasts aren't round), we made the implant slightly taller than it is wide, like a full, natural breast. We replaced the excessively sharp upper edge, which was sometimes noticeable, with a more rounded upper edge. Most importantly, using the tilt test, we filled the implant adequately to prevent upper-shell collapse and folding.

Anatomic, Silicone-Gel-Filled Implants

Simultaneously, we were looking at possible alternate fillers to silicone gel. Two main objections existed at that time regarding silicone gel: 1) When the implant ruptured, the gel was "gooey" and could be displaced into the breast tissue or other tissues, and 2) tiny amounts of the gel material could escape through the implant shell (gel bleed). We have always been interested in alternate fillers, including saline, peanut oil, polyethelene glycol (antifreeze), and several other possible fillers. But every alternate filler that we have ever seen has at least as many, if not more, trade-offs compared to silicone gel. While looking at alternate fillers, we thought, "Why not look simultaneously at silicone gel and try to correct its weaknesses (trade-offs 1 and 2 above)?" After all, we have over twenty-five years of medical data on silicone gel. Accumulating a comparable amount of data on any newer filler would require another twenty-five years.

Today's state-of-the-art, form-stable anatomic implants are manufactured by Allergan Corporation, the originator of modern anatomic
implants and the world's largest manufacturer of anatomic implants.
Other manufacturers, including Mentor Corporation and Silimed
Corporation (based in Brazil), have tried to emulate the Allergan
designs and introduce similar products in Europe and the United States,
but to date, none of the other designs incorporate all of the features of
the Allergan Style 410 and 468. Instead of the older, "gooey" silicone
gel, these new anatomic implants contain a newer, more cohesive
silicone gel. The gel in the Allergan Style 410 implant is so adherent to
itself and adherent to the implant shell that you can cut a pie-shaped
wedge out of the implant with scissors (see Figure 5-8 A,B) and then
squeeze the implant, and the gel does not migrate away from the
implant as pressure is applied. This is not necessarily true of other
implants that claim to be equally form stable or cohesive.

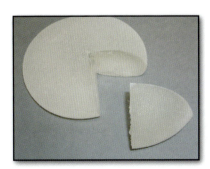 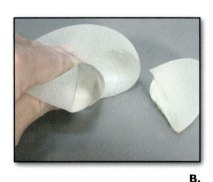

A.   **B.**

FIGURE 5-8

A major anatomic implant advance is a filler material (cohesive gel) that potentially reduces risks of gel migration following rupture of the implant shell.

Implant shell rupture can be caused by shell folding, a defect in manufacturing, surgical trauma, or trauma following surgery. All implant shells will eventually fail. A filler material that is less likely to migrate after shell failure is an advantage.

By putting an adequate amount of filler in the shell, the upper shell does not collapse or fold with the implant upright.

Another major advance is adequate fill to prevent shell folding.

This implant—the Allergan Style 410 anatomic, form-stable cohesive gel implant—has now been in clinical use for over fourteen years. Tens of thousands of Allergan anatomic, cohesive, form-stable gel implants have been used in countries other than the United States. Overall, aesthetic results have been excellent in a wide range of breast types.

The Allergan Style 410 cohesive, form-stable-gel anatomic implant makes three significant advances:

1. *adequate fill to attempt to optimally protect the shell,*

2. *a filler that is designed to reduce risks of gel migration, and*

3. *a filler designed to optimize aesthetic results by providing better control of upper breast fill.*

Premarket approval studies (PMA) for the Allergan Style 410 cohesive gel implant are scheduled to be completed in 2007 with data already submitted to the FDA. If the FDA approves the product, the Style 410 implant could become available to patients in the United States in 2007.

Anatomic, Saline-Filled Implants

Today's state-of-the-art, full height, anatomic, saline-filled implants are also manufactured by Allergan Medical Corporation. To prevent shell folding with a saline-filled anatomic implant, we needed to add slightly more filler to the implant compared to a cohesive gel-filled implant. Adding more filler to protect the shell makes the implant slightly firmer, but protecting the shell is more important, in our opinion, than a tiny increase in firmness. Fill issues are discussed in more detail later in this chapter. Figure 5-9 is an anatomically shaped, saline-filled Allergan Style 468 implant. Held upright during a tilt test (see Figure 5-10), the implant upper shell does not collapse and fold. At the same time, the upper shell stays full (necessary to maintain fullness in the upper breast), the upper shell does not bulge excessively, and it's more natural. It is not possible to achieve all of these objectives with any currently manufactured round implant, regardless of the filler material.

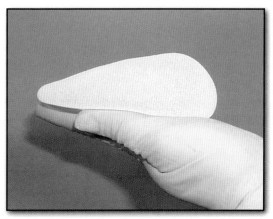

FIGURE 5-9

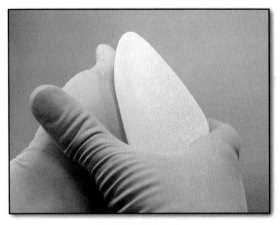

FIGURE 5-10

When we defined fill volumes for McGhan (now Allergan) anatomic saline implants, I insisted that McGhan define the fill volumes high enough to prevent upper shell folding. As a result, if you select a McGhan (now Allergan) saline-filled anatomic implant for augmentation, your surgeon does not need to overfill the implant above manufacturer's recommendations to prevent upper-shell folding and prolong the life of the shell. Before releasing anatomic implants, we set higher fill volumes compared to round implants. Because of its anatomic shape, we were able to put more filler in the implant without compromising the aesthetic result because of the shape of the implant. And, you can keep your warranty! Gone is the catch-22 of current round implants. When filled to Allergan's recommended fill, anatomic style 468 saline and 410 silicone anatomic implants do not experience upper shell folding (Figure 5-4 C) when subjected to the tilt test prior to implantation.

Allergan anatomic augmentation implants do not need to be filled past manufacturer's recommendations to minimize risks of shell folding.

With Allergan Style 468 anatomic-shaped, saline implants, you get shell protection, and you keep your warranty—no choosing between the two! No catch-22!

With round saline implants, you must overfill to minimize shell folding, and overfilling potentially voids current manufacturer warranties.

Trade-offs of anatomic gel and saline implants

As we have said, no implant is perfect. No implant shape is best for every patient. Anatomically shaped implants demand more of the surgeon. The pocket the surgeon develops to receive the implant must be much more precise with an anatomic implant compared to the pocket for a round implant. With an anatomic, the pocket should "fit" the implant. Because full height anatomic implants are taller than they are wide, if the pocket fits the implant in a side-to-side direction, the implant does not rotate or malposition unless the tissues stretch excessively. When a pocket is made to "fit" the implant, that does not mean that the implant does not move normally. When tissues relax and stretch in the first few weeks and months following surgery, patients in studies reported that their implant felt and moved naturally.[1-4]

What about surgeons who don't offer anatomic implants or who advise patients that anatomic implants have higher malposition rates?

Some surgeons find the additional demands of anatomic implants too technically challenging or time consuming, so they don't offer anatomic implants to their patients. When surgeons are unable or unwilling to create accurate pockets and select implants that best match patient tissue characteristics, or if they have little or no experience with anatomic implants, they may advise patients that anatomic implants are more prone to malposition compared to round implants. We have conclusive data from over 1,600 patients with up to seven-year follow-up published in the most respected professional journal in plastic surgery that prove otherwise.[1-4] The fact is that both round and anatomic implants can experience malposition, and malposition rates for full-height, saline-filled anatomic implants are no higher,[1-7] and in many cases, lower compared to rates reported for round implants.[1-4] In fact, in Table 5-1, earlier in this chapter, data reported to Health Canada (the equivalent of the FDA in the United States) show that implant malposition occurred much more commonly with round saline or gel implants compared to the anatomic, form-stable Allergan Style 410 implant.

In many cases that require reoperation, patients' tissues can become so thin and stretched (especially if they previously had large implants) that a surgeon cannot assure that the pocket will fit the implant. In reoperations (in contrast to first-time augmentations), until a surgeon has considerable experience with anatomic implants, the surgeon (and the patient) are probably better served using round implants, regardless of the trade-offs. If a patient has very thin tissues and requests very large implants (in general, larger than 350 cc), the weight of the implant will almost always stretch the patient's thin tissues and cause the implant pocket to enlarge. If the pocket enlarges substantially, an anatomic implant may rotate. Hence, round implants are probably a better option when a very thin patient requests a very large implant.

Anatomic implants may not be the best option for reoperation cases until a surgeon has gained considerable experience.

Anatomic implants are ideal for a majority of first-time augmentation patients.

Anatomic implants may not be the best option for thin patients who request excessively large implants larger than 350 cc.

All inflatable implants currently manufactured in the United States, whether round or anatomic, have a valve that is used to put filler (usually saline) in the implant. A valve is a device that is separate and additional to the implant although it is incorporated into the implant. Any device has a failure rate, so adding any valve to any implant theoretically increases the failure rate of the implant. All saline implants, not just anatomics, need to be adequately filled to minimize risks of visible shell folding or rippling, audible sloshing, and shell folding that risks early rupture.

Importance of the surgeon's experience

If a surgeon has minimal or no experience with anatomic implants, the surgeon may not offer you this option, or the surgeon may offer the option but discourage you with negative comments. Always ask your surgeon specifically how much experience the surgeon has with each type of implant. Ask to see pictures of results. Remember that *you can't necessarily distinguish a round from an anatomic implant in a picture*—a round implant can be underfilled and the result can look quite natural, but the shell may be collapsed or folded even if you can't see shell folding or rippling. If a round implant looks natural following augmentation, chances are that the shell is collapsed or folded.

My personal experience began with round implants. I used round implants exclusively for ten years until anatomic implants became available. Today I have twenty-six years of experience with round implants and fourteen years of experience with anatomic implants. I use both. I simply present patients all options and discuss those options with respect to each individual patient's tissues. The patient and I together choose the implant based on her wishes, her tissues, and the trade-offs she is willing to accept.

A question that patients frequently ask a surgeon is how many augmentations have you done? A better question (though difficult to ask in a tactful manner) is how many augmentations have you done well? I personally know surgeons with smaller case numbers who consistently deliver better augmentation results compared to certain surgeons with much larger case numbers. Surgeons are like every other professional. Some surgeons are more skilled than others. Some are more demanding of themselves compared to others. Numbers of cases are less important than the surgeon's self-critical pursuit of perfection.

ARE ALL ANATOMIC IMPLANTS SIMILAR OR THE SAME?

Absolutely not! Following the introduction of the full-height Style 410 cohesive gel and 468 saline anatomics in 1994, the popularity and track record of the products encouraged other manufacturers to attempt to develop similar products. The first such product was the Mentor contour profile Gel (CPG) implant, technically a shaped implant, but an implant that had a drastically different height-to-width ratio compared to the Allergan 468 or 410 full-height anatomic. The Mentor contour profile implant is a reduced-height anatomic implant with a shell texturing that is much less "textured" compared to the Allergan implants.

FULL-HEIGHT anatomic implants such as the Allergan style 468 saline and 410 full-height cohesive gel may be much less prone to implant malposition compared to reduced-height anatomic or shaped implants.

It is our belief based on our surgical experience, clinical experience and input that we have obtained from other surgeons and patients that **reduced-height anatomic or shaped implants may have a higher risk of rotational malposition compared to full-height anatomic implants**, especially if the implant has less aggressive texturing and the surgeon is unable to very precisely control implant pocket dimensions.

Full-height anatomics (Allergan styles 468 and 410) are taller than they are wide, and if pocket width fits the width of the breast, the height of the implant makes rotation almost impossible. If implant selection and pocket creation are optimal, risks of rotational implant malposition with the style 468 full-height anatomic are less than one-half of 1 percent.[1-4, 7] The same may not be true of reduced-height anatomic implants because they are not taller than they are wide and may be more prone to rotational malposition.

Any implant, round or anatomic, may malposition if tissues stretch excessively following surgery, and tissue stretch is a factor that no surgeon or patient can control, other than avoiding excessively large implants.

CURRENTLY PUBLISHED SCIENTIFIC DATA INDICATES THAT FULL-HEIGHT ANATOMIC SALINE IMPLANTS (ALLERGAN 468) HAVE LESS THAN A 0.5 PERCENT RISK OF ROTATIONAL MALPOSITION
(when optimal implant selection and surgical techniques are used).

SMOOTH OR TEXTURED SHELL? IMPLANT SHELL CHARACTERISTICS

It Won't Make Sense Unless You Know the History

Early generations of implants had smooth outer shells. Textured implant shells were developed to help reduce risks of capsular contracture. When any device is implanted in the human body, the body forms a lining or capsule around the device. This capsule forms around every implant in every patient, but the capsule can behave differently from patient to patient. All capsules tend to contract or tighten around any device. If the capsule around a breast implant tightens excessively, the capsule squeezes the implant. This can make the implant feel too hard and can push it out of position, usually upward. The term *capsular contracture* describes a breast after augmentation that is excessively hard, often misshapen, and often displaced. A typical statement from a patient with a capsular contracture is "My implants got hard." Actually, the implant itself does not become hard. If it were removed from the capsule that is squeezing it, it would feel soft. The pressure of the capsule surrounding and squeezing the implant causes the implant to feel hard in the breast. Cases of capsular contracture are illustrated in chapter sixteen.

With older, smooth-shell, silicone-gel-filled implants, capsular contracture was very common. Rates vary in reported studies, but a 30 percent capsular contracture rate was probably common. (One out of every three patients developed some degree of excessive breast firmness.) With all smooth-shell implants, surgeons learned to make the pocket to receive the implant very large, so that the capsule could theoretically contract a lot before it began squeezing the implant. Motion exercises were commonly prescribed for patients with smooth implants. The theory was that moving the implant could keep the pocket open against the tendency of the capsule to contract. Good idea, but you usually can't overcome Mother Nature. The body's healing mechanisms were often more powerful than motion exercises. Despite motion exercises, capsular contracture was still very common with smooth-shell implants. Patients hated capsular contracture. Surgeons hated capsular contracture. Both still hate capsular contracture. Patients with significant contractures required reoperations to soften the breast. If the capsule was removed, and smooth implants put back in, a large percentage developed recurrent contracture.

Enter polyurethane-covered implants. A polyurethane covering was cemented to the outer surface of the implant silicone shell. The reduction in capsular contracture rates was astounding. In my personal series of patients undergoing first-time (primary) augmentations, capsular contracture rates fell to less than 2 percent (2 out of 100). Incredible. But polyurethane-covered, silicone-gel- filled implants became unavailable in the United States when gel-filled implants were banned by the FDA. Additionally, questions were raised with regard to one of the breakdown products of polyurethane (TDA) as a cause of cancer in mice. Subsequent studies have shown that TDA levels in humans with these implants are so low that the risk of any carcinogenic effect is insignificant. When polyurethane implants became unavailable, surgeons wanted another alternative to smooth shells to reduce risks of capsular contracture. Implant manufacturers responded to the question: If a rougher, polyurethane surface retarded capsular contracture, why not produce a silicone shell with a textured outer surface?

Textured silicone shell implants were developed as an alternative to smooth shell implants to reduce the risk of capsular contracture.

You don't need to know all the scientific data with regard to capsular contracture or smooth versus textured shells. You just need a summary. The summary that follows is my current best judgement based on twenty years of experience:

Textured surface implants have a lower risk of capsular contracture than smooth-shelled implants if the implants are filled with silicone gel.

The difference between smooth- and textured-implant capsular contracture rates is more pronounced with silicone-gel-filled implants than with saline-filled implants.

Other filler materials have not been adequately tested in large enough numbers with adequate follow-up to make a valid judgement regarding smooth versus textured shells.

Textured or Smooth—How Do You Choose?

Shell texturing and risks of capsular contracture

With saline-filled implants, the difference in capsular contracture rates between smooth and textured implants is not as significant compared to silicone-gel-filled implants. But even if the capsular rate is only slightly lower with textured surface saline implants compared to smooth surface, you might prefer a textured surface implant.

The most important question: If you choose a smooth shell implant, saline or silicone filled, and you later develop a capsular contracture, are you going to look back and ask if it might have been avoided with a textured surface implant?

Or if you develop a capsular contracture and your surgeon recommends replacing the smooth shell implant with a textured surface implant, the obvious question is "Why not use a textured surface to begin with?" If you are then unlucky enough to develop a capsular contracture, there is no looking back and asking, "What if I'd chosen a textured implant?"

Current scientific data indicates that with *silicone-gel-filled implants*, capsular contracture rates are lower with textured than with smooth shell implants.

Current scientific data indicate that with *saline-filled implants*, there is less difference in capsular contracture rates with textured versus smooth shell implants, but our experience is that there is still a difference, with textured surface implants having a slightly (1–3 percent) lower capsular contracture rate compared to smooth implants.

Shell texturing and potential implant malposition

A textured surface helps maintain optimal positioning of an anatomic shaped implant in the pocket.

If you choose an anatomic implant, it should be textured to help maintain implant position in the pocket.

A common misconception is that the textured surface of an anatomic implant must adhere to adjacent tissues to minimize risks of implant malposition.

This misconception is simply not true. Many anatomic implants, even heavily textured implants, do not adhere to surrounding tissues, and the implant does not necessarily rotate! Texturing on the implant is helpful because the friction of the texturing contacting adjacent tissues helps maintain implant position as the capsule (tissue lining that forms around every implant) forms. Once the capsule forms, the capsule also helps maintain implant position. One of the most important and overlooked factors that maintains anatomic implant position (especially full-height anatomics) is implant design and gravity. Because the fullest, and therefore, the heaviest portion of the implant is in the lower portion, gravity pulls the lower part of the implant downward when standing.

Another common misconception is that anatomic implants should be positioned straight up and down and that if they are not, they are "malpositioned."

Wrong again! One of the advantages of an adequately filled, full-height anatomic implant (Allergan Styles 468 saline and 410 cohesive gel) is that the upper pole of the implant can be rotated slightly inward or outward to compensate for irregularities in the rib cage or to optimally shape the upper breast. No other currently available implant has this advantage! In fact, we rarely position a full-height anatomic implant straight up and down behind the breast because we can achieve a more optimal aesthetic result by rotating it slightly one way or another. *So malposition is not necessarily malposition!* It can be used to advantage with full-height anatomic implants.

If you choose a *round* implant, the implant can be smooth or textured. If you choose a round implant in the United States today, you can choose round saline or old style silicone gel as the filler material.

Why would anyone choose a smooth-shelled implant today in a first-time augmentation? Smooth-shelled implants are a no-brainer for the surgeon. Make a pocket. Drop it in. The implant always falls to the bottom of the pocket. Even if it is underfilled and the shell folds, it's often unnoticeable from the outside because the smooth implant with a collapsed shell falls downward, and shell folding is often hidden by the patient's breast tissue. Great! Easy and great! Even if the shell collapses and folds with underfilling, the patient doesn't see rippling or shell folding and complain. Wait a minute! Great for who? Maybe great for the surgeon, who doesn't see or hear about rippling, but what about the patient with the folded shell? What's likely to happen to the folded shell with time? A folded shell can lead to shell stresses and potentially cause shell rupture. In many cases, because the implant falls to the bottom of the pocket, neither patient nor surgeon can see the folded shell by looking at the breast. If the shell folding were visible on examination, the surgeon could replace the implant before rupture occurred.

Shell texturing and how it might affect whether you can "feel" your implant

Textured surface implants have a slightly (a few ten-thousandths of an inch) thicker outer shell compared to smooth shell implants. As a result, many surgeons advise patients that they are more likely to feel the shell of a textured surface implant compared to a smooth shell implant. The facts are:

MOST PATIENTS WHO ARE RELATIVELY THIN WILL BE ABLE TO FEEL SOME PORTION OF THE SHELL OR EDGE OF THEIR IMPLANTS, REGARDLESS OF WHETHER THE IMPLANTS ARE TEXTURED OR SMOOTH. This is especially true with saline-filled implants but also applies to silicone-gel-filled implants.

IF YOU FEEL ANY PORTION OF YOUR IMPLANT, YOU WILL NOTICE FEELING IT! FEELING MORE OR LESS IS ABSOLUTELY NOT AN ISSUE TO THE MAJORITY OF OUR PATIENTS.

IF YOU THINK OR IF A SURGEON TELLS YOU THAT BY SELECTING A SMOOTH SHELL IMPLANT YOU WILL NOT FEEL YOUR IMPLANT, THINK AGAIN!

Rupture rates of textured versus smooth implants

Another misconception that seems to be arising on Internet chat boards and discussion groups (and in some cases fueled by competing implant manufacturers) is that textured surface implants have a higher shell failure rate compared to smooth shell implants. Some even quote "data" to support their claims. Problem is the data are selective and not scientifically valid in our opinion. Often the data apply only to *one type* of textured implant. **All textured implants are not the same.** For example, the Mentor Siltex textured surface implant has one of the highest shell failure rates of any implant available today—a 12 percent failure rate at seven years according to Mentor's recent advertisements. Data from our peer-reviewed and published studies of the Allergan style 468 implant, which has a very different Biocell™ textured surface, showed that the 468 had only a 0.78 percent shell failure rate at seven years compared to Mentor's Siltex 12 percent shell failure rate.[1-4] Disturbingly, Mentor issued no interim reports to surgeons or patients during the seven-year period indicating a known higher failure rate of Siltex textured implants.

Our experience with the Allergan style 468 full-height, textured anatomic saline implant indicates that this textured implant certainly does not have a higher deflation rate compared to smooth shell saline implants.[1-4]

In fact, the following data comparisons are interesting. Our deflation rate for textured Inamed 468s in combined studies totaling over 1600 reported cases with up to seven-year follow-up was 0.78 percent. In data submitted to the FDA in saline implant PMA submissions, even at a much shorter three-year follow-up, the deflation rate for Mentor's saline implants was 3 percent and for Inamed's salines 5 percent. We are currently requesting a breakdown of the textured versus smooth deflation rates in these studies from both manufacturers, but our own peer-reviewed and published data certainly support our belief that adequately filled, full-height anatomic saline implants have a lower deflation rate compared to both companies' round textured or smooth implants that we believe are underfilled at current recommended fill levels.

Implant shell texturing and visible rippling

You might also hear that rippling is more common with textured surface implants compared to smooth-shelled implants. **Not true.** Rippling results from either inadequate fill in an implant (underfill rippling) or an excessively large implant (smooth or textured) pulling downward on an excessively thin skin envelope (traction rippling). If a textured-surface implant adheres to the tissues around the pocket and if that same implant is underfilled, rippling may be more visible. But the problem that most often causes wrinkling is underfill or traction of an excessively large implant pulling on thin overlying tissues, not the texturing on the shell!

Earlier we mentioned that textured surface implants, including the Biocell™ textured surface on Allergan textured implants, does not necessarily adhere to adjacent tissues. Many surgeons, especially those with less experience with a wide range of textured implants, believe that tissue adherence always occurs and that the adherence is what causes the visible rippling. This belief is simply not true in the vast majority of cases. Tissues do not "grow into" the textured Biocell™ surface. They adhere only if a large implant is placed under tight tissues, because the adherence is mechanical—the large implant pushing against the tight tissues. In most patients, adherence occurs over only a portion of the implant and in some, not at all. In either case, implant underfill or implant traction on thin overlying tissues are much more common causes of visible rippling compared to tissue adherence.

Two myths that are not based on facts:

Myth: Textured surface implants have thicker shells and are more easily felt in the breast.

Fact: The thickness of your tissues over the implant is much more important than the minimal differences in shell thickness.

Myth: Smooth-shell implants have less rippling than textured surface implants.

Fact: Visible rippling is the result of underfilling the implant, traction, or inadequate soft tissue coverage, not the shell surface.

Three good reasons to choose a round, smooth shell implant:

1. You are having a reoperation, not a first-time augmentation.

2. Your surgeon has little or no experience with anatomic implants.

3. You are requesting an implant with a volume greater than 350 cc.

Other reasons that we feel are less valid:

4. You will feel the smooth shell implant less.

5. Smooth-shell implants have a lower rupture rate (not supported by valid scientific data in our opinion, and our published
   data are just the opposite).

Implant Projection—High-Profile, Medium Profile, and Low-Profile Implants

The projection of an implant is the distance from the front of the
implant to the back of the implant when the implant is upright.

You will undoubtedly encounter surgeons and manufacturers who
believe that a higher profile implant will consistently produce a more
projecting (sticks out more) breast result following augmentation. This
is often not the case, and trying to achieve a more projecting breast can
result in more shrinkage of your breast tissue or even cause chest wall
or rib cage deformities over time.

> ### Remember this: A more projecting implant does not necessarily (and often doesn't) produce a more projecting result. Why?

The difference in projection of most implants is only a few millimeters.
When a more projecting implant is placed in the breast, it pushes
forward on the existing breast tissue. Depending on how much breast
tissue is present and how much the overlying skin stretches, every
implant compresses the existing breast tissue to some degree. The
more projecting the implant is, the more compression of your breast
tissue the implant causes. Several millimeters of compression can occur
without moving the skin forward. If the skin doesn't move forward,
the result isn't more projecting, you lose breast tissue over time, and
pressure on the rib cage can cause rib cage depression deformities.

Higher projecting implants cause more shrinkage of existing breast tissue (parenchymal atrophy) over time compared to moderately or lower projecting implants in breasts with similar tissue characteristics.

Implant Filler Materials—silicone versus saline versus other fillers

Before the FDA banned silicone-gel-filled implants in the United States, over 90 percent of surgeons preferred and used silicone-gel-filled implants over saline implants. If silicone-gel-filled implants were widely available in the United States today, many experienced surgeons and many patients might choose silicone fill over saline. Why? Because silicone-gel filler is more natural, it is more predictable, it is safe, and current data suggest that gel-filled implants have a longer shell life.

Saline-filled implants cause more stretch of the breast envelope compared to silicone-gel-filled implants of comparable size and shape. Therefore, predicting and controlling the result is more difficult for most surgeons with saline compared to form-stable silicone-gel-filled implants.

The demand for silicone-gel-filled implants is very high in the United States today. Many women travel outside the United States to obtain state-of-the-art, form-stable silicone-gel-filled implants, sometimes compromising their care in the process. Women in the United States deserve a full range of options, provided the options are accompanied by a full range of information. How logical is it to approve older generation gel implants before approving more state-of-the-art form-stable gel implants with lower implant failure rates and lower reoperation rates? Beats us! We are supposedly experts in the field, and we are still at a loss to decipher this one!

Saline is harmless if an implant ruptures. So is silicone if it is properly used. Even saline implants have a silicone shell. Silicone is silicone is silicone. If silicone is so bad (and scientifically it is not), why is a silicone shell on a saline-filled implant okay? It makes no sense, but the decisions that determine which options are available to you are not currently based on science.

If you are concerned that you are not allowed a full range of options, tell your legislators. Tell the FDA. Tell them over and over. You willl need to shout louder than the lobbyists and "patient advocate" groups who are paid by plaintiff lawyers to bend the ear of your legislators and the FDA.

Our biases? We will gladly share them with you. Here is a list:

- Breast augmentation is medically unnecessary, and patients should be fully informed with realistic information.

- By definition, an augmented breast is not a natural breast and never will be. Patients must decide whether benefits outweigh potential risks and trade-offs.

- Reoperations are inherently undesirable because they increase risks and costs to patients.

- Every implant should last as long as possible to minimize the number of reoperations for every augmentation patient.

- Adequate implant fill is important to minimize risks of upper implant shell collapse and folding that can shorten the life of the implant.

- Adequately filled (to minimize shell collapse), full-height ana-tomic implants currently offer the best solution to minimizing shell collapse while optimizing aesthetic results.

- Most informed patients are willing to trade-off some degree of naturalness in hopes of achieving better implant durability and longevity.[1]

- Patients deserve choices.

- Surgeons are responsible for informing patients of all available alternatives with the realistic potential benefits and risks of each alternative.

- Fully informed patients have the right to choose any implant or surgical alternative, provided they confirm their understanding and acceptance of trade-offs in informed consent documents.

- Patients deserve constantly improving implant solutions and surgical solutions.

- It is our responsibility to seek improved implant and surgical solutions for patients.

- Any "new" product should be thoroughly tested and have a substantial clinical track record of safety and efficacy before being offered to patients.

Because we are involved in implant design, our implant designs are one of the options that we offer patients. To date, our anatomic implant designs have become the most widely used anatomic implant designs in the history of breast implants. We have published the largest amount of scientific data in the most respected peer-reviewed journal in plastic surgery with respect to these products. In addition, we have published the most extensive information for colleagues and patients regarding clinical advances in breast augmentation in the last two decades. We receive financial gain directly or indirectly from sales of products (primarily implants and surgical instruments) we have designed, and we receive financial gain directly or indirectly from consultation fees paid by medical device companies and others. We prioritize our patients' welfare above any and all financial considerations.

TODAY'S PICKS (THEY WILL CHANGE WITH TIME; I GUARANTEE IT.)

First-time Augmentations

If I were a woman having a first-time augmentation or if my wife asked my best opinion for her choice of implants, I would advise: If you want a near-natural breast, choose anatomic, form-stable silicone-gel implants if you can get them (if they become available in the United States, if you live outside the United States, or if you are willing to travel abroad and accept the trade-offs). Saline textured anatomic implants are a very close second choice. If you are having a first-time augmentation by a surgeon who is experienced using anatomic implants, you won't notice a significant difference between a saline and a silicone-gel-filled anatomic implant. Hundreds of thousands of first-time augmentation patients are very happy with anatomic-shaped, saline-filled implants.

Since older type silicone-gel implants have recently again become available in the United States, then round, non-form-stable silicone-gel implants are an option if: you are not concerned about potential earlier shell failure with what we believe are under-filled designs of all round gel implants; you are aware of and accept a higher capsular contracture rate with current silicone gel-filled implants; you are fully informed and sign informed-consent documents.

REOPERATIONS . . .

If you need a reoperation, something wasn't ideal the first time around, or your body is making things difficult (capsular contracture, excessive tissue stretch, or other problems)! The first operation is the best chance for success. Augmentation surgery never gets easier the second, third, or fourth time around. Results are less predictable, trade-offs are greater, and risks are higher with each reoperation.

Don't expect any implant to necessarily solve a problem that requires a reoperation. Implants usually don't solve problems, especially when the quality or thickness of patient tissues is not optimal.

Don't waste your time looking for a "magic" implant to solve a problem. It doesn't exist. Look for an experienced surgeon, get second opinions, and at some point, don't beat the dead horse (remember what you get—a beaten, dead horse).

Need a reoperation? Select a round implant, smooth or textured, unless you have a surgeon who is very experienced with anatomic implants. All current round gel implants are underfilled, so beware of shell folding and possible early shell rupture. Until the newer form-stable, cohesive-gel anatomic implants become available in the United States, I would prefer a round, saline-filled implant adequately filled to protect the shell (forget the warranty or ask the manufacturer for an exception), and I would accept a slightly firmer, more globular breast. Many patients and surgeons would disagree and select an underfilled, round, smooth-shelled gel implant, but I would have to question their logic. Haven't we been down that road before? Did we not learn anything from the breast implant crisis? Instead of making bad team decisions, why don't we focus our efforts on bringing all options to women of the United States?

144

"Forget natural, even large and natural. I want really big, round breasts. . . ."

If naturalness is not a major concern, and you want very large, round breasts (implants larger than 350–400 cc), assuming you have accepted the trade-offs and future consequences, I would select a large, round, smooth shell, saline-filled, or older design gel-filled implant, provided you accept the trade-offs. Don't waste your money on large, in most cases over 350 cc, anatomic implants. They are more expensive, about $350 more per pair. You are not desiring a natural look anyway, and with a round implant, you avoid risks of anatomic implant malposition after your tissues stretch (and they will definitely stretch). Enjoy them while you can, save your money, and plan for a reoperation sometime in the future. You may look awesome—for a while.

"I don't want huge, but I want a full upper breast . . ."

If your main goal is beautiful fullness of the upper breast but not necessarily huge breasts, don't be misled by those who tell you that a round implant produces more upper fullness in the upper breast compared to an anatomic implant. **It's not true.** Remember that most round implants collapse unless they are overfilled. If they collapse vertically, they shorten. You lose upper fill. Allergan style 468 saline and full-height style 410 form-stable gel anatomic augmentation implants do not collapse, so they maintain their vertical height. Full-height anatomics are also taller than they are wide. With a properly selected anatomic implant, you have a better chance of getting and maintaining upper fill. Regardless of the shape of implant, all breasts, augmented or not, lose upper fill over time as the lower breast stretches (unless you develop a capsular contracture). But a full-height anatomic implant that is adequately filled to minimize upper shell collapse maintains upper breast fill better than any other currently available implant.

An Allergan Style 410 or 468 anatomic implant can maintain fill in the upper breast better than a round implant of equal size because the upper pole of the anatomic implant doesn't collapse—it maintains its vertical height.

Allergan style 410 and 468 full-height anatomic implants are taller than they are wide.

But remember—the larger the implant, whether round or anatomic— and the thinner your tissues, the more and faster your breast envelope will stretch. When the lower skin envelope stretches, the upper fill (regardless of implant shape) will decrease. No implant can overcome the effects of gravity on your tissues over time. With time, aging, and larger implants, you will eventually lose some upper fullness in almost any case. Many patients and surgeons fall into the trap of thinking that a larger implant will produce and maintain upper fullness. A larger implant will almost always create upper fullness, but it usually won't maintain that upper fullness over time because that same implant will inevitably stretch the lower skin envelope. With only a little bit of stretch, you'll lose the upper fullness. It isn't magic—the bigger the breast or the implant, the less likely it will maintain upper fullness over time.

WHAT'S NEW, AND WHEN CAN I GET IT?

Previously, we discussed some of the potential pitfalls of "new" products. Nevertheless, every patient needs to know all available options, so we will summarize currently available options again.

New Implant Designs

Interestingly, in the four years since the last edition of *The Best Breast*, three "new" implant designs—the Misti Gold implant, Trilucent™ soybean oil-filled implant, and PIP prefilled saline implant have, for all practical purposes, disappeared.

The Allergan styles 468 saline anatomic remains available, and the Allergan style 410 anatomic form-stable gel is currently undergoing study follow-up, anticipating approval in 2007. Since we have knowledge and experience of the design, clinical testing, and requirements for FDA regulatory approval for new implant designs, we believe that no other truly new implant designs currently exist that have any realistic chance of obtaining FDA approval within at least five years and, more likely, ten years in the United States. However, we fully expect that due to the lack of new products in the pipeline, several old design products will be resurrected and recycled during this decade. Patients should carefully examine the history, track record, and peer-reviewed scientific data regarding each new product before selecting it for augmentation.

We have already discussed the latest implant designs that are currently available today—the Allergan Style 410, cohesive-silicone-gel-filled, textured anatomic implants. But until they are available in the United States (perhaps in 2007), the nearest and best saline filled alternative is the Allergan style 468 textured, anatomic, saline-filled implant. In the rest of the world and, hopefully, by 2007 in the United States, the initial style 410 anatomic, form stable, cohesive gel implant will have been expanded to include a matrix of anatomic implant designs designed to offer surgeons more flexibility and options in tailoring implant needs to patients' tissues (Figure 5-11). The style 410 FM and MM (full height and moderate height) designs are optimal for more than 90 percent of breast augmentations. The other designs of the matrix are more appropriate for breast reconstruction or special needs patients.

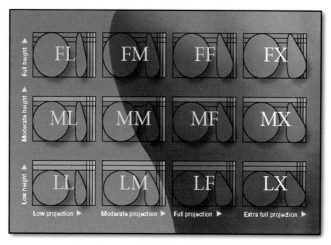

FIGURE 5-11

New Filler Materials

What about new filler materials? At the time of this writing, there is no radically new or better filler material that is likely to be available in the United States in the next two years. Peanut oil or soybean oil appeared promising from a mammogram standpoint, but the initial Trilucent™ soybean oil implants had significant rippling problems, the filler material odor was objectionable to some patients and surgeons, and the British equivalent of the FDA raised questions about possible carcinogenic breakdown products of the filler material and advised all patients who received the implants to have them removed. All other filler materials that I am aware of at this time are still in preliminary testing phases, and clinical availability is most likely many years away. We have seen several "magic, new" implants with "magic, new" filler materials come and go in the past few years. Each one is advertised as the holy grail, but mysteriously, once it is used in a significant number of patients, suddenly it isn't so magical. Problems appear.

When betting on new implant materials and fillers, don't place your bets until the product has at least a five-year track record.

History is replete with magic implant solutions that failed in the first two to three years of widespread use.

After closely watching and participating in this field for the past twenty-four years, my opinion has not changed since the first edition of this book in 1999:

Don't discard silicone- and saline-filled implants (in that order) until there is a proven alternative that has at least five years of followup in a large number of patients.

While you are thinking about what's new, remember what's important.

Just because a breast implant design or filler is new, it's not necessarily better—no matter how promising it may seem.

If it's really good, it will stand the test of time.

We continually learn. If you are the first to get a new device or if you fall for premarketing that is not substantiated by long-term clinical experience and scientific date, you may be the first, but your long-term result may not be the best. Think carefully before jumping on new bandwagons!

Implant choices: Marketing games the manufacturers play, and implant choices truly backed by scientific data.

Most patients are not aware that implant manufacturers can market and sell some types of implants that, although FDA approved, have never really been tested thoroughly in FDA studies. When the FDA approves a category of breast implants such as the recently approved old style, conventional silicone-gel-filled implants, they are approving a *range of implants*, some of which were not directly tested during the PMA study.

Implant manufacturers like to be able to use their marketing hype and strategies instead of thorough research to constantly "invent" new breast implant products, when in reality they are making changes in an FDA approved implant model that may or may not affect the performance of the device. By making changes that stay within FDA tolerances for categories of devices, creating gimmicky new names and marketing campaigns, and telling surgeons and patients that the altered device is new and better, manufacturers can create new products without spending the tremendous time, efforts, and money required to do valid scientific studies on each new implant design they create.

Similarities exist among many different implant types. Manufacturers use these similarities to convince the FDA that making changes in a device that is similar to an approved device is okay. The question is okay for whom, and how okay? Seemingly minor changes in the characteristics or design of an implant can make substantial differences in how the implant performs in patients. Interestingly, manufacturers are not currently required by the FDA to publicly and transparently disclose and report complications and implant device failures *by specific product* code and by implant size. In other words, by lumping a large number of implant types together (for example, all textured surface implants or all smooth shell surface implants), manufacturers can avoid reporting certain specific types or sizes of implants that may have a much higher failure or complication rate. If surgeons and patients do not have this information, they often continue to use products that may cause patients more problems or require more reoperations due to device failures.

If patient safety and optimal patient outcomes are the priority, only the specific product type and sizes that have been tested in an FDA PMA study should be available to patients.

"Substantially equivalent" or similar implant products are often nothing more than a design that was invented by the manufacturers' marketing department. Many of these modified designs have never been tested independently in the equivalent of an FDA PMA study.

Breast implant manufacturers should be required to report all complications and reoperation rates by specific implant product code and implant size, not by broad categories of implant products. Without this information, surgeons and patients cannot make optimal decisions that impact patient safety and outcomes.

FDA premarket approval (PMA) studies are the most stringent and scientifically valid of all breast implant studies worldwide. These studies are supervised by independent clinical review organizations (CROs) that review medical records of every patient in every surgeon investigator's office. The data from United States FDA PMA breast implant studies are the most rigorously scrutinized data according to scientific standards of all clinical studies, even if the clinical studies are peer-reviewed and published.

In every PMA study, only a certain number of specific implant devices are tested. The data from those tests are evaluated scientifically to base decisions about the safety and effectiveness of the implant category. After approval, depending on the range of tolerances the manufacturer has negotiated with the FDA, manufacturers can claim that a much wider range of implants, with designs that have not actually been tested in scientifically valid studies, are substantially equivalent to the implants that really were tested. This practice allows manufacturers to "invent" many "new" implant designs that are nothing more than some modification of an existing design, usually based primarily on marketing considerations, and offer them to surgeons and patients when those design modifications may affect safety or performance of the implant, but were never actually tested in an FDA study.

What types of modifications can manufacturers make within FDA tolerances that may affect the performance of breast implants? The most common modifications usually involve changes in implant shape or projection, or changes in the characteristics of the implant filler material, especially when the filler material is silicone gel.

When manufacturers really do not have a truly new implant product to sell, history suggests that they will create a "new" product, even if it is not really new. Examples include 1) the reintroduction of high-profile implants as new products, when high-profile implants were available over two decades ago, 2) the notion that all silicone-gel-implant filler is "cohesive," when vast differences exist in the degree of cohesiveness among silicone-gel implants, and 3) modifications to implant shells or gel filler materials that are touted as making the implant more "natural," when those changes are modifications that often make the new product perform more like older generation implants. Each of these three types of modifications can potentially affect the life of the implant shell, possible consequences to the patient when the shell fails, and effects of the implant on patients' tissues over time.

Amazingly, a majority of the surgeon market buys into manufacturers' marketing campaigns without thoroughly questioning the science behind each specific product offered to patients. History proves this statement by 1) comparing reoperation rates of various devices from data in FDA PMA studies over the past three decades and 2) reviewing the sales records of various implant products during the same period. (It is difficult to compare sales records because manufacturers rigidly protect this "proprietary" information.) Equally amazingly, some surgeons are quick to blame problems on a wide range of implants such as textured surface implants, when the problems are really caused by a specific model or type of the implant, not by the entire category of implants. If surgeons do not carefully question the scientific validity of data for any "new" implant product or design modifications, patients are unlikely to recognize that what may sound "new" and "better" in marketing programs may not really be either new or better.

Don't buy into a "new" or "better" implant design just because an advertisement sounded good or because you want to be sure you get the latest and greatest. Insist that the exact implant design you are choosing was an exact product type, design, and product code that was tested in the FDA PMA study for that type device.

When considering any type of breast implant, ask your surgeon if that exact model or type of implant was included in the FDA premarket approval study that resulted in FDA approval of the device.

If you have any doubts, ask the implant manufacturer to provide you a written answer to the question you asked your surgeon.

The manufacturers' practices that are described in this chapter have been consistent for the past twenty-nine years that I have been in practice. Surgeons are required by law to offer patients all currently available alternatives for treatment, including all types of breast implants, and advise patients of the potential benefits and trade-offs of each type. To assure the highest levels of safety and the best outcomes with the lowest reoperation rates for patients, surgeons must insist that manufacturers provide all known data on complications and failures by specific product code and size, and relay that information to patients. Further, surgeons should advise patients of any subgroup of implant type that has not actually been one of the specific devices that was tested during the FDA PMA study that resulted in approval of the implant type.

IMPLANTS—WHAT'S BEST?

If You Ask a Surgeon

When you ask a surgeon which type of implant is best, the surgeon will usually have an opinion based on that surgeon's experience. If the experiences were good, the surgeon likes the implant. Bad experiences, the surgeon doesn't like the implant. What if a surgeon never used a certain type of implant? The surgeon may, nevertheless, have an opinion. It's just not based on experience. If something bad occurs, surgeons sometimes blame the implant—sometimes justifiably, usually not justifiably. If a surgeon's opinions are based on experience, it's important to know what types of implants that surgeon has used. How many? Over what period of time? How long did the surgeon follow the patients to really know the long-term results?

The best opinion about implants is an opinion based on experience.

If a surgeon has minimal or no experience with a certain type of implant, the surgeon should preface any opinion with "I've never used that implant, but here's what I think of it."

You will rarely hear a surgeon admit lack of experience with any type of implant. Most surgeons will give you an opinion without specifying their experience, so it's your job to ask. Would you let someone operate on you if they said, "I've never done that operation, but would you like for me to try it on you?" Probably not. Do patients accept the first implant suggestion from a surgeon without knowing their options? Every day. You certainly want to listen carefully to your surgeon's recommendations, but you deserve to know all of your options before making choices. **Become informed.**

**If a surgeon has experience with only one type of implant, that's likely the implant the surgeon will recommend.
We hope.
It's scary to think about the alternative. The more experience a surgeon has with a variety of implant types, the more options the surgeon can offer you and the better the surgeon can put those options into a realistic perspective for you.**

If you ask a patient who has had a breast augmentation . . .

Most patients who have had an augmentation will tell you that the type of implant they have is best. Otherwise, why would they have it?

When a patient tells you her type of implant is best, ask why. Find out how much she really knows.

Ask what types of implant options she considered. Ask which implant options her surgeon offered. Ask why she and her surgeon chose her current implant. Even though the implant she has is "best," ask her to explain its trade-offs because every implant has trade-offs.

The more a previous patient knows, the more in-depth information you will get. But don't be disappointed if you don't get much. Many patients are never offered options. Many patients don't learn about options on their own.

Does that mean that they have a bad result or that they are unhappy with their result? Absolutely not. If you can be happy without knowing, is it really necessary to know a lot about implant choices and the trade-offs inherent to any implant? Only if you want to know. Only if you want to make the best choices. You can hope to be lucky, or you can become knowledgeable. We are assuming you want to know.

If a patient has a bad experience with a certain type of implant, is it the implant's fault? Possibly, but usually not. Many factors can affect the result: patient tissue, patient choices, surgeon skill, surgeon experience, and healing factors, just to name a few. The implant is easy to blame, but it's often not the only cause of problems. So, when you ask your friends their opinions about implants, weigh the opinions, considering their knowledge and your knowledge. The issues aren't simple. Neither are the answers.

Our Personal Opinion about What's Best . . .

Every surgeon and staff have biases when it comes to implants. We are no exception. Our biases are based on twenty-nine years of experience performing augmentations using virtually every type of implant that has been available in the United States since 1977. Based on this experience, we have some very strong beliefs (many of which we mentioned earlier when we listed our biases):

A breast implant should be as safe as possible.

A breast implant should last as long as possible.

No single type of breast implant is best for every patient.

Every patient deserves information and choices.

What's best for you depends on 1) what you want, 2) what your tissues will allow you to have, and 3) which set of benefits and trade-offs you are willing to accept.

Most of these statements are common sense. Safety should be a paramount concern when you are considering placing a device inside your body for an extended period of time. We know that breast implants are medically safe. How can we make them safer? By making them last longer and minimizing reoperations. The longer any implant lasts (before the shell wears out), the fewer times any woman will need a reoperation. The fewer reoperations, the fewer risks, trade-offs, potential complications, and costs. Make sense? You bet! So our personal, number one concern is maximizing the longevity of breast implants. To the extent that we can prolong the life of your implant, you are less likely to need reoperations with risks, trade-offs, possible complications, and costs.

IMPLANT LONGEVITY—THE MOST IMPORTANT ISSUE AND THE FACTORS THAT AFFECT IT

The longer an implant lasts, the fewer reoperations you will need during your lifetime.

Reoperations involve additional risks (more than the initial operation), costs, and recovery time; and the results are less predictable.

Over the past fourteen years, we have made implant longevity our primary concern. We have done this by making implant design changes, improving surgical techniques, and educating surgeons and patients about issues that affect implant longevity. Implant designs and materials will continue to change, but regardless of the design or material, the longer any implant lasts, the better for the patient. That's why we will continue to focus on implant longevity. That's why we want you to understand the issues, so that you can make informed decisions.

Naturalness versus Durability

Notice I said naturalness versus durability. With currently available materials that we are using and researching, I can assure you that

There are definite trade-offs between naturalness and durability when it comes to breast implants.

If you want your implant to last longer, you will need to accept some trade-offs in naturalness.

The only natural breast is a natural breast. Natural breasts don't contain a breast implant. If you want a totally natural breast, don't have an augmentation.

What is natural? It depends on who you ask and when you ask. Is "natural" the firm, perky, full breast in a typical eighteen-year-old woman, or is "natural" the less full, softer, slightly saggier breast of that same woman after three children when she is forty years old? If this woman chooses to have an augmentation when she is forty to refill her upper breast and improve the sagging, her implanted breasts will be firmer. They will feel more like the breasts she had when she was eighteen before pregnancies. So are they unnatural? Compared to what? Yes, they are unnatural compared to softer, saggier, and empty at the top. But are they acceptably natural to her? You would have to ask, but I would bet the answer is yes. This scenario illustrates common changes that occur in many women's breasts with pregnancy and aging and points out that

Naturalness is relative. It depends on what a woman has, what a woman wants, and what a woman is willing to accept in trade-offs.

What Makes an Implant Feel More Natural or Less Natural?

How natural an implant feels is determined by four main factors:

1. The thickness of the implant shell,

2. The thickness of your tissues that cover the implant,

3. The amount of filler material in the implant,

4. The amount of your own breast tissue covering the implant.

The *thinner* the outer shell of an implant, the less you can feel the implant in the breast. From the standpoint of naturalness, a thinner implant shell is better. But with current implant shell materials, thinner is weaker. Thinner is less durable. Most implants manufactured today have thicker shells compared to the shells of implants made twenty years ago. The twenty-year-old implants may be more natural, but they are less durable. Today's implants generally have thicker shells to increase durability and, hopefully, increase shell and implant longevity. Notice, I said "hopefully." Many factors affect the life of an implant shell, not just the thickness of the shell, but a thicker shell is a first step toward making your implant last longer.

How thick is thick? You will possibly hear different implant companies touting that their shells are thicker or less thick, depending on how you and your surgeon feel about naturalness versus durability. Surgeons don't like to hear patients complain about being able to feel their implants, so many surgeons will select or recommend implants with thinner shells. Question is did your surgeon discuss all of the issues with you that affect naturalness? Did your surgeon ask which you would rather have, an implant that feels more natural or an implant that lasts longer? These are important questions, important issues to resolve before choosing an implant.

The thickness of an implant shell is not the only factor that affects whether you may be able to feel your implants. The thickness and characteristics of your tissues are at least as important. Since you can't change your tissues, you should clearly understand the limitations and trade-offs your tissues will impose.

If you are thin and you can feel your ribs beneath your breast with your fingertip, you will probably be able to feel the edges or shell of any state-of-the-art implant in the world today, regardless of its shell thickness.

If you have thin tissues, you have thin tissues. You can't change that. Your surgeon can't change that.

The thinner you are, the more likely you will feel some portion of your implants after your augmentation.

Since you can't change your thin tissues (gaining weight won't change them enough), if feeling your implant is unacceptable to you, don't have an augmentation.

Feeling some portion of your implant is one thing—usually no more of an issue than feeling your ribs. Seeing the edges of the implant is a bigger problem to most patients. If you are thin, there are specific surgical options such as placing the implant behind muscle (more about that in chapter 6) that can often help prevent your seeing an implant edge. But no technique or pocket location can consistently overcome thin tissues and guarantee that you won't be able to feel some portion of the implant.

Thin is in. Many women spend considerable time, effort, and money to get thin and stay thin. In our practice, a large percentage of patients are thin. Thin patients are just as happy with their augmentations as patients with thicker tissues. We almost never hear a thin patient complain about feeling her implants. Why? Partly because we did everything surgically possible to cover the implant. Largely because we discussed the issues and the patient made the choices and accepted the trade-offs before her surgery.

Why Is the Amount of Filler in Your Implant Important?

The amount of filler material in your implant, regardless of the type of filler, saline or silicone, is critically important and is an issue that is frequently overlooked by patients and some surgeons:

The amount of filler in an implant largely determines whether the shell of that implant folds or collapses when the implant is in your breast.

If any implant shell (using today's materials) collapses or folds, this causes stresses on the shell that may make the shell wear out sooner.

If an implant shell folds, it increases your risks of feeling or seeing rippling in your breast.

Assume for a moment that you are holding an empty implant shell. The size doesn't matter. The shell material doesn't matter. Even the filler material you are going to put in the implant doesn't matter. As you gradually add filler to the implant (like filling a balloon with liquid), the shell expands. When only a small amount of filler is added, the implant feels soft, but the shell is floppy. If you tilt the implant upright, the shell collapses and folds. The more filler you add, the more the shell expands and the less likely the shell will fold when you tilt the implant upright.

With any implant and any filler material, the following occur:

The more filler you place in the implant, the less risk of shell folding.

The more filler you place in the implant, the firmer the implant—slightly firmer is a trade-off for durability.

Exceeding the capacity of an implant shell can cause distortions of the shell.

Let's illustrate these points by actually filling an implant shell. The round, saline implant shell is empty and collapsed in Figure 5-12. The manufacturer recommends placing 300–330 cc of saline (salt water) into this shell as an optimal amount of fill. In Figure 5-13, we have added 250 cc of saline. Looks pretty good on the table, right? But when we place the implant in our hand and support (not pushing) the lower implant with the other hand and tilt it upright (see Figure 5-14), what happens? The upper shell collapses and folds. Shell folding can cause visible rippling in your breast and can cause the implant shell to rupture.

Any folding or collapse of an implant shell should worry you if you want the shell to last as long as possible.

So let's add saline up to the manufacturer's recommendations and see what happens. Even after we reach the 330 cc the manufacturer recommends (see Figure 5-15), the shell still folds when we perform the tilt test! So let's see how much saline it takes to prevent the shell from folding when upright. We continue adding saline in small amounts until the shell first experiences no collapse or folding when upright (Figure 5-16). How much total saline was necessary to eliminate folding with the implant upright? 360 cc! So why doesn't the manufacturer recommend more fill to prevent shell folding? An excellent question! To demonstrate that excessive overfilling creates problems, we continue adding saline until we create distortion and scalloping of the shell (Figure 5-17) at 390 cc, so it's obvious that, at some point, excessive fill creates problems.

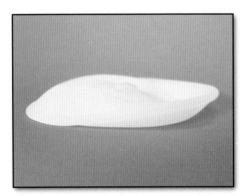

FIGURE 5-12

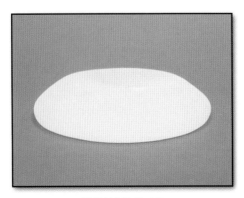

FIGURE 5-13

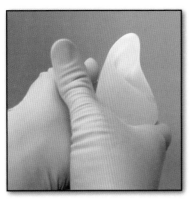

FIGURE 5-14

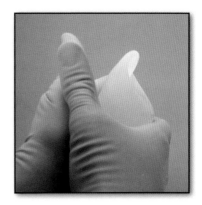

FIGURE 5-15

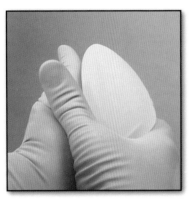

FIGURE 5-16

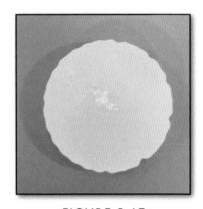

FIGURE 5-17

Optimal fill volumes and implant shape (Round or Anatomic)—
how do they relate?

*All of today's round saline implants are underfilled if
filled to manufacturer's recommendations.*

*With virtually all of today's round implants, regardless
of the filler material or the size of the implant, shell
collapse and folding occur if the implant is filled to the
manufacturer's recommendations!*

Can't happen, shouldn't happen, you say? Most surgeons instinctively acknowledge this fact. Having experienced problems with patients having visible rippling and wrinkling with saline implants filled to manufacturer's recommendations, some surgeons overfill saline implants past manufacturer's recommendations to prevent patients' having these problems. Problem solved? Not quite. Overfilling voids the manufacturer's warranty on the implant! Sound like a catch-22? It is. If a surgeon fills the implant enough to prevent shell folding and protect the shell, no warranty. If the surgeon fills to manufacturer's recommendations to protect the warranty, the patient has a greater risk of experiencing visible rippling or premature implant rupture. So why don't the manufacturers just define fill volumes higher for round implants?

The same is true for all of the older design round implants filled with the old type of non-cohesive silicone gel. They are all currently underfilled according to the tilt test and experience various degrees of upper-shell collapse and/or folding with the implant upright. These implants may become available again in the United States in 2008, but the fill volumes of silicone gel in these implants to date has not been increased significantly to minimize upper shell collapse or folding.

Manufacturers have not defined fill volumes higher for round implants, both saline and silicone gel filled, possibly because

Manufacturers believe that surgeons won't use and, therefore, won't buy round implants with more fill because the surgeon feels that the implant is too firm.

Historically, manufacturers respond to the pressures of their market like most successful companies.

Surgeons feel that firmer implants (even a tiny bit firmer) are unacceptable to patients.

Often they make this assumption without ever having used a significant number of firmer implants or asking patients which they would prefer, a slightly firmer breast or a reoperation sooner?

We now have a peer-reviewed clinical study in a large series of patients that indicates a majority of patients, if fully informed about fill issues, prefer an implant with a greater percentage fill to minimize potential shell collapse even if it means that the implant is slightly firmer.[1]

When round implants are filled adequately to prevent shell folding, they look very round, and the upper breast can look excessively bulging, even having a sharp, bulging stepoff.

Although some patients request an unnatural, excessively bulging upper breast, most don't.

These principles apply to all round implants, regardless of the filler material in the implant.

Older, round, silicone gel-filled implants were definitely softer than today's implants, but none of them could pass the tilt test. Examples include the Misti Gold implant, the Trilucent™ soybean oil filled implant, and the PIP prefilled saline implant, all of which experienced unexpectedly high shell failure rates, and all of which are now off the market. All of these, as well as the old type silicone-gel implants that were approved by the FDA in 2006 were softer because they were underfilled. Perhaps some older implants ruptured sooner because they were underfilled and had folded shells. No way to know, no way to prove the point retrospectively. But enough of a question that I would think we should consider simple ways to increase shell longevity— like just filling the shell adequately! Even today, eight years after we raised this issue in the first edition of *The Best Breast* and ten years after we raised the issue in the most respected professional journal of the specialty,[7] the issue is not adequately addressed by many manufacturers and surgeons.

Anatomic-shaped implants are more like a natural breast, fuller at the bottom, full and tapering at the top.

Because of the tapering upper pole, an anatomic implant can be filled adequately to prevent shell folding—without producing an unnatural appearing upper breast.

Allergan has defined the fill volumes of their style 468 saline and style 410 cohesive-gel anatomic implants higher at the outset—so there is no need for the surgeon to overfill the implant to protect the shell!

What Can You Do to Influence Surgeons and Manufacturers to Protect the Shell of Your Implant?

If you want the shell of your implants to be protected by assuring adequate fill and if you would like to avoid visible wrinkling and rippling after your augmentation, we suggest that you

Require that any implant placed in your body pass the tilt test before it is implanted, regardless of the type, shape, or filler material. Ask your surgeon to perform the test.

This basic, simple test doesn't answer every possible question about factors that affect implant shell life. But the tilt test is something you or your surgeon can easily do, it's logical, and it's probably better than any other test currently available that can be applied in or out of the operating room. How do you do it? If your surgeon is unfamiliar with the tilt test, refer them to reference number seven at the end of this chapter.

WHAT ABOUT NEW IMPLANTS AND THE FDA?

As a patient, you will hear about every new "wonder implant" that might ever hit the market. In fact, you will hear about it long before it's a reality, long before it's adequately tested. (That's called premarketing.) Excellent examples include the highly touted Trilucent™ soybean oil-filled implant. Another example is the PIP prefilled saline implant— no valve on the implant. Both of these highly touted and premarketed products are now gone. There will be countless more. Companies want you to be ready for new when it comes; they want you to want it even before it comes.

Did any of the ads for soybean oil implants ever mention shell wrinkling or rippling, or the possibility that underfill might compromise shell longevity? In at least five academic presentations by surgeons using peanut or soybean oil implants, I saw large, prominent folds in the shells in patients' mammograms following augmentation. Did any surgeon mention the folded shell? No, they were emphasizing how well X-rays could pass through the implant. Improving mammograms is important, but so is adequate fill to protect the shell. Now we know that these underfilled Trilucent™ and PIP implants experienced unusually high premature shell failures. Unfortunately, patients and surgeons who rushed to choose both the Trilucent™ and PIP prefilled saline implants are paying a price—more reoperations to replace prematurely failed implants. If only they had read *The Best Breast*, perhaps some reoperations might have been avoided.

In the first edition of *The Best Breast* more than eight years ago, I mentioned my concerns with the PIP prefilled saline implant manufactured in France and sold in the United States. I had heard the company tout the softness of its implant compared to other implants. When I performed a tilt test on the implant, guess what? It didn't pass; the shell folded significantly. Yes, it's a bit softer because it's underfilled, as shown by the tilt test. Any company can produce a softer implant— just underfill it. But remember, an underfilled implant may cost you a reoperation! Today, we know the price that patients are paying for underfilled implants. Trilucent™ and PIP prefilled implants are off the market. Is underfill the only issue with these implants? No, but it is one very important issue.

Want more food for thought? The FDA, after telling women that silicone implants were potentially dangerous (now proved scientifically not the case) and removing them from use for augmentation in the United States, is now allowing studies using the same gel implants that they said were so bad in the first place. Surgeons and patients who were glad to have more options have participated in the studies. Will any of these implants pass the tilt test? I encourage you to try it. So, why would the FDA allow studies on underfilled implants? Ask them. Perhaps, up to ten years after we published scientific articles about these issues, the FDA is still not aware of the fill issues, or perhaps the FDA doesn't consider them important. Why would manufacturers want to study the same implants that got them into litigation a few years back? The only plausible answer is that manufacturers must sell implants to be able to provide implants to American women. American women need and deserve more state-of-the-art for augmentation, and they deserve adequately filled implants to maximize the life of the implant shell and prevent reoperations.

But why regress? Why not progress? Why study an old design, under-filled silicone-gel implants of the type that the FDA banned initially, especially when newer, more advanced options are available? Why not approve new, cohesive-gel implants with a new filler material that are available in most of the rest of the world and have been used in over 40,000 patients? These implants will pass the tilt test, and you can cut a pie-shaped wedge out of this implant with scissors, squeeze the implant, and the gel won't migrate (figure 5-8)! We designed these cohesive gel, anatomic implants because we believe that they are safer and will last longer, and they are the implants I would unquestionably recommend over all other implants I have ever used (and I've used almost every type). Are cohesive gel implants perfect? No. Nor is any implant perfect. Is it best for every patient? No. But it is a step forward compared to most other implants. Now we are working on the next generation after cohesive gel, but if you are an American woman, you can't even get the current generation of the Allergan style 410 cohesive gel implant in the United States before 2007 under the best case scenario! We will continue to be committed to the design and development of newer, better implants for our patients. Our goal is to be able to provide patients with implants that will last a lifetime. We're not there yet.

Is the amount of filler in an implant important? We believe it is very important! Should we adequately fill all implants regardless of the design or filler material to prevent shell collapse and folding? No doubt in our minds! Otherwise, every woman who receives an underfilled implant may require a reoperation sooner than she would were it adequately filled. More reoperations mean more risks and more costs.

Which would you prefer: softer, more natural with a folded shell or slightly firmer with a protected shell and less chance of reoperation? You choose. It's your body.

WHO MAKES AND GUARANTEES MY IMPLANTS?

This is a critical question that many patients never ask. Why does it matter? Because you may be placing a device manufactured by a company in your body for many years. How good is the design? How good are the manufacturing processes? How good is the quality control? What happens if you have a problem? Who is there to support you? Does the company have the majority of its financial assets in the United States where its commitment is backed up by its money and large support staffs? All are questions that you should consider before selecting an implant or before allowing your surgeon to select an implant for you.

United States Companies

At the present time, two major companies manufacture breast implants in the United States, Allergan Medical Corporation and Mentor Corporation. Both are first-class companies committed to first-class patient care and state-of-the-art products. Both stand behind their products with strong guarantees, strong patient support, and commitments to research that advances the safety and efficacy of their products. Both companies are available when you need them and attempt to provide excellent service to patients and surgeons. Although we have worked more closely with McGhan Medical (now Allergan) Corporation, we have the utmost respect for both companies, and we use implants manufactured by both. We also encourage both companies to constantly prioritize patients and continue to improve their practices and their products.

Foreign Companies

Foreign-based companies sell breast implants in the United States. Amazingly, the FDA allows foreign companies to sell breast implant products in the United States based on foreign data that may or may not conform to the standards that the FDA demands domestically of Mentor and Allergan. Does that mean that the products are not up to standards? Not necessarily. But a foreign-based company is often not subject to the same pressures, risks, and demands of a United States–based company. If the majority of a company's assets (capital) are located outside the United States, you could have a substantially more difficult time recovering money from that company if you had a problem with its product.

Ask the following questions of any company, foreign or domestic:

- How long have you been in business?

- Are you a publicly traded company in the United States? Are most of your assets in the United States? Ask for documentation.

- How long have you been selling breast implants in the United States?

- How much money have you spent on breast implant research and development? Ask for documentation.

- What are the terms of your guarantee on your breast implants? Do you cover all of my expenses for my lifetime with respect to implant replacement and surgery in the event of implant failure? Listen carefully to the answers, and ask for written documentation.

- How many salespeople and support staff do you have in the United States? Where are they located? Ask for documentation.

The company that manufactures your breast implants doesn't matter until you need to replace its implants.

It's easier to assure that you will have a company's support when you need it before you put its product in your body.

Look into the company that manufactures your implants before you have an augmentation—or don't complain later.

When is an implant doomed to disappoint me?

Any implant will disappoint you if you expect it to do something that an implant can't do.

An implant is likely to disappoint you if . . .

You are very thin and expect that you won't feel some portion of your implant.

You have extremely saggy breasts and think an implant alone will solve the problem. (It may, more about that later, but it may not; it depends on several factors.)

You select excessively large implants that your tissues can't support over time.

You don't realize that your tissues won't get better with time and select your implants accordingly.

THE NEXT STEP

Now that you are knowledgeable about implants, let's examine different surgical options.

References

1. Tebbetts, J. B. Patient acceptance of adequately filled breast implants. *Plast. Reconstr. Surg.* 106(1): 139-47, 2006.

2. Tebbetts, J. B. Dual plane (DP) breast augmentation: Optimizing implant-soft tissue relationships in a wide range of breast types. *Plast. Reconstr. Surg.* 106(1): 273-290, 2002.

3. Tebbetts, J. B. Achieving a predictable 24-hour return to normal activities after breast augmentation, part I: Refining practices using motion and time study principles. *Plast. Reconstr. Surg.* 109(1): 273-290, 2002.

4. Tebbetts, J. B. Achieving a predictable 24-hour return to normal activities after breast augmentation, part II: Patient preparation, refined surgical techniques and instrumentation. *Plast. Reconstr. Surg.* 109(1): 293-305, 2002.

5. Tebbetts, J. B. A system for breast implant selection based on patient tissue characteristics and implant-soft tissue dynamics. *Plast. Reconstr. Surg.* 109(4): 1396-1409, 2002.

6. Tebbetts, J. B., and Adams, W. P. Five critical decisions in breast augmentation using 5 measurements in 5 minutes: The high five system. *Plast. Reconstr. Surg.* 116(7): 2005-2016, 2005.

7. Tebbetts, J. B. Achieving a zero percent reoperation rate at 3 years in a 50 consecutive case augmentation mammaplasty PMA study. *Plast. Reconstr. Surg.* 118(6): 1453-1457, 2006.

8. U. S. Food and Drug Administration. Product labeling data for Mentor and Allergan/Inamed core studies of saline-filled implants. http://www.fda.gov/cdrh/breastimplants/labeling/mentor_patient_labeling_5900.html. Accessed December 5, 2006; FDA web site updated November 17, 2006.

9. U. S. Food and Drug Administration. Product labeling data for Mentor and Allergan/Inamed core studies of saline-filled implants. http://www.fda.gov/cdrh/breastimplants/labeling.html. Accessed December 5, 2006; FDA web site updated November 17, 2006.

SURGICAL OPTIONS:

OVER/UNDER MUSCLE, IMPLANT SHAPE AND SIZE, INCISION LOCATION

"No set of surgical options or implant options is perfect for every patient— every option has trade-offs."

Many different surgical options exist in breast augmentation. To be able to offer you options, a surgeon must be familiar with different approaches and implants and have the experience and skill to apply those options confidently.

No specific set of surgical options is best for every patient.

If you are offered only one set of options, that may be the only options a surgeon can offer—consult other surgeons.

Every patient tends to think that the options she chose are also the best options for someone else. That isn't true because no two women are exactly alike. Your tissues are definitely different!

No surgical option is perfect.

No surgical option is without trade-offs.

The question is whether you know the relative benefits and trade-offs and pick the options that best maximize the benefits and minimize the trade-offs.

If you and your surgeon don't discuss your tissues and how your tissues influence the best choice of implant for you, you will need to blame something or someone for the consequences.

You will probably blame the implant or the surgeon, when it's really you who's largely responsible.

Retromammary Placement   **Partial Retropectoral**

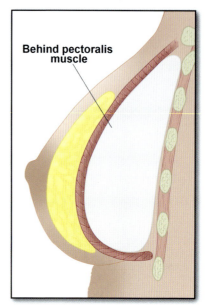

FIGURE 6-1   FIGURE 6-2

LOCATION OF THE POCKET FOR THE IMPLANT

Over or Under Muscle?

The most important priority in selecting a pocket for the implant is to assure *optimal tissue coverage over your implant for your entire lifetime.* Optimal tissue coverage means assuring that all portions and edges of your implant are covered by the *most tissue available,* given your body characteristics.

If your tissues are thin in the areas that cover your implant (and we will show you how to measure later), you may need to put the implant partially behind muscle, especially in the upper and middle areas of the breast, to assure adequate tissue cover over the implant. If you don't, you run more risks of seeing the edges of your implant and seeing visible traction rippling later, both of which are usually uncorrectable. But there is much more to making the decision.

Dual Plane Placement

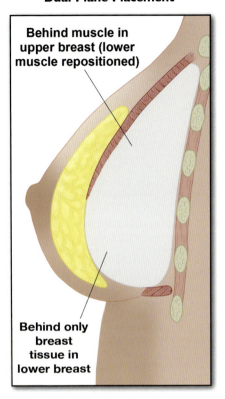

Behind muscle in upper breast (lower muscle repositioned)

Behind only breast tissue in lower breast

FIGURE 6-3

Breast implants in the past have been placed in one of **two locations:**

1. Behind your breast tissue but in front of your pectoralis muscle—**retromammary placement** (Figure 6-1), or

2. Partially behind your pectoralis muscle—**partial retropectoral** placement (Figure 6-2).

Now there is a new and frequently *better* option: *dual plane*[1]—behind muscle in the upper breast and behind breast tissue in the lower breast—the best of both worlds (1 &2) above, while minimizing the trade-offs of each! (Figure 6-3)

When silicone-gel-filled implants were available and widely used in the United States, surgeons began placing implants partially behind the pectoralis muscle because silicone-gel implants had a lower risk of capsular contracture (excessive firmness) when they were placed partially behind the pectoralis. With today's saline-filled implants, the risk of capsular contracture is about the same whether the implant is placed in front of the muscle or behind the muscle. So, what difference does it make, and how do you choose? The choice is based on the thickness of your tissues—how much thickness you have to cover your implants.

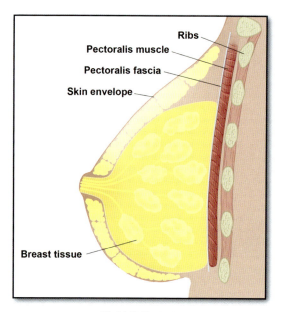

FIGURE 6-4

What Muscle, and Where Is It?

Let's review our anatomy from the Introduction. Figure 6-4 shows a cross-sectional side view of the upper body. Let's look at the layers of tissue beginning with the skin over the breast. Beneath the skin is a layer of fat—variable from patient to patient. The skin and fat layer make up what we call the "skin envelope" of the breast. The skin envelope covers the breast tissue, the next deeper layer. Beneath the breast tissue is the pectoralis major muscle that lies on top of your ribs. Implants can be placed behind the breast tissue but in front of the pectoralis (retromammary), or they can be placed behind the breast tissue and behind the pectoralis muscle (partial retropectoral), OR behind muscle in the upper breast and behind breast tissue in the lower breast (dual plane[1]). To understand why we use the term "partial" retropectoral, let's look at a front view of the anatomy.

Retromammary Placement   **Partial Retropectoral**

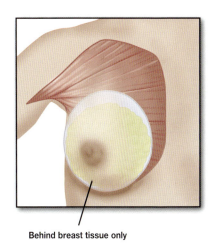

Pectoralis Muscle

Behind breast tissue only

"Partial" retropectoral because this area is not covered by pectoralis muscle

FIGURE 6-5   FIGURE 6-6

The pectoralis muscle lies beneath the upper half or upper third of the breast. When an implant is placed *in front of the muscle*, the implant is covered in the lower portion by breast tissue and in the upper portion by only skin and fat (Figure 6-5). When an implant is placed *behind the pectoralis major muscle*, the upper portion of the implant is covered by muscle, but the lower portion (especially the lower, outside portion) of the implant is still covered only by breast tissue (Figure 6-6). Hence, the term "partial" retropectoral—the implant is only partially behind muscle in the upper breast. In the lower breast, the implant is not totally covered by muscle.

Partial retropectoral placement means that the upper portion of the implant is partially covered by the pectoralis major muscle and that attachments of the pectoralis muscle along the fold under the breast are left intact. In dual plane, some of these attachments are released to decrease the amount of pressure the muscle puts on the implant in the lower breast (more about that later).

Below and to the side of the pectoralis muscle is the serratus muscle. Although this muscle can be lifted to provide total muscle coverage of an implant, this option is best reserved for difficult reconstruction cases, not for augmentation. When an implant is totally covered by muscle (total submuscular), the shape of the lower breast is seldom as good and never predictable. The fold beneath the breast (the inframammary fold) is flatter and doesn't stretch as predictably with time. The additional pressure of the serratus muscle on an implant can also cause upward displacement of the implant, requiring reoperation. These trade-offs generally mean that:

Although technically possible, total muscle coverage is never the best option for a first-time augmentation.

Rare exceptions exist where total muscle cover may be a good choice, but only in very, very thin patients who will accept all of the trade-offs listed above.

Retromammary (Behind Breast Tissue Only) Placement— Benefits and Tradeoffs

The goal of augmentation is to produce the best breast. The implant helps produce the best breast by putting pressure on the overlying breast tissue and skin envelope to fill and shape the breast.

An implant placed in front of the muscle (behind breast tissue, retromammary) can sometimes control breast shape more predictably, but . . .

If you are thin, placing the implant in front of muscle in the upper and middle edge of the breast may not provide enough coverage to prevent your seeing the upper edge of the implant, now or in the future.

Newer dual plane techniques allow surgeons to provide you the best coverage for your implants AND provide you an optimal aesthetic result.

From a practical standpoint, what are the advantages of retromammary (behind breast only) placement?

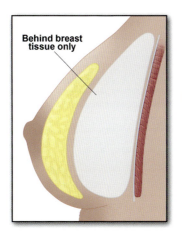

Behind breast tissue only

Retromammary Placement

FIGURE 6-7

Advantages of Retromammary Placement

Historically, surgeons have believed that advantages of placing the implant only behind breast tissue and not behind muscle (Figure 6-7) included the following:

More precise control of cleavage—the distance between your breasts,

More precise control of upper breast fill—especially upper fill toward the middle of your chest,

Less chance of muscle pressure pushing your implants to the side over time, widening the distance between your breasts,

Less chance of distorting your breast shape when you tighten (contract) your pectoralis muscle,

More rapid recovery following surgery? (This is no longer true.[2, 3])

With all these supposed advantages, why in the world would you ever put an implant behind muscle? There's one overwhelming reason—to provide optimal, long-term soft tissue coverage over the implant so you don't see the edges of the implant or see visible traction rippling in the future when the weight of the implant pulls on thin, overlying tissues. The best news is that now, with the development of dual plane techniques, you can have virtually all of the advantages of submammary placement, and at the same time provide muscle coverage in the upper and middle areas of the breast . . . and be out to dinner the same evening in most cases.[2, 3]

If you are thin and you place your implants only behind breast tissue, you will have a greater risk of feeling or seeing an edge of the implant. How thin is thin? How do you determine when "thin" is "too thin"? In a moment, we'll tell you. Another issue with placing implants only behind breast tissue and not behind muscle has to do with mammograms. More about that later. For starters, memorize this one:

The number one priority in breast augmentation is providing optimal soft tissue cover over an implant for your lifetime.

If you are very thin, adequate tissue cover is more important than all of the advantages of retromammary placement combined and is always the first priority.

The main trade-offs of retromammary placement are:

1. This location may not provide adequate soft tissue cover to prevent your seeing the edges of your implant or developing visible traction rippling as you age, especially if you are exceedingly thin.

2. This location may make your mammograms more difficult (more about this later). This placement potentially exposes your implants to more bacteria that are present in every woman's breasts.

Subfascial Placement—Benefits and Tradeoffs

The pectoralis major fascia is a very thin layer of tissue that lies beneath the breast tissue but in front of the pectoralis muscle (Figure 6-8). Recently, some surgeons have promoted placing implants behind this layer instead of just behind breast tissue as a superior alternative to deeper submuscular or dual plane locations (discussed later in this chapter).

The pectoralis fascia is less than one millimeter thick at its thickest portion, and much thinner than one millimeter in many areas. No surgeon has ever proved that it is possible surgically to accurately lift this

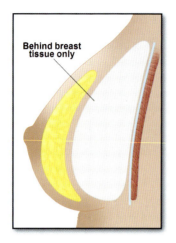 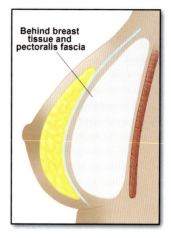

Subfascial Placement

FIGURE 6-8

fascia intact or keep it intact to cover an implant. Most surgeons who promote subfascial placement claim that its benefits are essentially the same as the retromammary pocket discussed previously in this chapter. These same surgeons claim that patients have less pain and a faster recovery with implant placement under pectoralis fascia compared to placement under the muscle itself. Unfortunately, none of these claims is verified by valid scientific data, and subfascial placement is really no different than retromammary placement.

Later in this chapter, we will discuss a modification of placement under muscle, called dual-plane placement,[1] that offers more than ten times the amount of additional soft tissue cover compared to the paper thin pectoralis fascia. Patients having dual plane placement routinely go to dinner the evening of surgery and resume full, normal activities within twenty-four hours.[2] No surgeon using subfascial placement has ever demonstrated or published equivalent rapid recovery. Long-term follow-up of large numbers of patients using dual plane techniques has demonstrated an overall reoperation rate lower than is reported in any equivalent peer-reviewed and published studies.[1-4] No comparative results with subfascial placement have ever been published.

Subfascial pocket placement adds less than one millimeter of additional soft tissue coverage over your implants.

A one millimeter or less amount of additional coverage is totally insignificant long-term as you become older and your tissues become thinner.

No long-term, scientifically valid comparative study has ever demonstrated any difference between submammary (retromammary) and subfascial placement.

No objective study for speed of recovery has ever matched the twenty-four-hour recovery we have demonstrated with dual-plane placement.[1,2]

Partial Retropectoral (Behind Pectoralis Muscle, Figure 6-9) Placement—Benefits and Trade-offs

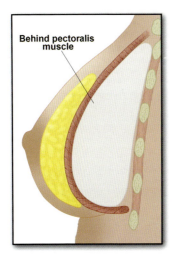

Subpectoral Placement

FIGURE 6-9

Advantages of retropectoral placement

You already know the main advantage of putting an implant partially behind muscle—to prevent seeing an edge of the implant and to prevent visible traction rippling in areas where tissue coverage is thin.

The major advantage of placing an implant behind muscle is to prevent implant edge visibility and visible traction rippling.

This does not mean that you may not feel portions of the implant, especially in the fold under the breast and the outside portion of the breast.

A second stated advantage of subpectoral placement is better reduction of risks of capsular contracture compared to retromammary placement, especially with silicone-gel-filled implants.

Historically, differences in capsular contracture rates are more marked with silicone-gel implants than with saline implants. With saline implants, risks are about the same.

Better mammograms? Maybe, but a soft breast that can be pulled away from the chest for mammography is also important.

A third stated advantage of retropectoral placement is that some radiologists believe that placing the implant behind muscle improves mammogram interpretation. Although this concept is well-established in the medical literature, it's not an absolute. (Remember, most medical "facts" are shades of gray.) One of the most important requirements for getting a good mammogram is that the breasts are soft (no capsular contracture). If the breasts are soft, it's easier for the technician to pull the breast tissue forward (away from the implant) to get a better picture. Other factors can significantly affect mammograms: the skill of the technician performing the mammogram, the skill of the person interpreting the mammogram, and the consistency and characteristics of your breast tissue—just to name a few. Also, mammograms are not perfect, with or without implants. Earlier, we told you that a significant number of breast cancers may not show up on a mammogram. A mammogram is not the only way to assess a breast. Your personal exam and your physician's exam are equally important. Remember, every implant interferes with mammograms to some degree. If you have a strong family history of breast cancer (mother and grandmother), don't have a breast augmentation. Ask your surgeon about mammogram issues with implants; then make your own decisions.

Trade-offs of retropectoral placement

When an implant is placed behind the pectoralis muscle using conventional submuscular techniques (not the newer dual plane techniques), the following trade-offs can occur. They may occur to different degrees in different patients, but you should be willing to accept them, if necessary, in exchange for minimizing risks of upper implant edge visibility and possibly for better mammography. The pressure of the pectoralis muscle overlying the implant causes the following:

Distortion of breast shape when you tighten (contract) your pectoralis muscle—this varies tremendously from patient to patient and is not predictable.

Shifting of the implants to the side over time, widening the distance between the breasts—this also varies

tremendously but is usually worse the thinner your tissues, the thicker your pectoralis, and/or the larger your implant.

Less control of upper breast fill, especially upper and toward the middle—the pressure of the pectoralis on the upper implant reduces control of fill in these areas.

Increased risk of upward displacement of the implant— this is related to the surgical techniques used. With optimal surgical technique, it is rare unless capsular contracture occurs and closes the lower pocket, pushing the implant upward.

Newer, dual-plane techniques provide virtually all of the tissue coverage benefits of muscle coverage, while drastically reducing or eliminating each of the trade-offs listed above for traditional retropectoral placement. Since the number one priority in breast augmentation is assuring optimal soft tissue coverage for a patient's lifetime, minor trade-offs to achieve that goal are logical and essential to making good decisions.

By choosing the DUAL-PLANE pocket location (a combination of retromammary and retropectoral) instead of purely retropectoral or retromammary, at least 80 percent of the trade-offs listed above for partial retropectoral pockets are substantially reduced! You still get the upper coverage you need, but with dramatically fewer trade-offs.

Dual-Plane (Behind Pectoralis Muscle Above, Behind Breast Tissue Only Below) Placement—Benefits and Trade-offs

Realizing the importance of assuring adequate tissue coverage over all breast implants, but also wanting to reduce the trade-offs of traditional "behind muscle" placement, in April of 2001, in the journal of *Plastic and Reconstructive Surgery,* we published results of a clinical study of 426 patients whose implants were placed in the "dual-plane" position—a new pocket location that optimized coverage by placing implants beneath muscle in the upper breast, while minimizing the trade-offs of traditional "behind the muscle" placement by repositioning the lower border of the muscle and allowing the implant to lie in front of muscle, or behind breast tissue only, in the lower breast (Figures 6-10 and 6-11).

Dual-Plane Placement

Dual-Plane Placement

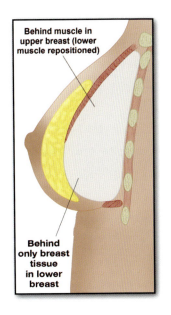

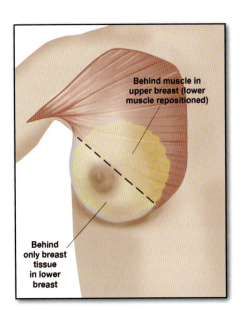

FIGURE 6-10

FIGURE 6-11

For the first time, surgeons can now offer patients the dual-plane pocket location (behind muscle in the upper breast and behind only breast tissue in the lower breast—optimizing tissue coverage while minimizing trade-offs).

The dual-plane pocket location has revolutionized the traditional approach to implant pocket location by assuring adequate coverage while optimizing implant-tissue relationships to assure patients fewer trade-offs.

Advantages of dual-plane placement

Maximal soft tissue coverage in the upper breast to reduce risks of implant edge visibility or visible traction rippling:

Allows the implant to optimally shape the breast without excessive pressure from the overlying pectoralis muscle in the lower breast,

Makes the location and shape of the fold beneath the breast more predictable and more accurate and allows the fold to form final contours earlier,

Reduces pain by decreasing tension on the muscle by the underlying implant,[2]

Allows over 95 percent of patients with dual-plane pockets to return to full normal activities in twenty four hours following augmentation and allows over 80 percent to be out to dinner the evening of their surgery,[2,3]

Allows patients to have muscle cover over their implants and not have more pain or a longer recovery as they formerly experienced with traditional behind-the-muscle placement,

Reduces pressure of the pectoralis muscle distorting breast shape when the muscle contracts,

Reduces pressure of the muscle that tends to displace the implants to the sides and widen the gap between the breasts.

Trade-offs of dual-plane placement

Slightly less thickness of muscle cover along the fold beneath the breast (and therefore not optimal for exceedingly thin patients who have a pinch thickness of skin and fat at the fold that is less than 0.5 cm (5mm).

No other trade-offs of dual-plane placement are scientifically documented at this time.

Feeling or Seeing an Implant Edge

If you place an implant under the pectoralis muscle, you have done all that is possible to prevent seeing the upper edge of the implant. What about feeling the implant? The muscle only covers the upper and middle portions of the implant, not the lower and outside portions. In the lower and outside portions of the breast, if you are very thin and can feel your ribs with your finger, you will almost certainly be able to feel the edge or shell of your implant, especially in the fold under the breast or at the outside of the breast. And don't let anyone tell you that you won't feel a smooth shell implant compared to a textured shell implant. If you're thin, you'll likely be able to feel either one. It you feel it, you feel it—you either do or you don't, so fear of feeling an implant edge is not a good reason to avoid textured surface implants.

You can't see the area under the fold of the breast (when standing), no matter how thin you are, so seeing an implant edge under the breast isn't much of an issue.

At the outside part of the breast, if your skin envelope is extremely thin, you may be able to see an implant edge in certain body positions—no matter what implant, no matter how much skill a surgeon may possess! Why? Because you can't change your tissues, and the only tissues covering the implant at the sides (laterally) are skin and fat. If skin and fat are thin, you may see or feel an edge of the implant! No way around it! If the surgeon tries to cover the lower, outer areas with muscle, you'll have other trade-offs described previously.

ABOVE MUSCLE, BELOW MUSCLE, OR DUAL PLANE (A COMBINATION OF ABOVE AND BELOW)—WHAT IS THE DECISION BASED ON? THE THICKNESS OF SKIN AND FAT ON YOUR CHEST ABOVE YOUR BREAST TISSUE.

If you are thin (and we'll tell you how to measure it) and don't want to see the upper edge of your implants, put them behind the pectoralis muscle.

If you want to avoid many of the trade-offs of traditional behind-the-muscle placement, select the DUAL-PLANE option, which combines the best of both worlds.

Your assessment of the relative benefits and trade-offs of placing implants above or below muscle: Nothing is perfect. You'll have to accept some trade-offs with either location.

How thin is thin? That's a tough question to answer! At what degree of thinness do risks of seeing an implant edge become significant? An even tougher question! The answers to these should not be—based on subjective opinions (yours or your surgeon's) but should rely on objective measurements.

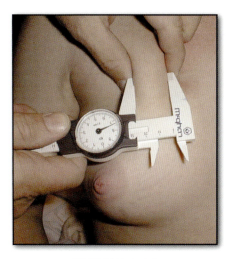

FIGURE 6-12

We use a simple, quantifiable pinch test to determine whether soft tissue coverage will be adequate with retromammary placement, or whether the tissues are so thin that retropectoral placement is a better option. You can do it yourself if you have a caliper. Isolate the breast tissue (parenchyma) by pinching to pull the breast tissue down and forward. Above the breast tissue, firmly pinch the skin and underlying fat, and measure the thickness with a caliper (Figure 6-12). If the thickness is greater than two centimeters (cm), your tissues are thick enough that retromammary or subfascial placement is an option, with minimal risks of seeing an implant edge. On the other hand, if the pinch thickness is two cm or less, you should definitely place your implants in the partial retropectoral position (traditional "behind the muscle") or dual plane (under muscle in the upper breast, not under muscle in the lower breast).

If the pinch thickness of your tissues above your breast tissue is less than two cm, retromammary or subfascial placement of an implant is not the best option for best tissue coverage. If you put your implant under inadequate soft tissue cover, don't be surprised and don't complain when implant edges are visible and you develop an uncorrectable tissue deformity.

Don't try to cheat on this! It truly isn't worth it! With the innovations of the dual-plane pocket, you can optimize soft tissue cover in the upper breast and reduce the possible consequences of placing your implants under inadequate soft tissue cover: visible edges, visible traction rippling or wrinkling, visible implant shell—and the list goes on. If you are thin, measure your pinch thickness. If you measure less than two cm on the pinch test, and a surgeon recommends retromammary (behind breast tissue only, in front of muscle) placement, ask why. Also ask the surgeon about the risks listed above, and ask if the surgeon is familiar with the dual-plane pocket location that has all of the advantages of retromammary placement, while improving implant coverage in the upper breast. If a surgeon tells you that some "magic" type of implant can be placed only behind breast tissue and not be visible, be careful. Did the surgeon measure your tissue thickness? What kind of guarantee is the surgeon providing that you won't see traction rippling when that implant weight pulls on thin overlying tissues? Providing optimal tissue coverage is always best, regardless of the type of implant.

One more time for emphasis:

1. **If you are extremely thin (less than two cm pinch thickness above your breast), you should put the implant either dual plane (fewer trade-offs) or traditionally behind muscle (more trade-offs) to assure adequate tissue cover over the implant.**

   If you don't, you run more risks of seeing the edges of your implant, seeing visible traction rippling, and risking other long-term problems that may be uncorrectable.

2. **If you have adequate thickness of tissues (more than two cm pinch thickness above your breast), weigh the advantages and trade-offs listed above, and choose above or below the muscle based on your preferences and your surgeon's recommendations.**

Myths about Muscle . . .

You may hear some popular myths about muscle, so let's mention them:

MYTH 1

Under muscle prevents capsular contracture.

Not true. You can definitely develop a capsular contracture whether your implants are above or below muscle. Only with silicone-gel implants does over or under muscle make a significant difference.

MYTH 2

Under muscle supports the implant better.

Not true. The theory here is that the attachments of the pectoralis muscle to the ribs (near the fold beneath the breast) act as a sling to support the implant. In fact, when these attachments are all left intact, they tend to cause two problems: Upward implant displacement (a high riding implant with excessive upper bulge) and more lateral (to the side) displacement of the implants, widening the gap between the breasts.

MYTH 3

Over muscle is never good.

Not true. In fact, provided you have adequate soft tissue cover, over muscle allows your surgeon better control of breast shape and fill, but dual plane offers equal control of breast shape and better coverage in the upper breast.

MYTH 4

Under muscle is never good.

Not true. If the pinch thickness of your tissues (above your breast tissue) is less than two cm, dual plane or under muscle is always better.

INCISION LOCATIONS

Figure 6-13 illustrates four commonly used incision locations for augmentation.

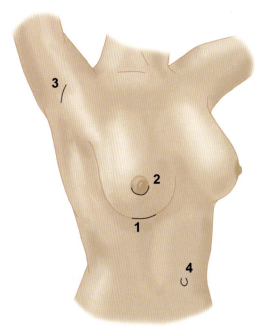

INCISIONS
1 - Inframammary
2 - Periareolar
3 - Axillary
4 - Umbilical

FIGURE 6-13

Based on twenty years of experience with all incision locations, I am convinced of the following:

Most patients worry far more about incision location before the surgery than they care after the surgery (provided they have a good result).

If an incision is on you, you will notice it!

If you have a beautiful breast, neither you nor anyone else will care where the incision is located.

Every patient thinks that the incision location she has is best.

Incision location is a common way that surgeons use to market their augmentation practice. If a surgeon touts the 'X incision'" as unquestionably the best, and states, "I am the expert at the "X incision," run the other way. No incision is best, and the likely message is that the surgeon doesn't know how to do it any other way.

If a surgeon is experienced with all incision locations, the surgeon will offer you all options.

If you hear negative comments about an incision location from another patient or surgeon, it's usually because neither has much experience with that incision location.

No incision location is always best. Each location has advantages and trade-offs.

Every woman's breasts, at some time in her life, are likely to acquire a blemish, a stretch mark or a biopsy scar. A well-executed incision scar is usually no more noticeable than these other blemishes, and if the breast is beautiful, who notices? Who cares?

Just because your friend had a certain incision doesn't mean that incision location is best for you. In most cases, it doesn't matter. A few, very rare breast deformities are best addressed through a certain incision, and when these deformities occur, we don't hesitate to tell a patient, "With this specific breast deformity, a specific incision location gives us better control over your operation, and, hopefully, we'll get a better result." But in over 90 percent of patients that we see, we offer the patient a choice of incision locations. If a surgeon is experienced in all incisional approaches, the surgeon is less likely to recommend one location over another. Instead, the surgeon will give you a full range of options.

What's really most important about incision location?

- How much control it gives your surgeon over your operation.

- How much it allows your surgeon to minimize trauma to your tissues.

- How far the incision location is from the implant pocket.

- How much normal tissue your surgeon must go through before getting to the implant pocket. The greater amount of normal tissue your surgeon has to go through, the more trauma, bleeding, pain, length of your recovery, and possible other complications you should expect.

- How many critical structures (mostly nerves and blood vessels) are located near the incision or on a path from the incision to the pocket.

Don't form an opinion about incision location until you know about all the alternatives! Incision location is one of the LEAST important decisions you'll make in augmentation. Each incision location has relative advantages and trade-offs.

What about Scars?

We've said it once, and we'll say it again. No scar location is necessarily always better than another. Let's examine some myths about scars:

MYTH I

For patients with minimal or no breast tissue, a scar under the breast isn't a good choice.

Not necessarily. If the scar is properly positioned exactly in or very slightly above the crease beneath the breast, it will be minimally noticeable.

We've heard from more than one patient, "My boyfriend (a medical student on a medical fact finding mission, I'm sure) said that he saw a scar on a topless dancer that was up on the breast, and it was terrible. I don't want that incision." The facts? Topless dancers have more inframammary incisions than any other incision. The reason the scar was more noticeable was that it was improperly located. If the scar is placed too high above the fold, it's in an area where it is maximally stretched by the pressure of the implant. If it were kept exactly in the fold or very slightly above the fold, there's less stretch, and the scar would be narrower. A popular misconception I've heard from surgeons is that inframammary scars should be placed well above the fold "so that it won't show when she raises her arms in a bikini." Fact is, less than 1 percent of a woman's life is spent in a bikini. Fact is, a good scar exactly in the fold is far better than a widened scar that occurred because it was placed too far above the fold. If a surgeon is experienced in all incision locations, you can just choose! If you don't like one (incision or surgeon), choose another!

MYTH 2

One incision location is less noticeable than another.

Not true. It depends on the patient's body position, who is looking, how long after the surgery (whether the scar is mature and faded), and the quality of the scar (largely dependent on each patient's healing tendencies). What is always less noticeable is a better quality scar, regardless of its location.

MYTH 3

A shorter scar is always better than a longer scar.

Not true. The quality of a scar is much more important than its length. A short, ugly scar is always more noticeable than a slightly longer, thin, faded scar. Experience has taught many surgeons that when you make an incision too short to minimize scar length, you often stretch that incision and "traumatize" the incision edges excessively during surgery. The scar does not heal as well, often stays redder longer and becomes wider. The result is a shorter scar, but also an uglier scar. A better quality scar, even if it is slightly longer, is far better than a short, ugly scar.

MYTH 4

If you can put the incision off the breast in the armpit or the belly button, it's always better.

Not true. We'll cover specific advantages and trade-offs of each incision location later in this chapter, but there are definite trade-offs for both the axillary (armpit) and umbilical (belly button) approaches that may not appeal to some patients. Fact is, after surgery, scar location usually becomes a nonissue if the patient has an excellent result.

MYTH 5

One scar location or another always preserves breast sensation better.

Not true. We formerly believed the axillary (armpit) incision preserved sensation better than other approaches, but after many more years' experience, we don't think that is necessarily true. The factors that most affect sensation are 1) surgical technique—the more the surgeon directly visualizes the anatomy and the less bleeding, the less risk of nerve compromise, and 2) the size of the implant—the larger the implant, the larger the pocket required, the more nerves are likely to be cut, and the more stretch the implant places on nerves; hence, the greater the chance you'll lose more sensation.

MYTH 6

Surgeons pick scar locations because they think one is best.

Not necessarily true. Surgeons usually pick scar locations based on their experience. If they have a lot of experience with different scar locations, they'll offer you all options and discuss the trade-offs. If they've only done augmentations one way (or even the majority one way), that's the scar location they will most likely suggest.

THE INFRAMAMMARY INCISION

Located in the fold beneath the breast, the inframammary incision is the most widely used incision in augmentation and is the standard against which all other incision locations must be judged. The reasons? It gives the surgeon excellent access for augmentation in a wide range of breast types, offers better control of the operation in many instances, places the incision closest to the pocket compared to any other incision, requires the surgeon to go through less normal tissue compared to any other incision, has no critical adjacent structures (nerves or blood vessels), and is a "gold standard" that most surgeons learned during their residency training. More women have had (and continue to have) augmentation through an inframammary incision compared to all other incision locations combined.

The greatest advantage of an incision beneath the breast is the degree of control it allows the surgeon in a wide range of breast types and the fact that it minimizes damage to normal tissues and potential damage to adjacent critical structures.

More augmentation patients have had this incision location than all other incision locations combined.

The only trade-off of an inframammary incision is the presence of a scar in the fold beneath the breast.

The trade-off of the inframammary incision is the scar beneath the breast. Properly placed in a patient with normal healing, after the scar matures, the scar is less noticeable than the imprint of your bra on your skin when you remove your bra. A very small percentage of patients form less than optimal scars (more about that later). If you have formed very heavy scars on your chest area in the past (that did not improve with time), you may want to consider another incision location. No test can predict the quality of scar you will form. But for the vast majority of patients (well over 90 percent) , the inframammary scar location is an excellent choice.

So why would patients consider other incisions? In our experience, two main reasons:

1. If a patient has a "head trip" or preconceived negative ideas or concepts about an inframammary scar without understanding the trade-offs of other scar locations, or

2. If a patient has a personal friend or acquaintance who has had another incision approach and is happy with it. It's human nature to think that if your friend is happy with a certain incision approach, you should choose that approach. In fact, that's not true at all once you're really informed.

THE PERIAREOLAR INCISION

This incision is placed around the edge (or just within) the areola, the pigmented skin surrounding the nipple. In most instances, the skin around the areola is thinner than the skin in the fold beneath the breast. There is some evidence that, all other things equal, thinner skin forms better scars than thicker skin. Some surgeons tout a periareolar (around the nipple-areola) scar as less visible than a scar beneath the breast. Is that true? Not necessarily. It depends on the quality of the scars in the two places, and that's not totally predictable.

The greatest advantage of an incision around the areola is that it's located in thinner skin that usually heals well.

The greatest trade-offs of a periareolar incision are increased trauma to breast tissue, increased exposure of the implant to bacteria normally found in the breast, and if you develop a bad scar, the scar is located in the most visible location on the breast.

A periareolar scar is located on the most visible area of the breast. As long as the scar is good—great. But if it's not so good, and we don't know who may form a bad scar, it's not so great. It's true that the skin of the areola area usually heals well, but if it does not, the less than optimal scar is noticeable every time you look at the nipple or areola.

Another stated advantage of the periareolar incision is that it's easier for the surgeon to reach all parts of the breast from a central incision. Truth is, a skilled surgeon can reach all parts of the breast under direct vision by all incisions (with the exception of the belly button incision where a portion of the dissection is usually "blind").

Trade-offs of the periareolar approach? If you have a very small areola, incision length can be inadequate without extending the incision onto breast skin which forms less optimal scars. When you cut skin, you cut nerves. When you cut nerves, most grow back, but not all, and not predictably. You might think that an incision around the areola would always make patients lose more sensation compared to other incisions, but it doesn't! Why not? We don't know! Probably because sensory loss is very unpredictable and may be more related to how the surgery is done (more about that later) or the size of the implant (the larger, the more stretch on nerves and potential sensory loss).

Every woman's breast tissue contains bacteria. These bacteria live on the skin of healthy women and enter the breast through the nipple. They don't usually cause infection because the body is accustomed to their presence in the breast. But put a large foreign object, your breast implant, in the area, and the bacteria can sometimes produce problems. When an implant is inserted through a periareolar incision, the breast implant is more directly exposed to breast tissue compared to other approaches. With more exposure to bacteria, you might think that infection rates would definitely be higher with this approach, but increased infection risk has not been scientifically documented. Even if an implant doesn't get infected, bacteria around the implant are probably a major factor contributing to capsular contracture, so you might expect a higher risk of capsular contracture with a periareolar incision. Again, not scientifically confirmed, but in our practice, we've seen a slightly higher incidence of capsular contracture in patients who select the periareolar approach.

If you happen to form bad scars (and this can happen, regardless of your history of scars), the areola would not be an ideal place to have a bad scar. Bad scars are very rare in any location, but to date, we have no way of reliably predicting which patients will develop bad scars.

THE AXILLARY INCISION

Placed in the deepest area of the armpit, the axillary incision is probably the least conspicuous of all augmentation incisions. Proper incision placement is critical. If placed in the highest portion of the armpit hollow, the scar is unnoticeable in virtually any body position. Even with arms fully raised, and even before the scar fades, losing its pink color, the incision looks like a normal crease. Once the scar is mature, it is almost impossible to detect in most patients, even with the arms raised. Another stated advantage of the axillary approach is better preservation of sensation in the breast. Actually, sensory preservation is quite variable and is more likely related to the type of dissection performed and the size of the implant.

The greatest advantage of an incision in the armpit is that its location makes it the least visible of all scars for augmentation.

The greatest trade-offs of axillary incisions are that a surgeon must be experienced, the operation time is usually slightly longer if the surgeon uses state-of-the-art techniques, and the patient must tolerate more potential nuisances in the armpit and upper arm areas postoperatively.

With older axillary techniques, after making the incision in the armpit, the surgeon used various types of blunt instruments to "blindly" create a pocket for the implant. The development of an instrument called an endoscope (Figure 6-14) allows surgeons to see inside the body on a television screen to more precisely control the operation. With the advent of modern endoscopic instrumentation, surgeons can see to precisely create the pocket for the implant instead of bluntly, blindly tearing tissues. This minimizes bleeding, maximizes accuracy, and shortens recovery. The longer operation time required for endoscopically assisted axillary augmentation is more than compensated by increased accuracy and control. A slightly longer operating time can mean more costs but should not increase any risks associated with the operation. Ask your surgeon.

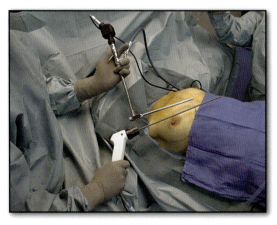

FIGURE 6-14

The axillary approach using endoscopic instrumentation is technically more demanding of the surgeon compared to periareolar and inframammary approaches and is difficult for some surgeons to learn. If you are considering an axillary approach, be sure that your surgeon is experienced in endoscopic techniques and that the surgeon minimizes blunt, blind dissection.

The axillary approach traverses more normal tissue enroute to the pocket compared to the inframammary approach, and there are more critical structures (nerves and blood vessels) located in the armpit area compared to any other incision approach. Risk of injury to these critical structures is exceedingly small in the hands of an experienced surgeon, but nevertheless deserves consideration. Finally, minor nuisances around the incision (swelling, numbness, tiny bands of tissue beneath the skin, etc.) that can occur with any incision are usually somewhat more noticeable and bothersome to patients who have axillary incisions compared to other incision locations.

Regardless of a surgeon's expertise, making an incision and tunnel through the armpit area requires that patients accept the fact that postoperatively, they may be dealing with one or more of the following:

- Enlarged lymph nodes in the armpit area,

- Fluid collections beneath the skin in the armpit area,

- Areas of numbness or tingling in the armpit and upper inner-arm areas,

- Potential permanent numbness in areas of the armpit or upper inner arm,

- A ridge where the incision is located for several weeks that requires care when shaving,

- Possible formation of small bands in the armpit area that may limit arm lifting movements. (These usually resolve spontaneously in a few weeks.)

All of these potential nuisances are manageable, and many patients experience few of these nuisances, but if you are considering an axillary incision approach, you should know that these nuisances are possible.

The axillary approach is not ideal for reoperations to correct postoperative complications or problems because it limits a surgeon's direct vision and control. A second incision, usually inframammary, may be required to address postoperative problems or complications. Although it is technically possible to treat an excessively tight capsule (capsular contracture) via the axillary approach, the inframammary approach affords the surgeon much more control, more complete removal of capsule, and better control of bleeding, and it avoids traversing breast tissue (required with the periareolar approach).

THE UMBILICAL INCISION

Umbilicus is the medical term for your belly button. The incision for the umbilical approach is placed in and around the belly button. I use the terms "in" and "around" because, to some degree, the location of the incision depends on the size of the belly button. Most women's belly buttons are small, and the incision required is one inch or more in length. The surgeon may not make the initial incision one inch, but the instruments required for the operation usually stretch the incision, and portions of the incision can sometimes extend outside the boundaries of the belly button.

The main advantage of the belly button incision is that it is located off the breast. The belly button incision sounds very acceptable to many women because they are familiar with other endoscopic procedures in the abdomen that use similar incisions, such as ligation of the fallopian tubes (tubal ligation). Actually, the incision required to insert a breast implant through the umbilicus is much larger than that required for many abdominal procedures.

The main advantage of an incision in and around the belly button is that the incision is located off the breast.

The main disadvantages of the umbilical incision compared to other incisions are:

- It offers the surgeon the least direct vision and control compared to other incisional locations and, therefore, the least predictable results.

- It is located farther from the breast, and more normal tissues must be traversed enroute to the implant pocket, increasing tissue trauma, potential pain and bleeding, and recovery time.

Access to the breast is created by bluntly pushing a one-inch-diameter tube from the umbilicus to each breast through the tissues of the upper abdomen.

The pocket for the implant is developed by inserting an uninflated implant, blowing it up, then pushing it vigorously side to side to tear a pocket to receive the implant. The surgeon cannot see inside the pocket to create the most precise pocket with the least bleeding.

When the pocket is created by any method other than direct vision, the pocket is less accurate, bleeding is potentially increased, control is less, and tissue trauma is potentially greater.

Most surgeons who use the umbilical approach do not offer implant placement behind muscle. If you are thin, dual plane or traditional behind muscle is better long term.

Precise dual-plane pocket development and pectoralis muscle positioning is currently not an option if the umbilical approach is selected. No currently published studies indicate that patients having augmentation via the umbilical approach can routinely experience comparable recovery to the inframammary and axillary approaches we have published.[2,3]

The umbilical approach is not ideal for reoperations to correct postoperative complicatioins or problems because it limits a surgeon's direct vision and control. A second incision, usually inframammary may be required to address postoperative problems or complications. Although it is technically possible to treat an excessively tight capsule (capsular contracture) via the umbilical approach, the inframammary approach affords the surgeon much more control of capsule removal, more complete removal of capsule, and better control of bleeding.

So why would anyone want to use this approach? It sounds good, until you really look at it objectively. Does this mean that you can't get a good result through this incision? No. It just means you should be able to expect an even better result in the same patient through an axillary approach, with a faster recovery by avoiding additional tissue trauma when passing through the abdominal tissues and avoiding blunt, blind dissection. The armpit incision satisfies the advantage of moving the incision off the breast. The armpit incision is much closer to the breast, so much less normal tissue is traumatized getting to the breast, and the risk of depressions or troughs in the abdomen from bluntly pushing a large tube through the fat are avoided. From the armpit, the entire pocket can be created precisely and bloodlessly under direct vision for a more accurate, more controlled pocket with less bleeding. Your surgeon can also easily place the implant above or below muscle via the armpit, depending on your tissue needs.

Why would any surgeon want to use the umbilical approach? The umbilical approach allows some surgeons to differentiate themselves from other surgeons by advertising: "I can do it, and they don't. Come to me." The umbilical approach can be appealing from a marketing perspective, but I challenge any surgeon to debate me in a scientific forum on the logic of why it is really better. There is no scientific study that indicates that recovery (the best indicator of tissue trauma and bleeding) after umbilical augmentation can compare to the twenty-four hour return to normal activities we have confirmed for patients via inframammary, periareolar, and axillary approaches.[2,4,5] We have many patients who are interested in umbilical augmentation—until they learn the facts and compare recovery to the other approaches. As long as surgeons are performing umbilical augmentations using blunt, blind dissection techniques, the umbilical approach offers no comparison to other approaches if precision, control, minimal tissue trauma and bleeding, and the most rapid recovery are objectives. In fairness, I hope that one day the umbilical approach will be able to offer the same level of control as other approaches and avoid unnecessarily traumatizing a normal area of the body (the abdomen) to get to the breast. When it can, and when a surgeon can create the pocket without using blunt, blind dissection, I'll be happy to endorse the approach. We can always use more options—provided they make sense.

IMPLANT SHAPE AND IMPLANT SIZE

Much of the information you need about implant selection and size is included in Chapter 5. Some of the information is worth repeating, and you'll need some new information that relates implant choices to the surgical choices previously discussed in this chapter.

The Implant Selection Process

A few guiding principles first:

Implant selection is ideally a team decision between you and your surgeon.

Assuring optimal soft tissue cover (selecting the pocket location, above or below muscle) is more important than implant selection.

When selecting implant shape (round or anatomic), think about the potential risk of shell folding and how that could affect the life of your implants.

Remember that all anatomic, or shaped, implants are not the same. Full-height anatomic implants with adequate fill to minimize risks of upper-shell collapse or folding while maintaining upper-breast fill are quite different compared to reduced-height or underfilled shaped implants.

When selecting implant size, the larger the implant, the more trade-offs and risks you'll encounter, especially long term.

Incision location is less important than implant selection. Both are less important compared to optimal tissue coverage.

Don't worry too much right now about selecting your implant. Wait until you visit with surgeons and determine which surgeon best understands what you want and can best explain in detail your tissue characteristics and how they will affect your augmentation. Listen carefully to your surgeon's implant recommendations and the reasons. Then make your decision.

Implant, Pocket Location, Implant, and Incision: Combinations That Are Available

The following table shows you that almost any implant can be put in almost any pocket location through almost any incision—provided you select an experienced, qualified surgeon. This table shows you the options that are currently available. A "yes" means that this is an accepted combination that has been scientifically confirmed and presented. A "no" means that although someone may be doing it, the jury is not in yet.

Implant Shape	Implant can be placed: Retromammary (over muscle)	Implant can be placed: Partial retropectoral or dual plane (partially under muscle)	Implants can be placed: over or under muscle through all incisions
ROUND			
Smooth	Yes	Yes	Yes
Textured	Yes	Yes	Yes
ANATOMIC			
Textured	Yes	Yes	No - Not as predictably and accurately compared to other approaches

TABLE 6-1

If anyone tells you that a combination labeled "yes" is not available, keep searching. I assure you that the options are there for you if you find a surgeon with experience in all approaches.

HOW THE SURGEON CREATES THE POCKET FOR YOUR IMPLANT

You'll undoubtedly hear discussions about surgical techniques in your quest for the best breast. Most patients are not qualified to judge the details of surgical techniques. That's what you're paying your surgeon to do. But some basics are worth knowing.

There's a difference between doing things because they're easier and doing them because they are better.

Surgeons are human. Some surgeons do things because they are easier and may even convince themselves that they're better. It's possible to achieve easier and better, but it requires surgeon commitment to increasing technical skills, time, and effort.

In surgery, better is usually more difficult until you learn more; then better is easier.

If I as a surgeon don't know any better, I simply don't know any better. That doesn't mean that better doesn't exist or can't exist.

Surgical techniques evolve, and most get better with time. There's always something new. The new things that are really better survive the test of time. The list of "new, better" implants and techniques that have disappeared is long, because time and scientific studies proved their weaknesses. Do all "better" surgical techniques become widely accepted? Absolutely not. In fact, a small minority prove their worth! When better things are more difficult, it almost always takes much longer for them to become widely accepted, sometimes until a new generation of surgeons comes along.

A good example is techniques used to create the pocket to receive a breast implant. Traditionally in surgery, sharp instruments, scalpels or scissors, were used to cut tissues. Problem is, when tissues are cut with sharp instruments, they bleed. Blood covers and stains adjacent tissues and obscures details that allow a surgeon to be more accurate. Blood loss, even if it is not life threatening, is messy, wastes time, and compromises accuracy. Blood soaks into your tissues and causes more inflammation, more pain, and a longer recovery time.

If a technique is easier or faster, I guarantee it will find its way into many surgeons' bag of tricks. Blunt dissection, a technique used to create the pocket for the implant, is an example. Basically, a blunt dissector is an 18" round rod about the diameter of a ball point pen that is bent into a curve at one end (Figure 6-15). This instrument is used to tear, rather than precisely cut tissues. After the surgeon inserts the instrument, the remainder of the pocket dissection is "blind." The

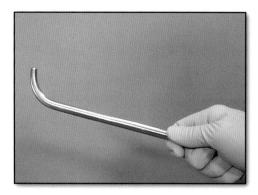

FIGURE 6-15

surgeon is not looking inside the tissues as the instrument sweeps from side to side, tearing and separating tissues to create the pocket. During my residency training twenty-nine years ago, I was taught to use blunt dissection to create a pocket for a breast implant. Blunt and blind are not an optimal combination to create a pocket if the goal is to reduce tissue trauma and avoid bleeding. Blunt and blind have never been optimal, but blunt, blind dissection techniques still predominate today. It works, and it's fast, but it's also very traumatic to tissues and causes a lot of bleeding. Surely, there had to be a better way! I started searching, and I found the electrocautery. Scientific studies we have published[1,2,5] now prove that precise electrocautery dissection techniques offer patients dramatically shortened recovery times—less tissue trauma, less bleeding, less pain, and hence a faster, easier recovery!

Electrocautery instruments use electrical current to cut tissue and to stop (coagulate) bleeding vessels (Figure 6-16). With electrocautery dissection, tissue cutting and blood vessel coagulation occur simultaneously! Incredible benefits! Dramatically less bleeding! The surgeon can see. The surgeon can be more accurate and spends less time stopping bleeding. Sound great? You bet! So everybody uses it to create pockets for implants, right? Wrong. A lot of surgeons still use blunt, blind dissection.

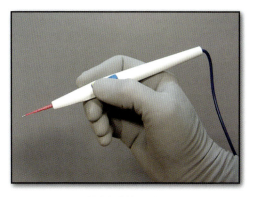

FIGURE 6-16

Blunt, or blunt and blind, dissection techniques for creating the implant pocket cause more tissue injury, tear tissues, create more bleeding, and result in a longer recovery time compared to state-of-the art electrocautery-dissection techniques.

During the seven years that I used blunt dissection, most of my patients (especially when the implant was placed beneath muscle) could not return to normal physical activities for at least ten to fourteen days. Today, over 95 percent of our patients (even with submuscular, dual-plane augmentations) return to normal activities within twenty-four hours![2] Why? No more blunt dissection! No more BLUNT AND BLIND dissection. More precise techniques using direct vision for control and to minimize bleeding and tissue trauma.

Compared to special, precise techniques of electrocautery dissection, creating a pocket by blunt dissection injures tissues more than precise electrocautery dissection, prolongs recovery, and carries a higher risk of complications such as bleeding and capsular contracture.

Having used all types of dissection, I can't bring myself today to sharp dissect or blunt dissect a pocket! Thank goodness for progress! Our patients' experience is totally different, with a return to normal activities that has previously been unthinkable. Think of the difference between a two-week recovery and, potentially, a one-day recovery! No surgeon can guarantee 100 percent of patients a one-day recovery, but avoiding blunt dissection dramatically shortens recovery times and allows over 95 percent of patients to return to normal activities within twenty-four hours.[2,3]

All electrocautery dissection techniques are not the same.

1. There are people who can play a piano, and there are concert masters. It's not just *whether* a surgeon uses electrocautery dissection. It's all about *how* that surgeon uses the instruments. Details of surgical technique make a massive difference in bleeding and tissue trauma and determine your recovery and your chances of many potential problems.

2. If you ask a surgeon if he or she uses electrocautery dissection, and they answer yes, the next question should be, when will I be able to return to full normal activities without any bandages, special bras, drains, or pain pills? Recovery will tell you just how well they can do it.

3. Electrocautery dissection has become a buzzword, but remember, it's not *whether a surgeon does it, it's how the surgeon does it!* Just because a surgeon uses the buzzword doesn't necessarily mean that the surgeon optimally uses the instruments and techniques!

4. Asking about *recovery* will give you the answers you need. If you don't have an overwhelming chance to return to normal activities within twenty-four hours, something isn't optimal, no matter what a surgeon tells you or what buzzwords a surgeon uses.

THE NEXT STEP . . .

Now you know about different surgical options. The next step is learning about the problems that can occur in breast augmentation, regardless of the options you choose.

References

1. Tebbetts, J. B. Dual plane (DP) breast augmentation: optimizing implant-soft tissue relationships in a wide range of breast types. *Plast. Reconstr. Surg.* 107: 1255, 2001.

2. Tebbetts, J. B. Achieving a predictable 24-hour return to normal activities after breast augmentation, part I: Refining practices using motion and time study principles. *Plast. Reconstr. Surg.* 109: 273-290, 2002.

3. Tebbetts, J. B. Achieving a predictable 24-hour return to normal activities after breast augmentation part I: Refining practices using motion and time study principles. *Plast. Reconstr. Surg.* 109: 293-305, 2002.

4. Tebbetts, J. B. Patient acceptance of adequately filled breast implants. *Plast. Reconstr. Surg.* 196(1): 139-147, 2000.

5. Tebbetts, J. B. Achieving a zero percent reoperation rate at 3 years in a 50 consecutive case augmentation mammaplasty PMA study. *Plast. Reconstr. Surg.* 118(6): 1453-57, 2006.

chapter seven

NOTHING IS PERFECT:

TRADE-OFFS, PROBLEMS, AND RISKS

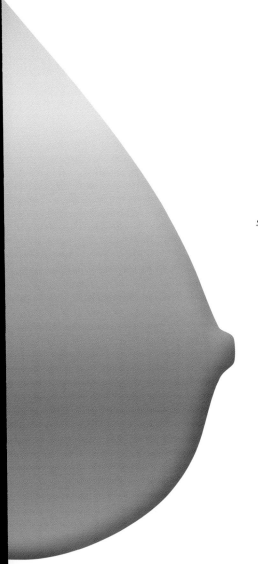

"Every choice in augmentation has trade-offs. Good team decisions before surgery are the best way to reduce risks and trade-offs."

Don't fool yourself. Nothing in life is perfect; nothing is without trade-offs. Augmentation is no different. You can't choose a set of options for breast augmentation that doesn't come with a package of trade-offs. Trade-offs are compromises that you accept when you select an implant, a pocket location, an incision location, or any other option in augmentation. You will accept trade-offs whether you know it or not. The more you know about trade-offs of each option, the better choices you can make.

In our practice, any surprise that occurs in augmentation is a problem. We don't want surprises. We certainly don't want problems. Our goal is to inform and educate you to help us make the best possible decisions.

The better we help you understand what to expect before surgery, the more you know, the fewer surprises, and the fewer problems.

When you decide to have an augmentation, you are deciding to take risks. Every medical procedure requires that you take certain risks to potentially gain certain benefits. Every cosmetic surgical procedure is totally elective. You choose it. You don't require it. There is no medical reason that requires you to have it. For any procedure that you want but don't really need, the potential benefits should far outweigh any potential risks. To decide whether a set of risks is reasonable and justifiable, you must first know what the risks are and how likely it is that those risks will occur.

TRADE-OFFS

The following table lists trade-offs that are associated with common options available in augmentation. This list is not comprehensive; other trade-offs can occur. The purpose of this overview is to emphasize that:

No option or set of options in augmentation is without trade-offs.

The potential benefits of each of these options are described in chapters five and six for comparison with the trade-offs.

TABLE 7-1

OPTION	POTENTIAL TRADE-OFFS
I. Implant Shape	
a. Round implant	Less natural appearance (if filled to minimize shell collapse or shell folding)
	Increased risk of shell collapse or folding if filled to manufacturer's recommendations
	If overfilled to minimize shell collapse or folding, not covered in manufacturers' written warranties
b. Anatomic implant	More expensive
	More demanding of the surgeon
	Can rotate or malposition if pocket is not accurate or if tissues stretch excessively (risk less than 2 percent with optimal techniques and implant selection[1-3])
c. High profile implant	Additional weight for any given implant width
	Applies more pressure to surrounding tissues (breast tissue over the implant and ribs and muscle beneath the implant)
	May cause permanent thinning and shrinkage (atrophy) of your breast tissue over the implant.
	May cause depression or deformity of the chest wall beneath the implant
	If tissues shrink (atrophy) due to added pressure, result may not be more projecting
2. Implant shell surface	
a. Smooth-shell-surface implant	Higher risk of capsular contracture with conventional silicone-gel-filled implants
	No characteristics or influences to reduce risks of capsular contracture
	No characteristics or influences to control implant position
	No characteristics or influences to help support weight of implant
	Implant always falls to bottom of pocket created for the implant—no control of distribution of fill in the breast
	Implant may shift excessively to the side when lying down

OPTION	POTENTIAL TRADE-OFFS
b. Textured-shell-surface implant	Some surgeons believe that a slightly thicker shell is easier to feel in very thin patients (shell thickness only varies a few ten thousandths of an inch from smooth to textured, and a thicker shell may be more durable).
	Some surgeons believe that small particles of silicone can shed from textured surfaces (never demonstrated to have any effects in a large studies of augmentation patients)
	Textured surfaces vary from manufacturer to manufacturer.
	Implants with the Siltex textured surface manufactured by Mentor Corporation have been shown to have a substantially higher deflation rate at seven years compared to their round smooth implants.
	Large studies with long-term follow-up show that the Biocell textured surface on Allergan/Inamed Style 468 implants had an very low deflation rate (0.8% at up to seven year follow-up) compared to other types of implants.[1-3]

3. Implant Pocket Location

OPTION	POTENTIAL TRADE-OFFS
a. Retromammary pocket (behind breast tissue, not behind muscle)	Possibly more exposure to bacteria in the breast tissue (but no scientific study proves a higher infection rate)
	Possibly higher risk of capsular contracture with silicone-gel-filled implants (no higher risk with saline implants)
b. Partial retropectoral pocket (behind the pectoralis muscle)	Distortion of breast shape with muscle contraction
	Less control of upper-breast fill (especially upper toward the middle)
	Tendency of implants to shift to sides over time, widening distance between the breasts (worse in thinner patients or with larger implants or with thicker pec muscles)
	Longer recovery when muscle is manipulated
c. Dual plane	Slightly less implant coverage at the fold beneath the breast compared to previous under muscle techniques

4. Implant Pocket Creation Technique

OPTION	POTENTIAL TRADE-OFFS
a. Sharp dissection to create the pocket	More bleeding, obscures anatomy detail during surgery
	More bruising after surgery
	More risk of fluid or blood collection around implant
	More inflammation and pain from blood in tissues
	Longer recovery
b. Blunt dissection to create the pocket	More traumatic to tissues
	More bleeding, blood in tissues, bruising
	More inflammation and pain
	Longer recovery
c. Electrocautery dissection to create the pocket	Can cause tissue charring if electrocautery is improperly set
	Requires specific technical skills of the surgeon
	Requires special instrumentation
	Technique that enables most rapid recovery at present[1-3]

OPTION	POTENTIAL TRADE-OFFS

5. Incision Location

a. Inframammary incision location (under the breast)

Scar located under the breast
Scar more visible lying down compared to axillary (armpit)
If not positioned optimally, can locate higher on underside of breast where it can stretch and widen.

b. Periareolar incision location (around the areola)

Scar located around the areola
If suboptimal healing, scar is on the most visible portion of the breast
May interfere more with nipple sensation (though not scientifically proved)
May expose implant to more bacteria in breast tissue (not scientifically proved)
Transverses normal breast tissue enroute to implant pocket

c. Axillary incision location (in the armpit)

Technically more demanding of surgeon
If improperly positioned, scar can be visible without raising the arms (scar is least visible of all scars in all body positions when properly located)
Requires special instrumentation to perform optimally
Transverses normal tissue enroute to implant pocket
Adjacent to more critical anatomic structures (blood vessels and nerves) compared to inframammary

d. Umbilical incision location (in and around the belly button)

Visible scar in and around belly button
Least accurate control of all approaches
Injures abdominal fat tissues to gain access to the breasts
Traverses more normal tissue enroute to implant pocket compared to any other incision approach
Risk of visible troughs on abdomen, abdominal bruising after surgery
Pocket dissection is blind and blunt, no direct visualization during pocket dissection
Access is farthest from breast
Creates pocket by manually tearing tissues using an inflated device or blunt dissection

Trade-offs always depend on the details of each specific case.

The characteristics of your tissues can significantly affect the trade-offs.

The experience of your surgeon with different options can significantly affect the trade-offs.

After a surgeon examines you, be sure to ask about specific trade-offs and how they relate to your specific tissues and the surgeon's experience with different options.

PROBLEMS

If it's a surprise, it's a problem.

There are two kinds of surprises:

A surprise can be something you don't know about that confuses or frightens you,

Or

A surprise can be a medical complication that causes untoward medical events.

The first type of surprise, something you don't know about that confuses or frightens you, is potentially preventable. The second, a medical complication, can occur despite all best efforts by you and your surgeon.

Problems (Surprises) That Result from Things You Don't Know

Most people deal with the unknown problems better if they know what's coming. When you have an augmentation, your body will do predictable, and sometimes unpredictable, things in response to your surgery during the healing process.

The more you know about what to expect and what is normal, the less confused or frightened you will be when it occurs.

It's a team job to assure that you know what to expect after your surgery.

It's the responsibility of your surgeon and your surgeon's staff to provide information for you.

It's your responsibility to use it and assume responsibility for your choices, requests, and decisions.

If you don't receive comprehensive information from your surgeon, you never have an opportunity to read and digest it. The amount and quality of written and spoken information that you receive from surgeons is an excellent way to evaluate different surgeons. If you receive good information and you don't read and digest it, you aren't doing your job, and you are making your life more difficult during recovery. You can't possibly remember every detail about what to expect. That's why most surgeons will give you specific, written information to use as a reference. Keep it; use it. Despite good reference material, things can occur that reading an explanation just doesn't solve. Call your surgeon or the surgeon's staff. Helping you is their part of the team job.

Once usually isn't enough. After you read information, you should hear or read many of the same facts again from your patient educator or surgeon and see many items repeated in written documents you will sign. Surgeons who provide you information in stages and information that is repetitive are making the best effort to assure that you're receiving the most complete information and have the best chance of understanding the information.

Before your augmentation, be sure that all of your questions are answered. If you are the least bit unclear about anything, ask. Take notes, and spend time going over them. The more you know, the more comfortable you'll be, the fewer surprises you'll have, and the fewer problems there will be. If you can't get your questions answered and feel that you thoroughly understand, stop until you do!

Problems (Surprises) That Result from Medical Complications

The other type of problems that can occur fall into the category of medical risks, untoward events that can occur following any type of surgery. These problems can be very significant, and you should understand and consider all medical risks very thoroughly before deciding to have breast augmentation surgery.

RISKS ASSOCIATED WITH BREAST AUGMENTATION —THE BASICS

Every breast augmentation operation carries inherent risks.

Medical complications are not totally preventable by you or your surgeon.

Do not have an augmentation unless you thoroughly understand and accept the potential risks and trade-offs of the procedure.

When you are first learning about risks, be sure that you thoroughly understand exactly what the risk involves. Secondly, ask how often each risk occurs. A risk can sound terrible, but if it only occurs once in every 100,000 cases, it's logical to be informed but not excessively worried about that particular risk. In other words, try to put all risks into perspective. How bad is it, what are the possible consequences, and how often does it occur? In this chapter, you'll learn the basics, but **always ask your surgeon three basic questions:**

Exactly what does the risk involve?

What are the possible consequences?

How often does the problem actually occur?

The risk of your developing a specific problem or complication is usually expressed as a percentage. For example, the risk of your developing a hematoma (collection of blood inside the pocket around the implant) may be 2 percent. That means that this problem occurs in approximately two out of every one hundred patients. When you are trying to decide whether to have an augmentation based on risk factors, it's logical to always consider the worst-case scenario. Always ask if the quoted risk factor is an *average figure reported in the medical literature* (averages that are derived from large scientific studies). Risk figures derived from large scientific studies more closely represent a possible worst-case scenario compared to figures based on a surgeon's personal experience.

Let's consider an example from our practice. Over the past twenty-seven years, I am aware of only five patients out of more than 3,000 cases who experienced bleeding (hematomas) following augmentation that required additional surgery. However, in all of my literature and discussions with patients, I quote the risk of hematoma as one or two in every 100 cases, 1 percent or 2 percent. My personal rate of hematomas is much lower, but every patient should base her decision about whether to have surgery on the higher number and assume that she has at least a 1 percent or 2 percent risk of developing a hematoma after augmentation.

DETAILS OF BREAST AUGMENTATION RISKS—FROM THE FDA

In 2000, the FDA updated their information for the public that details augmentation risks that the agency thinks are important. The entire text of FDA information for patients regarding augmentation is available from the FDA's Web site at http://www.fda.gov/cdrh/breastimplants/indexbip.html

For each category of risk, the text is from the FDA's Web site information. Our comments regarding each FDA statements immediately follow each statement and are labeled "JT."

FDA BREAST IMPLANT RISKS FROM FDA's WEB SITE

The Institute of Medicine (IOM) completed its independent, unbiased review of all past and ongoing scientific research study of silicone breast implant safety in June 1999.[4] Among the major findings from this study were that local complications with silicone breast implants were the primary safety issue with breast implants, that these have not been well studied, and that information on these complications is crucial for women deciding whether or not they want breast implant surgery. The IOM report said:

First, reoperations and local and perioperative (right after surgery) complications are frequent enough to be a cause for concern and to justify the conclusion that they are the primary safety issue with silicone breast implants. Complications may have risks themselves, such as pain, disfigurement, and serious infection and they may lead to medical and surgical interventions, such as reoperations, that have risks. Second, risks accumulate over the lifetime of the implant, but quantitative data on this point are lacking for modern implants and deficient historically. Third, information concerning the nature and the relative high frequency of local complications and reoperations is an essential element of adequate informed consent for women undergoing breast implantation.

There are risks or complications associated with any surgical procedure, such as the effects of anesthesia, infection, swelling, redness, bleeding, and there are complications specific to breast implants. These complications are described below.

JT—What the FDA doesn't say in the statement above is that the same IOM study they quote found no scientifically valid evidence that silicone gel implants or saline implants cause any specific disease in humans. The IOM findings emphasize that the major concern with breast implants is the rate of reoperations and local complications that can occur. We couldn't agree more. The IOM study did not assign any specific responsibility for the occurrence of reoperations and local complications to either surgeons, patients, or implant manufacturers. We believe that our peer-reviewed and published clinical studies[1-3, 7] of over 1,600 reported cases with up to seven-year follow-up conclusively demonstrate that the rates of local complications and reoperations quoted by the IOM and FDA can be drastically reduced by 1) more thorough patient education and informed consent, 2) basing decisions about implant type and size on individual patient tissue characteristics, 3) utilizing optimal surgical techniques to minimize tissue trauma and bleeding, and 4) selecting adequately filled implants that pass the tilt test to reduce rates of implant shell failure resulting from shell collapse, shell folding, and shell fold fatigue.

Table 5-1 in chapter five compares rates of problems that occurred in our studies with those reported in the largest studies to date of saline implants reported to the FDA.

1. FDA—Capsular Contracture

Capsular contracture occurs when the lining or capsule that normally forms around the implant tightens and squeezes the implant. It may be more common following infection, hematoma (collection of blood), and seroma (collection of watery portion of blood). There are four grades of capsular contracture:

Capsular Contracture. Grades I through IV.

Grade I	the breast is normally soft and looks natural
Grade II	the breast is a little firm but looks normal
Grade III	the breast is firm and looks abnormal (visible distortion)
Grade IV	the breast is hard, painful, and looks abnormal (greater distortion)

Additional surgery may be needed to correct capsular contracture grades three and four. This surgery ranges from removal of the implant capsule tissue to removal (and possibly replacement) of the implant itself. Capsular contracture may happen again after this additional surgery.

In a prospective FDA PMA clinical study of saline-filled breast implants conducted by Mentor, the cumulative, three-year, by-patient rates of a first occurrence of capsular contracture Grades III and IV were 9 percent for the 1,264 augmentation patients and

30 percent for the 416 reconstruction patients. In a prospective FDA PMA clinical study of saline-filled breast implants conducted by McGhan, the cumulative, three-year, by-patient rates of a first occurrence of capsular contracture Grades III and IV were 9 percent for the 901 augmentation patients and 25 percent for the 237 reconstruction patients.

JT—Our rates for first occurrence of capsular contracture in 1,645 reported cases of patients who received McGhan (Inamed) style 468, full height anatomic implants, followed for up to seven years[1-3] (a larger series with longer follow-up compared to the FDA studies) were 1.28 percent compared to Mentor's 9 percent and McGhan's 9 percent for augmentation patients.

FDA—"A randomized controlled study comparing silicone gel-filled and saline-filled implants in women undergoing reconstruction reported a 54 percent contracture rate of Baker Grades III and IV in the silicone gel group after six months.[5]

"A retrospective study by Gabriel et al. indicated that 131 of 749 (17.5 percent) women had at least one surgical procedure over an average of 7.8 years because of capsular contractures. This would not include capsular contracture that may have been severe but did not result in surgery. This study included women who had implants for cosmetic and reconstruction purposes, most of whom had silicone gel-filled breast implants."[6]

JT—Both of the studies listed immediately above indicate capsular contracture rates that we believe are excessive and largely preventable as indicated by our data in Table 5-1.

A capsule or tissue lining forms around every device implanted in the human body. Capsular contracture is not a medical complication—it's a normal body response to a foreign body—but there is too much of that response in some women! In most women, the capsule surrounds the implant but does not squeeze excessively on the implant, even if the capsule contracts a bit. Problems occur when the capsule contracts or tightens excessively, squeezing on the implant, making it feel hard, and sometimes pushing it out of position, distorting breast shape. The implant itself doesn't become hard. If you removed it from within the capsule, it is still soft. The breast feels hard because the capsule is squeezing on the implant.

There is no medical test and no other method to predictably identify patients who are prone to form excessively tight capsules. No surgeon can totally predict or prevent a patient forming an excessively tight capsule or capsules. This is a real risk and is one of the most significant risks patients should carefully consider.

With current saline-filled implants, we advise patients that the risk of capsular contracture is roughly three to five percent. Our data in Table 5-1 of our own patients with McGhan (Inamed) style 468, textured anatomic implants reflects an actual rate with one- to seven-year follow-up of 1,645 patients of 1.25 percent.[1-3]

Our preferred correction of capsular contracture is to completely remove the existing capsule surgically and replace the implant. Most surgeons would suggest a textured surface implant, especially if replacing a silicone-gel implant.

We take a much stronger stand than many surgeons with respect to capsular contracture, especially recurrent capsular contracture. Because we have no test to predict which patient will develop capsular contracture, and we don't know definitive causes or methods of predictably preventing it, we always worry about it. Fortunately, today's implant technology (textured shells and a shell barrier to silicone gel bleed) has substantially reduced the risks of capsular contracture. Most patients who develop capsular contracture will develop it in the first year following surgery, but a small percentage can develop it much later. My advice to patients today prior to surgery is this: If you develop significant capsular contracture, we will go back to the operating room, remove as much of the capsule as possible, and replace your implant. If you develop a second capsule, I will recommend that you remove your implants and not replace them. I can't force you to do this, but your body is giving us a message—you are a capsule former. Surgical procedures don't change your body's predisposition to form capsules. Since we don't know how to predictably prevent another capsule in patients who tend to form capsules, removing your implants reduces or removes all the risks, costs, and trade-offs of additional operations in the future. If you're not willing to agree to this good team decision up front, I'd rather refer you to another surgeon.

While technology has made giant strides, a small percentage of patients will form capsules and continue forming capsules despite everything we know today. It's better to remove implants than reoperate because each reoperation adds additional risks and causes additional trauma and irreversible changes to tissues that are permanent. Patients almost never want to part with their implants, and surgeons try to please their patients. Sometimes bad team decisions result, and the consequences are rarely satisfactory. Repeated operations are one of the most common causes of severe problems.

2. FDA—Deflation/Rupture/Leakage

Breast implants are not lifetime devices and cannot be expected to last forever. Some implants deflate or rupture in the first few months after being implanted and some deflate after several years;

others are intact ten or more years after the surgery.

a. **Silicone-Gel-Filled Breast Implants**—When silicone-gel-filled implants rupture, some women may notice decreased breast size, nodules (hard knots), uneven appearance of the breasts, pain or tenderness, tingling, swelling, numbness, burning, or changes in sensation. Other women may unknowingly experience a rupture without any symptoms (i.e., "silent rupture"). Magnetic resonance imaging (MRI) with equipment specifically designed for imaging the breast may be used for evaluating patients with suspected rupture or leakage of their silicone-gel-filled implant.

JT—We've already told you that no device lasts forever, especially breast implants. Many factors affect the life of a breast implant. The implants that are available today are technologically the best implants in history, but their life span is not predictable. Assume the worst—if you needed to replace an implant in the first few months after surgery, is it worth it? Both Allergan and Mentor currently guarantee their implants. See their informational literature for details.

Rupture means that the outer shell of the implant disrupts in a major way, allowing most or all of the filler material in the implant to leave the implant. If you have a saline implant, the breast usually decreases significantly in size, making rupture easy to recognize. Since saline implants are inflatable, the term *deflation* is used synonymously with rupture—the shell disrupts. Remember that your body forms a capsule around every implant. If your capsule is intact, with saline implants, the body absorbs the saline. With silicone implants, provided you did not have a closed capsulotomy (squeezing on the implant and capsule to break the capsule) and provided the capsule is intact, most or all of the silicone remains inside the capsule and is removed when the implant is replaced. With older silicone-gel-filled implants even if a closed capsulotomy was not performed, it is possible for silicone gel to escape from the capsule into the breast or adjacent tissues, but in my personal experience, escape of significant amounts of silicone through an intact capsule is exceedingly rare.

Leakage refers to escape of smaller amounts of filler from an implant without gross disruption of the implant shell. Leakage is a very poorly defined term. If a saline implant "leaks," it usually deflates, partially or totally. All silicone-gel implants experience some leakage—trace amounts of silicone can escape the shell of the implant. This phenomenon is called "gel bleed." The key questions are: How much escapes? What is the result? With gel bleed, only trace amounts of silicone escape. What is the result? The answer depends on whom you ask. Silicone is contained in many cosmetic products that women use every day. Many antacid preparations contain simethicone. Silicone has been used for decades in a variety of implantable devices from lenses in the eye to shunts in the brain. And even needles and syringes used every day in most fields of medicine are lubricated with liquid silicone!

FDA—Silicone gel which escapes the fibrotic capsule surrounding the implant may migrate away from the breast. The free silicone may cause lumps called granulomas to form in the breast or other tissues where the silicone has migrated, such as the chest wall, armpit, arm, or abdomen.

JT—Migration of significant amounts of silicone gel (enough to cause granulomas) is exceedingly unusual if a patient's breast has not been previously squeezed to try to correct capsular contracture (closed capsulotomy). Trace amounts of silicone gel (gel bleed) may occur from any current silicone gel implant. Current state-of-the-art silicone-gel implants manufactured by Allergan and Mentor contain a barrier coating designed to minimize gel bleed. Gel bleed is one of many factors that may influence the development of clinically significant capsular contracture, but a causal relationship has not been scientifically proved.

FDA—Plastic surgeons usually recommend removal of the implant if it has ruptured, even if the silicone is still enclosed within the scar tissue capsule because the silicone gel may eventually leak into surrounding tissues. If you are considering the removal of an implant and the implantation of another one, be sure to discuss the benefits and risks with your doctor.

FDA completed a retrospective study on rupture of silicone-gel-filled breast implants.[6] This study was performed in Birmingham, Alabama, and included women who had their first breast implant before 1988. Women with silicone-gel-filled breast implants had an MRI examination of their breasts to determine the status of their current breast implants. The 344 women who received an MRI examination had a total of 687 implants. Of the 687 implants in the study, at least two of the three study radiologists agreed that 378 implants were ruptured (55 percent). This means that 69 percent of the 344 women had at least one ruptured breast implant. Of the 344 women, 73 (21 percent) had extracapsular silicone gel in one or both breasts. Factors that were associated with rupture included increasing age of the implant, the implant manufacturer, and submuscular rather than subglandular location of the implant. A summary of the findings of this study is also available on FDA's Web site at http://www.fda.gov/cdrh/breastimplants/studies/biinterview.pdf and http://www.fda.gov/cdrh/breastimplants/studies/birupture.pdf.

JT—This study is highly controversial for several reasons. Implants diagnosed as ruptured by MRI are not necessarily ruptured. The only proof of rupture is surgical exploration. Implants can rupture during the process of opening the breast and examining an implant. In our twenty-seven-year clinical practice, rupture rates of even the oldest generation silicone gel implants were much lower compared to this study, and our data for rupture of the Allergan/Inamed style 410, form-stable gel implant was 0 percent at three years[7], and less than 1 percent at five-year follow-up.

FDA—Robinson et al. studied 300 women who had their implants for one to twenty-five years and had them removed for a variety of reasons.[9] Visible signs of rupture in 51 percent of the women studied were found. Severe silicone leakage (silicone outside the implant without visible tears or holes) was seen in another 20 percent. Robinson et al. also noted that the chance of rupture increases as the implant ages.

Other studies indicate that silicone may escape the capsule in 11 to 23 percent of rupture cases.[10,11,12,13]

JT—All patients in each of the studies listed above had old-design, round silicone-gel implants filled with noncohesive silicone gel—all were underfilled, would never pass the tilt test, experienced massive shell collapse and folding with the implant upright, predisposing them to shell fold fatigue and shell failure. These studies support our belief that adequate fill of a breast implant to minimize shell collapse and folding is critical to reducing rates of implant shell failures and reoperations. Interestingly, the FDA has approved and manufacturers have reintroduced a large variety of underfilled, conventional silicone gel implants in the United States. If you choose to have round, silicone-gel-filled implants filled with noncohesive gel, you should be aware that because these implants remain underfilled and experience shell collapse and folding when upright, they may experience a higher rate of shell failure compared to adequately filled silicone gel implants or implants filled with cohesive, form-stable silicone gel.

JT—The consequences of silicone gel implant rupture can vary widely depending on many factors. A key factor is whether the lining (capsule) surrounding the implant is intact. Provided another surgeon has not forcibly squeezed a hard breast to disrupt the capsule (a procedure called closed capsulotomy), I personally find it very easy to remove all visible gel from within the capsule and replace the implant. If the capsule and implant were broken while squeezing the breast to break a capsule, there is a greater risk of manually forcing silicone gel into adjacent tissues. When silicone gel remains in adjacent tissues, the body can form firm nodules (granulomas) around the gel.

Detecting a ruptured breast implant is similar in some ways to detecting breast cancer—there's no test that is 100 percent accurate. Even expensive MRI's are not totally accurate. The only sure way to know is to open the incision and take a look at the implant. Despite the nuisance and slight risks, it will answer the question definitively. Not knowing is the worst solution. If you don't want to open it and take a look, just how worried are you? If you're really worried, perhaps the best solution is to remove and not replace your implants.

b. **FDA- Saline-Filled Breast Implants**—Saline-filled breast implants deflate when the saline solution leaks either through an unsealed or damaged valve or through a break in the implant shell. Implant deflation can occur immediately or progressively over a period of days and is noticed by loss of size or shape of the implant. Some implants deflate or rupture in the first few months after being implanted and some deflate after several years. You should also be aware that the breast implant may wear out over time and deflate. Additional surgery is needed to remove deflated implants.

FDA PMA (pre markets approval) study data versus Tebbetts data

In a prospective clinical study conducted by Mentor,[14] the cumulative, three-year, by-patient rates of a first occurrence of deflation were 3 percent for 1,264 augmentation patients and 9 percent for 416 reconstruction patients. In a prospective clinical study conducted by McGhan/Inamed, now Allergan,[15] the cumulative, three-year, by-patient rates of a first occurrence of deflation were 5 percent for the 901 augmentation patients and 6 percent for the 237 reconstruction patients.

A retrospective study of saline breast implants by Gutowski et al. indicates that 10.1 percent of women followed for an average of six years had at least one implant deflated.[16]

JT—Our peer-reviewed, published scientific data presented in Table 5-1 of over 1,600 reported cases with one- to seven-year follow-up indicate an implant deflation rate for the McGhan (Inamed) adequately filled, textured, anatomic, style 468 saline implant of 0.87 percent compared to Mentor's three-year rate of 3 percent and McGhan (Inamed)'s three-year rate of 5 percent.[1-3,7] Our rates of shell failure at up to seven years was one-third as high as Mentor and one-fifth as high as McGhan's at just three years. Our data strongly support our belief that adequate implant fill and optimal surgical techniques are critical to reducing rates of implant shell failure and additional reoperations.

Saline-filled implants are not inherently "weak." I've actually filled implants, placed them on a hard floor, and stood on them to demonstrate the strength of the shell (and I'm a big guy). Any inflatable implant contains a valve. Every additional device added to the shell of an implant has a failure rate. Although we can't prove all the answers, the life span of saline implants is probably shorter than comparable silicone-gel-filled implants for several reasons: less cohesive filler that does not buffer movement forces transmitted to the shell, underfill (see chapter five), and the presence of a valve (an additional device). So many factors can affect the life of an implant that it will be difficult or impossible to ever precisely estimate implant life regardless of what type of study is done. The bottom line is if you're not willing to undergo replacement, regardless of when it becomes necessary, don't have an augmentation.

FDA—For silicone-gel- and saline-filled implants, some causes of rupture or deflation include

- damage by surgical instruments during surgery,

- overfilling or underfilling of the implant with saline solution (specific only to saline-filled breast implants),

- capsular contracture,

- closed capsulotomy (described below),

- stresses such as trauma or intense physical manipulation,

- excessive compression during mammographic imaging,

- placement through umbilical incision site,

- injury to the breast,

- normal aging of the implant,

- unknown/unexplained reasons.

JT—There is a serious error in the FDA statement above that implies that shell failure due to underfilling is unique to saline filled implants. This statement implies a serious lack of understanding or acknowledgement by the FDA that underfilling, whether done by the manufacturer when manufacturing prefilled silicone-gel implants (to make the implant softer) or by the surgeon in the case of saline implants, increases risks of shell failure. This lack of understanding is surprising in light of the studies the FDA quotes above that show extremely high shell failure rates for prefilled silicone-gel implants.

FDA—Closed capsulotomy is a technique used to relieve capsular contracture. It involves manually squeezing the breast to break the hard capsule. This has been implicated as a possible cause of breast implant rupture. Closed capsulotomy is not recommended by breast implant manufacturers.

JT—Closed capsulotomy has absolutely no place in the treatment of capsular contracture! We ceased performing any closed capsulotomies over twenty years ago, despite the fact that it was an accepted procedure at the time. Closed capsulotomy, in our twenty-seven-year experience, rarely, if ever, definitively solves the problems of capsular contracture, and the procedure carries very high risks of implant rupture, forceful gel migration into adjacent tissues, bleeding, and other potential problems.

3. FDA—Additional Surgeries

You should understand there is a high chance that you will need to have additional surgery at some point to replace or remove your implant(s) due to problems such as deflation, capsular contracture, infection, shifting, and calcium deposits. Many women decide to have the implants replaced, but some women do not. Those who do not have their implants replaced may have cosmetically undesirable dimpling and/or puckering of the breast following removal of the implant.

JT—You should also understand that the decisions that you and your surgeon make regarding type of implant, how much the implant is filled, whether the implant shell collapses or folds, and the surgical techniques used to place the implant **all significantly influence your risks of needing reoperations or implant removal in the future. You and your surgeon are responsible.**

FDA—In a prospective clinical study of saline-filled breast implants conducted by Mentor,[14] the cumulative, four-year, by-patient rates of a first occurrence of additional surgeries were 13 percent for the 1,264 augmentation patients and 40 percent for the 416 reconstruction patients. In a prospective clinical study of saline-filled breast implants conducted by McGhan,15 the cumulative, three-year, by-patient rates of a first occurrence of additional surgeries were 21 percent for the 901 augmentation patients and 39 percent for the 237 reconstruction patients.

JT—Compared to Mentor's three-year reoperation rate of 13 percent and McGhan's (Inamed's) three-year rate of 21 percent, our reoperation rate for 1,645 reported cases followed up to seven years was only 2.99 percent,[1-3] and 0 percent in another reported series from an FDA PMA study at three-years.[7] This massive difference in reoperation rates compared to the studies quoted by the FDA is confirmed by data from our peer-reviewed and published clinical studies using adequately filled textured, anatomic implants combined with implant-selection criteria and optimal surgical techniques. From our perspective, the point is clear. Our reoperation rates are less than those of Mentor and less than those of McGhan (Inamed) where predominantly round, underfilled saline implants were used. In our studies, full height, adequately filled, textured anatomic implants were used. The data from our studies strongly support our belief that adequately filled implants combined with implant selection criteria based on tissue characteristics and with optimal surgical techniques that allow twenty-four-hour return to normal activity can drastically reduce reoperation rates.

FDA—A retrospective study by Gabriel et al.[17] shows that 24 percent of women with breast implants experience adverse events resulting in surgery during the first five years after implantation (silicone and saline implants were studied together). According to this study, about one in three women getting breast implants for reconstruction may need a second surgery within five years, and about one in eight women getting breast implants for augmentation may need a second surgery within five years. These additional surgeries may result in the loss of breast tissue.

JT—Our peer-reviewed and published results document reoperation rates at up to seven years of approximately 3 percent,—one-eighth the reoperation rate reported in the Gabriel study! The Gabriel study also studied round, underfilled implants compared to our studies of adequately filled, full height, textured anatomic implants.

4. FDA—Pain

Women may feel pain of varying severity (degrees) and duration (length of time) following breast implant surgery. In addition, improper size, placement, surgical technique, or capsular contracture may result in pain associated with nerve entrapment or interference with muscle motion. You should tell your doctor if you have pain.

JT—Pain that occurs in the first three months following surgery is, in our experience, usually related to either excessively large implants in a tight tissue envelope or to the stretch of excessively large implants on nerves in the breast. When implant size is matched to a patient's tissue characteristics, pain is exceedingly rare. The fact that 95 percent of our patients can return to full normal activities within twenty-four hours as documented in our published study[3] supports this belief. Severe capsular contracture, which typically appears in the first three to six months but can occur later, can produce discomfort or pain at any time.

5. FDA—Dissatisfaction with Cosmetic Results

Dissatisfying results such as wrinkling, asymmetry, implant displacement (shifting), incorrect size, unanticipated shape, implant palpability, scar deformity, hypertrophic (irregular, raised scar) scarring, and/or sloshing may occur. Careful surgical planning and technique can minimize but not always prevent such results.

Additionally, for saline-filled implants that have a valve, you also might be able to feel the valve of the implant with your hand.

Repeated surgeries to improve the appearance of the breasts and/or to remove ruptured or deflated prostheses may result in an unsatisfactory cosmetic outcome.

JT—You need to know a lot more than you'll learn from the four sentences the FDA tells you that are reproduced above!

Visible wrinkling or rippling is usually caused by one or more of the following: 1) inadequate fill volume of an implant (underfill rippling) or 2) placing an implant under excessively thin soft-tissue cover (for example placing the implant only behind breast tissue and not dual plane or behind muscle in a patient with thin overlying tissues). The weight of the implant pulling on the thin overlying tissues can produce visible rippling (traction rippling). Underfill rippling is preventable (in the absence of a leak in the implant) by selecting an implant that passes the tilt test preoperatively. Traction rippling can occur with any type of implant, smooth or textured, round or anatomic, saline or silicone filled, but is largely preventable by placing the implant in a pocket location that provides thicker soft tissue cover and avoiding selecting an implant that is too large to match your tissue characteristics. Traction rippling often does not develop until months following surgery when the implant causes stretch or thinning or until tissues thin as a woman ages.

Incorrect size can mean many things. Most often it means that a patient wants a larger implant following her augmentation, a common occurrence that is never preventable by choosing larger implants for the first operation. Correct size is not some out-of-the-air bra cup choice or matching some picture of another woman. Correct size is matching the implant size to the dimensions and stretch characteristics of the breast and trying to balance that "correct size" to what a patient expects. Communication is critical during the patient education and informed consent process.

Approximately one-third of all reoperations in Mentor and McGhan's (Inamed) saline PMA studies was for *size exchange*. The data are staggering. A total of 254 patients (out of a total of 2,165 patients) had operations for size change within just five years! More than one out of ten patients (11.7 percent) had a reoperation for size change, and size change accounted for almost one-third of all reoperations. These statistics reflect poorly on patient education levels, informed consent methods, non-quantifiable implant selection methods, criteria for reoperation, and decision-making processes. Both surgeons and patients are responsible. One-third of all reoperations could be prevented by avoiding size change. Is it possible? Absolutely, and our data prove that reoperations for size exchange can be virtually eliminated by optimizing the factors listed above. In our combined, peer-reviewed, and published experience with 1,645 reported cases and seven-year follow-up (two years longer than Mentor and McGhan), instead of the 11.7 percent reoperation rate for size exchange they reported, we performed size exchange operations in only four patients (0.2 percent)[1-3,7]. The methods we have developed and shared with surgeons and patients have the potential to reduce current reoperation rates by almost one-third.

Unanticipated shape is also largely preventable if your surgeon measures your breast dimension and stretch, calculates an optimal fill for your tissue characteristics, and then helps you balance your expectations with reality—the limitations that your tissues and breast shape and size impose in every case.

Any currently available implant, and likely all implants in the future if they are designed to be durable, can be felt when you feel the breast. The heavier a woman is or the thicker the tissues overlying the implant, the less a patient may feel the implant. Sometimes this means feeling an edge of the implant in the area of the fold under the breast or at the side of the breast where the tissues are thinnest and are not covered by muscle even with sub-pectoral or dual plane pocket placement. In other instances, feeling the implant may mean feeling the shell of the implant "pop" back and forth when pressure is applied, often when the implant is filled with saline or other non cohesive filler materials and especially when the implant is underfilled.

Sloshing within the implant (in the absence of a leaking implant) is totally and completely preventable by adequately filling a saline implant or choosing an adequately filled silicone-gel implant that passes the tilt test preoperatively. Immediately following surgery, slight sloshing can occur due to fluid accumulation in the pocket around the implant. This fluid is usually rapidly reabsorbed by the body in four to ten days. If you choose to have a breast augmenta-tion, regardless of the type of implant you choose, you should expect to feel some portion of your implants. If you aren't able to feel any portion of the implant, wonderful, but no surgeon can assure you that you or the surgeon will be unable to feel a portion of your implant. Implanted breasts are not natural breasts, and feeling a portion of an implant is not a significant issue to patients who are informed before surgery that they are likely to feel some portion of their implants.

The FDA's statement that the problems listed in their paragraph are not totally preventable is correct. However, thorough patient edu-cation and informed consent, matching implant choices to tissue characteristics, optimal surgical planning, choice of pocket location, and surgical techniques can have a massive influence on the occur-rence of each of these problems. Check out our occurrence of these problems in Table 5-1 compared to the rates reported in Mentor and McGhan's (Inamed) saline PMA study results reported to the FDA.[14,15]

6.   FDA—Infection

Infection can occur with any surgery. Most infections resulting from surgery appear within a few days to weeks after the operation. However, infection is possible at any time after surgery. Infections with an implant present are harder to treat than infections in normal body tissues. If an infection does not respond to antibiotics, the implant may have to be removed, and another implant may be placed after the infection has cleared up.

In rare instances, toxic shock syndrome has been noted in women after breast implant surgery, and it is a life-threatening condition. Symptoms include sudden fever, vomiting, diarrhea, fainting, dizziness, and/or sunburn-like rash. A doctor should be seen immediately for diagnosis and treatment.

JT—The usual risk of infection is less than one in one hundred cases. We have been fortunate in our practice that in twenty-seven years performing first-time augmentations, we have had only four infections. In our published clinical series[1-3] of 1,645 reported cases, our infection rate was 0.15 percent of breasts. The problem is that infection is a real risk that is not totally preventable, even with the most state-of-the-art techniques and drugs. During that twenty-seven years, we had the opportunity to treat a larger number of patients with infection who were referred to us, and from that experience, we have developed criteria for infection treatment that are much more stringent compared to the FDA and compared to many other surgeons.

In our current practice, we advise every patient before augmentation that if they develop an infection, we recommend removing both implants, and we do not ever recommend replacing either implant.

Although this is a very hard position for both patient and surgeon, it definitively solves the problem, forever. Any attempt to salvage an infected breast implant is tenuous at best. No matter how long you wait after removing an infected implant, there is a significant risk of reinfection if you attempt to replace the implant, regardless of treatment techniques used. Even if a replaced implant does not become reinfected, there is a substantial risk of capsular contracture in the previously infected breast. Reinfection or capsular contracture both require additional surgery with additional risks, potential complications, costs, time off work, and possible permanent deformity. Fortunately, infection is very rare, but if it occurs, implant removal is the best option.

7. FDA—Hematoma/Seroma

Hematoma is a collection of blood inside a body cavity, and seroma is a collection of the watery portion of the blood around the implant or around the incision. Postoperative hematoma and seroma may contribute to infection and/or capsular contracture. Swelling, pain, and bruising may result. If a hematoma occurs, it will usually be soon after surgery; however, this can also occur at any time after injury to the breast. While the body absorbs small hematomas and seromas, large ones will require the placement of surgical drains for proper healing. A small scar can result from surgical draining. Implant deflation/rupture can occur from surgical draining if damage to the implant occurs during the draining procedure.

JT—A reasonable guideline is that hematomas occur in about one or two cases out of 100 (1 to 2 percent). In our published data summarized in Table 5-1, hematomas occurred in less than one-tenth of 1 percent of breasts (0.09 percent)! Hematomas are largely (not totally) preventable with state-of-the-art electrocautery dissection techniques and by eliminating all blunt dissection. Contrary to popular opinion, our data conclusively prove that early return to full, normal activities does not cause bleeding or hematomas,[1-3,7] and that compression devices such as tight wraps and special bras are also unnecessary, provided a surgeon uses optimal instrumentation and techniques.

If you develop a large hematoma, it should always be drained, and you may have a drain tube in place for several days. The risk of capsular contracture (excessive tightening of the capsule around the implant producing an excessively hard breast, sometimes misshapen) is substantially higher following a hematoma. If you have any history of abnormal bleeding, you *must* advise your surgeon. Avoid all medications that contain aspirin for at least three weeks before and after surgery, and ask your surgeon for a list of other medications to avoid, medications that could impair normal blood clotting. Smaller quantities of bleeding around an implant may not be detectable clinically by your surgeon, but can nevertheless cause increased inflammation and increase risks of capsular contracture or pocket closure that can result in implant displacement or distortion.

8. FDA—Changes in Nipple and Breast Sensation

Feeling in the nipple and breast can increase or decrease after implant surgery. The range of changes varies from intense sensitivity to no feeling in the nipple or breast following surgery. Changes in feeling can be temporary or permanent and may affect sexual response or the ability to nurse a baby. (Refer to the Other Illnesses section for more information on breast feeding.)

JT—What do we tell patients? "If you are like most patients, you will lose some sensation, and you will get some back. It's possible to lose all sensation, but this is exceedingly unusual. If you can't cope with that, don't have an augmentation. The larger the implant we use, the larger the pocket we have to make, the more nerves we have to cut or stretch, and the more sensation you're likely to lose." If you consider your breasts abnormal or unattractive before augmentation, that could also affect your sexual response, so tactile sensation isn't the only factor. Some factors relate to the breast; other factors relate to the brain. We have had patients who, even though they lost some sensation, told us that they felt so much more attractive following augmentation that the effects of their sensory loss were minor compared to the benefit of feeling much more attractive and sensual. Ultimately, every woman is different, but if you decide to have a breast augmentation, be sure that you are willing to possibly give up some breast sensation because sensory loss can occur. Less than 5 percent of our patients complain of any type of sensory loss six or more months following their augmentation.

Some patients actually experience some hypersensitivity (overly sensitive) following augmentation, but hypersensitivity usually subsides rapidly in a matter of days to weeks. We can't recall a patient who has had permanent hypersensitivity though theoretically it is possible.

9. FDA—Calcium Deposits in the Tissue Around the Implant

Deposits of calcium can be seen on mammograms and can be mistaken for possible cancer, resulting in additional surgery to biopsy and/or remove the implant to distinguish these deposits from cancer. Calcium deposits may be felt as nodules (hard knots) under the skin around the implant.

JT—In my experience, this is a rare problem and usually occurs around silicone-gel implants more than ten years old. Most calcium deposits that I have seen are immediately adjacent to, or contained as part of, the capsule surrounding the implant. Most are very easily removed with the capsule. Calcium deposits can, however, form in any scar tissue anywhere in the body, so theoretically, they could certainly form in areas of the breast that have been treated surgically

10. FDA—Delayed Wound Healing

In some cases, the incision site fails to heal normally or takes longer to heal.

JT- Delayed wound healing is rare, but can occur as the result of minor, localized infection, body reaction to suture material, smoking, certain drugs including Accutane and various steroids, some types of herbal medications that are not well defined, and other causes. In some cases, surgical revision of the incision area may be necessary. It is critically important that you make your surgeon aware of all types of drugs, including nicotine and herbal supplements, that you have taken prior to your surgery.

11. FDA—Extrusion

An unstable or compromised tissue covering and/or interruption of wound healing may result in extrusion of the implant, which is when the breast implant comes through the skin. The additional surgery needed to correct this complication can result in unacceptable scarring or loss of breast tissue.

JT—Implant extrusion is exceedingly rare and most commonly occurs when infection is present, especially if surgeon and patient delay implant removal by trying (sometimes repeatedly) to salvage the implants by drainage and antibiotic treatment. The longer infection is present, the more inflammation and tissue damage and destruction occur, increasing risks of permanent deformity. When infection is present, remove the implants—immediately—to minimize extrusion and tissue damage risks.

Implant extrusion can also occur from excessively large implants causing excessive stretch and thinning in the lower breast. Although rare, this disastrous complication is almost totally preventable by avoiding excessively large implants, especially in patients with thin tissues, and removing implants if excessive tissue thinning occurs.

Implant extrusion can also occur if steroids or similar drugs are injected into the implant pocket (historically in an effort to minimize risks of capsular contracture). We never recommend use of steroids in the pocket surrounding the implant.

12. FDA—Necrosis

Necrosis is the formation of dead tissue around the implant. This may prevent wound healing and require surgical correction and/or implant removal. Permanent scar and/or deformity may occur following necrosis. Factors associated with increased necrosis include infection, use of steroids in the surgical pocket, smoking, chemotherapy/radiation, and excessive heat or cold therapy.

JT—Necrosis of tissue surrounding an implant is exceedingly rare and usually caused by infection. The other possible causes listed by the FDA are important for you to consider.

13. FDA—Breast Tissue Atrophy/Chest Wall Deformity

The pressure of the breast implant may cause the breast tissue to thin and shrink. This can occur while implants are still in place or following implant removal without replacement.

JT—Three factors largely determine if you will experience shrinkage of your breast tissue following augmentation. The larger the breast implant, the more high profile (distance from front to back of the implant), or the tighter your skin overlying your breast, the more likely the risk of breast tissue atrophy. Trying to force tissues to a desired result with high profile or highly projecting implants significantly increases risks of breast tissue atrophy and/or chest wall deformity.

Two of these factors—the size of the implant and avoiding high profile implants just because you want a more projecting breast—are totally preventable! Think before you push implant size or order a more projecting breast, unless you have a specific breast deformity or condition they may require them. You can't control how tight your skin envelope is, but you can respect the fact that the tighter the skin envelope, all other factors equal, the more you need to limit implant size to avoid shrinkage or atrophy of your breast tissue.

14. FDA—Interference with Mammography

Interference with mammography due to breast implants may delay or hinder the early detection of breast cancer either by hiding suspicious lesions (wounds or injuries or tumors) or by making it more difficult to include them in the image. Implants increase the difficulty of both taking and reading mammograms. Some women who undergo reconstruction will have some breast tissue remaining, and some have all of their breast tissue removed. It is important that a woman with breast tissue remaining continue to have mammography of that breast, as well as of the other breast, to detect breast cancer.

Mammography requires breast compression (hard pressure) that could contribute to implant rupture. In addition to special care taken by the technologist to reduce the risk of implant rupture during this compression, other techniques are used to maximize what is seen of the breast tissue during mammography. These techniques are called breast implant displacement views, Eklund displacement views, or Eklund views after the radiologist who developed them. These special implant displacement views are done in addition to those views done during routine mammograms.

Because of the extra views and time needed, women with implants should always inform the receptionist or scheduler that they have breast implants when making an appointment for mammography. They should also tell the radiology technologist about the presence of implants before mammography is performed. This is to make sure that the technologist uses these special displacement techniques and takes extra care when compressing the breasts to avoid rupturing the implant.

The displacement procedure involves pushing the implant back and gently pulling the breast tissue into view. Several factors affect the success of this special technique in imaging the breast tissue in women with breast implants. The location of the implant, the hardness of the capsular contracture, the size of the breast tissue compared to the implant, and other factors may affect how well the breast tissue can be imaged.

A radiologist may have difficulty distinguishing calcium deposits in the scar tissue around the implant from a breast tumor when he or she is interpreting the mammogram. Occasionally, it is necessary to remove and examine a small amount of tissue (biopsy) to see whether or not it is cancerous. This can frequently be done without removing the implant.

JT—To my knowledge, there are no definitive scientific studies that conclusively prove that breast implants hinder the early detection of breast cancer by mammography. The FDA uses the word "may" in their statement. Many factors affect the accuracy of mammograms and the accuracy of breast cancer diagnosis. Nevertheless, breast implants are one of many factors that affect mammography, no doubt, and breast implants are medically unnecessary. If you are not willing to sacrifice some degree of mammogram accuracy, don't have a breast augmentation!

15. FDA—Galactorrhea

Sometimes after breast implant surgery, you may begin producing breast milk. In some cases, the milk production stops spontaneously or when medication is given to suppress milk production. In other cases, removal of the implant(s) may be needed.

JT—Galactorrhea following augmentation is rare and, in our experience, is more common when augmentation is performed within three months of cessation of nursing. As a result, we recommend that patients wait a minimum of three months following cessation of nursing before having an augmentation. If milk production begins, it usually subsides spontaneously or we will ask for your gynecologist's assistance in prescribing appropriate medications to decrease lactation. We have never experienced a patient who required implant removal, but removal is one theoretical treatment alternative.

16. FDA—Shifting of the Implant

FDA—Shifting of the implant: Sometimes an implant may shift from its original position, giving the breasts an unnatural look and possibly causing pain and discomfort. An implant may become visible at the surface of the breast as a result of the device pushing through the layers of skin. Further surgery is needed to correct this problem. Placing the implant beneath the muscle may help to minimize this problem.

Other problems with appearance could include incorrect implant size, visible scars, uneven appearance, and wrinkling of the implant.

JT—All of these things can happen. If an implant shifts from its original position AND causes pain and discomfort, the usual cause is capsular contracture. Implant "shifts" can also occur from skin stretch due to an excessively large implant under excessively thin tissues. No surgeon can accurately predict exactly how your tissues will respond to an implant or how much they will stretch. Excessive stretching and thinning can occur even with relatively small implants, but the risk definitely increases in our experience with implants larger than 350 cc in volume. Visible implant edges indicate inadequate soft-tissue coverage over the implant. Surgeons can best prevent visible implant edges or shell by measuring soft-tissue thickness before surgery and making decisions on pocket location (over or under muscle) based on those measurements. An excessively large implant in a patient with thin tissues is a setup for implant visibility and later visible traction rippling when the implant pulls on the thin overlying tissues. The implant further stretches and thins already thin tissue, and the implant becomes visible, or traction rippling develops. Once the problem of a visible implant or visible traction rippling occurs, it's exceedingly difficult or impossible to correct. Better to make the right team decisions before the first operation.

Choosing optimal implant size for your individual tissue characteristics is difficult for the most skilled surgeons and requires very careful, compulsive communication between you and your surgeon before your augmentation. A large percentage of augmentation patients, if questioned more than a year following surgery, state that they would like to be larger. Some surgeons, recognizing this predilection, rationalize, "Why not just make them bigger to begin with?" Decisions about breast size should be team decisions between patient and surgeon, based as much as possible on measurements that are quantifiable, not on subjective cup size. No method currently exists to precisely predict breast cup size. If you are not totally comfortable that your surgeon understands your "wants," don't proceed with augmentation. At the same time, be sure that you are honest with yourself and your surgeon about your true desires. Always remember: the larger the implant, the worse the potential compromises and the higher the risks long term as aging occurs. Also remember, you are responsible for the decisions and choices you make, now and forever. There's a good chance you're thinking more about now instead of tomorrow or forever. Carefully consider your wishes and the possible consequences on your tissues over time.

DEALING WITH PROBLEMS

The best way to deal with a problem is to deal with it—now!

All patients and all surgeons hate problems. But when they occur, it's best to deal with them, and the sooner, the better. Often it's a good idea to get another opinion to make everyone more comfortable and assemble as much brainpower and experience as possible.

There isn't a surgeon alive who wants an unhappy patient. Keep your lines of communication open.

No surgeon can solve a problem unless the surgeon is aware that a problem exists. Most of the best surgeons will encourage you to seek another opinion—don't hesitate to ask.

Try to keep the team together. Honesty is important. Communicate with your surgeon. Confront the problem, discuss the alternatives, get other opinions, if necessary, and then make joint decisions. If, for any reason, you aren't comfortable with your surgeon or vice-versa, try to stay friends and seek additional help. You'll almost always benefit from a nonadversarial approach. I haven't seen many lawyers solve complicated medical problems.

One principle is worth repeating: If you have any problem twice or if you have the same problem twice, remove your implants or don't complain later. If problems occur, seek additional information or other medical opinions, and use common sense.

You are partially responsible for what happens to you.

If problems occur, remember there are worse things than removing and not replacing implants.

THE NEXT STEP . . .

By now, you've digested a lot of information. You're informed about implants, different surgical options, and potential problems. The last step before consulting a surgeon is learning about recovery and the factors that affect recovery so you can ask the right questions and make the right decisions.

References

1. Tebbetts, J. B. Patient acceptance of adequately filled breast implants. *Plast. Reconstr. Surg.* 196(1): 139-147, 2000.

2. Tebbetts, J. B. Dual plane (DP) breast augmentation: optimizing implant-soft tissue relationships in a wide range of breast types. *Plast. Reconstr. Surg.* 107: 1255, 2001.

3. Tebbetts, J. B. Achieving a predictable 24-hour return to normal activities after breast augmentation, part I: Refining practices using motion and time study principles. *Plast. Reconstr. Surg.* 109: 293-305, 2002.

4. Safety of Silicone Breast Implants. Institute of Medicine National Academy Press. Washington, DC, (IOM Report).

5. Gabriel, S. E., Woods, J. E., O'Fallon, W. M., Beard, C. M., Kurland, L. T., and Melton, L. J. Complications leading to surgery after breast implantation. *N. Engl. J. Med.* 336: 679-682, 1997.

6. Brown, S. L., Middleton, M. S., Berg, W. A., Soo, M. S., and Pennello, G. Prevalence of rupture of silicone gel breast implants in a population of women in Birmingham, Alabama. *Am. J. Roentgenol.* 175: 1-8, 2000.

7. Tebbetts, J. B. Achieving a zero percent reoperation rate at 3 years in a 50 consecutive case augmentation mammaplasty PMA study. *Plast. Reconstr. Surg.* 118(6): 1453-57, 2006.

9. Robinson, O. G., Bradley, E. L., and Wilson, D. S. Analysis of explanted silicone implants: a report of 300 patients. *Ann. Plast. Surg.* 34: 1-7, 1995.

10. Vinnik, C. A. Migratory silicone—clinical aspects. Silicone in medical devices—conference proceedings. U. S. Department of Health and Human Services, FDA Publication. 92-4249: 59-67, 1991.

11. Duffy, M. J., and Woods, J. E. Health risks of failed silicone gel breast implants: a 30-year clinical experience. *Plast. Reconstr. Surg.* 94: 295-299, 1994.

12. Berg, U. A., Caskey, C. I., Hamper, U. M., Kuhlman, J. E., Anderson, N. D., and Chang, B. W., et al. Single- and double-lumen silicone breast implant integrity: prospective evaluation of MR and US criteria. *Radiology.* 197: 45-52, 1995.

13. Gorczyca, D. P., Schneider, E., DeBruhl, N. D., Foo, T. K. F., Ahn, C. Y., and Sayre, J. W., et al. Silicone breast implant rupture: comparison between three-point Dixon and fast spin-echo MR imaging. *Am. J. Roentgenol.* 162: 205-310, 1994.

14. U. S. Food and Drug Administration. Saline-filled Breast Implant Surgery: Making an Informed Decision (Mentor Corporation). http://www.fda.gov/cdrh/breastimplants/labeling//mentor_patient_labeling_5900.html. Accessed January 1, 2007.

15. U. S. Food and Drug Administration. INAMED - Making an Informed Decision Saline-Filled Breast Implant Surgery. Available at: http://www.fda.gov/cdrh/breastimplants/labeling/inamed_patient_labeling_5900.html. Accessed January 1, 2007.

16. Gutowski, K. A., Mesna, G. T., and Cunningham, B. L. Breast implants: a plastic surgery educational foundation multicenter outcomes study. *Plast. Reconstr. Surg.* 100: 1019-1027, 1997.

17. Gabriel, S. E., Woods, J. E., O'Fallon, W. M., Beard, C. M., Kurland, L. T., and Melton, L. J. Complications leading to surgery after breast implantation. *New Engl. J. Med.* 336: 679-682, 1997.

RECOVERY:

LEARN ABOUT IT BEFORE SURGERY

"Learning about your recovery can tell you a lot about a surgeon and the quality of your surgery. A more skilled surgeon usually offers you a simpler and faster recovery."

Learn about recovery before surgery? You must be kidding! Why not just worry about that when the time comes? Because . . .

Learning about recovery can potentially tell you more about a surgeon's skills than anything else you can ask a surgeon. It is almost impossible for any surgeon to exaggerate the surgeon's level of expertise if you ask the right questions about recovery.

Your experiences during recovery are a direct consequence of what happens during your surgery.

The less traumatic your surgical procedure, the easier and faster your recovery.

You can't see what your surgeon will do in the operating room, but you can quickly figure out how much trauma and bleeding you're likely to experience by simply asking in detail about recovery.

Would you like to have an easier and faster recovery? Would you prefer less time away from your normal activities? Less time off work? Less bruising? No drain tubes coming out of your body? No tight bandages or special bras? All of these things are possible, but only if you choose the right surgeon. In fact, all of these are routine in some augmentation practices. But not in all augmentation practices. The only way you'll know is to *ask about recovery before your augmentation!*

WHAT'S TO RECOVER FROM?

Tissue Trauma

Any operation causes some degree of injury (trauma) to your tissues. The more precise and delicate the surgery, the less trauma, but some tissue trauma is unavoidable. Your body responds to tissue trauma in predictable ways: pain, swelling, bruising, and stiffness after surgery.

The greater the amount of trauma to your tissues, the more discomfort and other symptoms you'll have after surgery.

The greater the trauma, the longer it takes your body to heal and the longer it takes for you to feel normal and return to normal activities.

The more trauma and bleeding you experience during surgery, the greater the likelihood you may develop problems such as capsular contracture or hematoma that require additional operations and can compromise the quality of your result.

To put an implant in your breast, the surgeon creates a pocket to receive the implant. The pocket can be behind breast tissue (retromammary), or behind breast tissue and behind muscle (partial retropectoral). If it's just behind breast tissue, the surgeon lifts the breast tissue off the pectoralis muscle to create the pocket. If you are thin and need more soft-tissue coverage, you need additional muscle cover over the implant, and the surgeon needs to create a pocket behind the muscle (submuscular) or partially behind muscle and partially behind breast tissue (dual plane). Traditionally, you could expect more discomfort, swelling, and a longer recovery. How much longer? It depends on your tissues, and it depends on how the pocket is created at surgery. Since we developed and published the first techniques in the history of augmentation that allow patients to return to full normal activities within twenty-four hours, you can now recover just as rapidly if an implant is placed behind muscle as if it were placed only behind breast tissue! Using our twenty-four-hour recovery surgical techniques, manipulating your pectoralis muscle to provide more coverage, if done properly, does not result in more pain or a longer recovery.[1, 2]

Recovering from a pocket created behind breast tissue is NOW THE SAME AS RECOVERING FROM A POCKET CREATED BEHIND MUSCLE, USING OUR TWENTY-FOUR-HOUR RECOVERY SURGICAL TECHNIQUES![1–2]

Why? We have now developed techniques that minimize trauma and bleeding when we manipulate your pectoralis muscle.

If you are thin and need muscle cover (or need it for other reasons), it is more important to have muscle cover than to avoid slightly more tissue trauma. You and your surgeon must decide based on your tissues. Even if a surgeon is unfamiliar with our twenty-four-hour recovery surgical techniques, you should prioritize assuring adequate soft-tissue cover over your implant.[3,4]

The more tissue trauma caused by your surgery, the longer and more difficult your recovery. Our published studies and techniques in the past few years[1–6] have completely redefined patient recovery, and it all results from techniques that minimize trauma to your tissues and minimize bleeding.

Ask about recovery and compare what surgeons tell you. The opportunity to return to full, normal activities within twenty-four hours following your augmentation tells you that a surgeon really can deliver less trauma and bleeding, not just say that he or she can. Longer recovery times usually imply more tissue trauma at surgery. No matter what a surgeon tells you about the surgeon's expertise or techniques, recovery tells the truest story.

Tissue Stretch—Another Form of Tissue Trauma

Your implant will stretch your tissues and also stretch nerves in and around your breast. The larger the implant or the tighter your tissues, the more pressure the implant exerts on your tissues. This pressure subsides over time (weeks to months) as your tissues stretch to accommodate your implant. But pressure of an implant (especially a larger implant in tighter tissues) can produce more discomfort, more stretch on nerves in the breast, and more temporary or permanent loss of sensation. The message? Some tissue stretch injury is unavoidable, but

Excessively large implants in excessively tight tissues can produce excessive stretch trauma that can cause more discomfort and temporary or permanent sensory loss.

Consider your tissues when selecting implant size.

Tissue stretch can produce temporary numbness, tingling, pin-prick sensations, and other weird feelings during the first few weeks of recovery. These sensations are a normal part of recovery. Sensation varies tremendously from patient to patient and is not predictable. If you select a large implant that stresses your tissues excessively, expect more sensory loss and a longer time for sensation to return to near normal.

Bruising and Swelling—What Causes It?

Bruising is blood within your tissues.

Bruising and swelling are caused by tissue trauma.

The more tissue trauma, the more bruising and swelling.

The more bruising and swelling, the longer your recovery.

The more bruising and swelling, the longer before you'll return to normal activities.

You can judge a lot about your upcoming surgery by asking:

Will I have bruising? For how long? What about swelling? When can I return to normal activities? Will I have drain tubes? Will I have any type of bandage or bra to compress my breasts?

TISSUE TRAUMA AND SURGICAL TECHNIQUE

In chapter 6, you learned about different surgical techniques, different methods that surgeons use to create the pockets for your implants. The technique a surgeon uses to create the pocket can significantly affect how much tissue injury occurs and, hence, can significantly affect your recovery.

Blunt dissection techniques cause substantially more trauma compared to specially developed electrocautery dissection techniques.

Sharp dissection techniques cause substantially more bleeding compared to specially developed electrocautery techniques.

Ask your surgeon specifically what technique will be used to create the pockets for your implants. If it's not twenty-four-hour[1] precise electrocautery dissection techniques and instruments, expect more bruising, swelling, and a longer recovery time.

TUBES COMING OUT OF YOUR BODY

No matter how tiny a tube, when you see it coming out through a puncture in your skin, it looks the size of a fire hose. You won't like it. You'll be told that it's necessary to remove fluid from around your implant and that if you don't have it, your chances of collecting blood (hematoma), fluid (seroma), and chances of capsular contracture are increased. True? Not necessarily. Using techniques we developed and published[1,2,4,6] in over 1,600 reported cases, hematomas occurred in only 0.09 percent and seromas in 0.06 percent. Optimal instrumentation and precise surgical techniques unquestionably make a difference.

All electrocautery dissection instruments and techniques are not the same and do not necessarily deliver the same results. A surgeon may tell you that he or she uses electrocautery dissection, but the real question is not *whether* the surgeon uses electrocautery dissection, but precisely *how* the surgeon uses it and whether the surgeon has the optimal instruments. The best way for any patient to judge is to simply ask about recovery! If a surgeon has optimal instrumentation and knows optimal techniques, the surgeon can offer you twenty-four-hour return to normal activities.

It is true that if substantial bleeding and tissue injury occur at the time of surgery, your body will release more blood and fluid into the pocket around the implant and that it's better to remove the fluid with a drain than to leave it there. But it's also true that:

In first-time augmentations (as opposed to reoperation cases), techniques now exist that make drain tubes completely unnecessary.[1-6]

Ask if you'll need drains. If the answer is yes, does that mean that the surgeon isn't good or isn't doing a good job? Not necessarily, but it should raise the question "Why do I need those?" Does it mean that the surgeon is doing something wrong? No. You should consider many factors in choosing a surgeon, but this is certainly one of those factors. Why does the surgeon need drains when other surgeons don't? Why does a surgeon need drains when there are peer-reviewed, scientific publications in the most respected journal in plastic surgery describing techniques that make drains obsolete in first-time breast augmentations? Get answers from different surgeons, and then you decide.

ANESTHESIA AND RECOVERY TIME

It's nice to have anesthesia when you're having surgery! Having anesthesia means that you will receive drugs. The longer the operation, the longer the anesthesia, and the more drugs you'll receive. When the drugs are discontinued following surgery, your body must break down (metabolize) the drugs before you will feel normal. Anesthetic drugs often cause some hangover. Hangover can be good if it eases your discomfort immediately after surgery. But once you're feeling better, a hangover that lasts longer is a nuisance because you don't feel normal as quickly.

Some people are prone to develop nausea following anesthesia. Even the best antinausea drugs don't totally prevent nausea in some patients. However, the fewer narcotic drugs you get, the less chance of your developing nausea. The shorter the anesthesia and the less tissue trauma during surgery, the fewer narcotic drugs you'll need.

The longer you need anesthesia and the more tissue trauma, the more drugs you'll need, the longer you'll be required to remain at the surgery facility, and the longer time before you'll feel normal.

Ask about surgery time, anesthesia time, time in the recovery room, and how long until you'll return home the day of surgery. All of these factors will tell you a lot about how much anesthesia you'll receive and when you can expect to feel normal.

There is no avoiding the fact that the shorter your surgery and the less tissue trauma, the fewer drugs you'll need, the less chance of nausea and hangover, and the more rapidly you'll return to normal.

I know I'm repeating, but I want to be sure you've got the picture!

In our peer-reviewed and published study of 627 patients in our twenty-four-hour recovery publications,[1,2] refining our anesthetic and surgical techniques resulted in documented recovery times that we previously considered impossible. All patients were operated on using general, endotracheal anesthesia, and here are the recovery results:

Time from the beginning of the augmentation procedure until patients left our accredited outpatient surgery facility to return home averaged less than ninety minutes! All patients scored maximum on recovery criteria, and all were able to raise their arms fully over their heads before leaving.

No patient required narcotic-strength pain medications at home.

An incredible 96 percent of the patients were able to resume full, normal activities within twenty-four hours!

Full, normal activities were defined as the patient's being able to do the following:

- Raise arms above the head with arms fully extended, three times every four hours

- Lie directly on the breasts

- Lift all normal weight objects

- Perform all normal activities

- Drive a personal car

- Go out for work, shopping, or entertainment

Specific instrumentation and techniques unquestionably minimize surgical trauma and bleeding and allow this type of recovery.

General Anesthesia Versus Local Anesthesia With Sedation— What's Best?

When considering anesthesia, what's best is what is safest and allows your surgeon the greatest degree of control during your operation.

Many people don't love the idea of being "put to sleep." It just has a bad ring to it. Everyone has heard about disasters that have occurred with anesthesia. All the disasters are reported, but you never hear about the hundreds of thousands of anesthetics daily that go without a hitch. So it's normal to think: "The less anesthesia the better. If I can have this surgery without being 'put to sleep,' that's better, right?" Wrong!

When problems occur with anesthesia, most fall into two general categories:

1. You have a totally unpredictable reaction to a routine anesthetic drug (an idiosyncratic drug reaction).

2. You regurgitate while you are asleep or heavily sedated, and instead of vomiting the material out of your mouth, you suck stomach acid down your windpipe into your lungs. Your lungs react violently, and reflexes usually cause your heart to react by developing abnormal heart rhythms—a very bad combination.

Both of these potentially dangerous events are exceedingly rare, but they can occur. The first, an idiosyncratic drug reaction, cannot be predicted or totally prevented. If it occurs, it's treatable. The second event (aspiration), however, is almost totally preventable by inserting a small tube with a balloon into your windpipe after you're asleep. When the balloon is inflated, it minimizes risk of stomach contents passing into the windpipe. The only trade-off is that your throat may be a little raspy from the tube for a few hours after surgery.

Endotracheal tubes can be lifesaving, but you won't enjoy having an endotracheal tube (the tube with a balloon in your windpipe) unless you're asleep. If you have local anesthesia, you are not asleep. More drugs combined with the local anesthesia will heavily sedate you, but technically you're still not asleep. Mainly, you're not asleep enough to tolerate an endotracheal tube. If you have local anesthesia injected, it deadens the tissues, but you'll need additional drugs to stay comfortable. If you get uncomfortable during surgery, your surgeon may need to stop while the person giving your anesthesia gives you more drugs. That slows things down. Remember, longer anesthesia, more drugs and more nausea result in a longer recovery. Does local anesthesia work? Usually, but those additional drugs that keep you comfortable can also interfere with your gag reflexes. If you regurgitate, you may be too sedated to gag and vomit, and the stomach acid can go down your windpipe because you don't have an endotracheal tube in place.

Local anesthesia with sedation (you're not asleep) usually does not allow you to have an endotracheal tube to protect you from aspiration.

There is no peer-reviewed scientific publication on a series of breast augmentation patients using local anesthesia that is even remotely comparable to the recovery results in our twenty-four-hour studies.[1,2] Local anesthesia simply doesn't measure up any more and is no longer state-of-the-art for breast augmentation.

General anesthesia (you are asleep) with an endotracheal tube in place better protects you against aspiration.

Optimal general anesthsia is unquestionably more predictable at keeping you asleep and comfortable, so you are less likely to remember events of your surgery, and your surgeon has more control over a larger number of factors that affect your outcome.

Some surgery facilities are not equipped and accredited to administer general anesthesia. You certainly don't want to have any anesthesia unless a facility is fully accredited and its personnel are equipped and optimally trained. Before surgery, ask your surgeon the following:

What type of anesthesia will I have?

Which is safer, local or general?

Which offers better control, local or general? Under local anesthesia with sedation, how am I protected against aspiration?

Can you offer me both options and let me choose?

Popular Misconceptions about Anesthesia and the Facts

A popular misconception that general anesthesia causes more nausea than local anesthesia is not necessarily true. Nausea relates more to the type and quantity of drugs you're given and how they are given. Some medical personnel administer anesthesia better than others. Ask your surgeon who will be giving the anesthesia. Is this someone the surgeon works with regularly? How regularly?

A second misconception is that general anesthesia requires giving you more drugs than local anesthesia. Again, not necessarily true, and our published studies and results now prove this fact beyond question.[1] By having you asleep and your surgeon having optimal control, your surgery can proceed more smoothly in a shorter time. General anesthesia can require fewer drugs because of more control and a shorter surgery time. Again, it depends on who is doing it and how they do it.

A third misconception is that it takes longer to recover from general anesthesia. Again, not true, as our peer-reviewed and published data prove.[1] Recovery depends on the amount of drugs you received during and after surgery. The longer the operation, the more drugs you'll receive. Well-done general anesthesia involves a shorter recovery than many local-anesthesia-with-sedation cases. If a surgeon does not have access to top-notch general anesthesia, local with sedation can be a better option.

You have a choice of surgeons and a choice of surgical facilities. No surgeon or facility can offer you risk-free anesthesia. It doesn't exist. But one of the major risks (aspiration) is almost totally preventable with general anesthesia. It's up to you to ask the right questions and make the best team decisions.

Bandages, binders, and special bras

Another aspect of recovery that can tell you a lot about your surgery is the use of special bandages, binders, and special bras.

Devices don't produce optimal results. Optimal surgery produces optimal results.

Key questions about any device you have to tolerate following augmentation are "Why is the device necessary in the first place?" and "If techniques to avoid all of these devices are now published in the most respected journal in plastic surgery,[1-6] why do many surgeons continue to use all of the postoperative devices?"

The more you rely on external devices to produce a result, the less predictable the result.

The biggest problem with devices is that you have to use and tolerate them.

How much do you like wearing things that are tight, uncomfortable, or a nuisance?

What do you often do with things you don't enjoy wearing? Take them off!

So when a surgeon depends on a device that you can wear or not wear, the result is not as predictable.

Does that mean that all external devices are a bad idea? Not necessarily. If a surgeon feels that a device is necessary after surgery, the surgeon should have a reason. You should ask for the reason and ask if there are published techniques to avoid all of those devices.

Bandages

Survey several surgeons, and you'll find that bandages vary from none to mummy-like, near-total body wraps. Why? Often because a surgeon was trained to use a certain type of bandage for augmentation and has used it ever since. During my residency training, I was taught that it was necessary to firmly wrap every augmentation patient with an elastic bandage that covered everything from the neck to the waist. The reason given was that the elastic wrap would put pressure on the breasts to reduce risks of bleeding and provide support to keep the patient comfortable. Sounded logical to me, so I did it. What they didn't know and didn't tell me was that with optimal instruments and techniques, bleeding requiring the wraps didn't occur, and compression was really unnecessary. Patients tolerated the compression wraps and garments for a couple of days because they thought it was necessary. But when I asked them how it felt, they all said, "Horrible. It's tight, it rolls up, it is hot, it itches, and I can't take a bath and wash my hair!" My patients have taught me that they would much rather be able to bathe and wash their hair and avoid the nuisance and expense of additional wraps or compression garments if they were really unnecessary.

Bandages to stop bleeding? Why not just do the surgery in a way that you don't have bleeding in the first place? How you do the operation is what determines the amount of bleeding. Not a bandage, not a wrap, not anything else. So by improving how we perform the operation, we've done away with bandages completely. No bandages on any patient for the past fifteen years! Any bleeding? Hematoma in less than one-tenth of one percent of patients.[1,2,4,6] Bleeding can occur after surgery—no matter what technique is used. But . . .

Bandages don't prevent bleeding as well as optimal instrumentation and precise surgical techniques do.

Bandages are a nuisance that prevent you from showering and washing your hair.

Bandages are largely unnecessary, provided certain surgical techniques are used.

Bandages to improve patient comfort? Ever been wrapped in an elastic bandage for a couple of days? Ever had adhesive tape pulled off? Ever been unable to bathe or wash your hair for a day or two? In some operations, bandages are necessary. Following augmentation, they are not necessary, provided specific surgical techniques are used.

Binder Devices, Straps

Quite an array of binder devices exists, mostly touted as essential aids to keep an implant in place or to push it somewhere: upward, downward, inward, outward. Surgeons utilize these devices in a variety of ways for a variety of reasons, usually due to a bad experience with implants "going" somewhere that neither the surgeon nor the patient likes.

Implants largely "go" where surgeons place the implants at surgery. If the pocket to receive the implant is substantially larger than the implant, the implant can move. When implants are put under the muscle, you'll hear from some surgeons and patients that the implants tend to ride up. Behold, an opportunity for a device, some type of strap or binder across the upper breast to hold them down.

The tendency of implants to ride up is usually due to one of four causes:

1. Excessive tissue forces are pushing on the lower implant,

2. The implant was positioned too high at surgery,

3. The implant chosen was too large for the patient's tissues, or

4. The distance between the nipple and fold beneath the breast was set inappropriately relative to the width of implant placed in the breast.

The most common reason for excessive tissue pressure on the lower implant is that the implant is too large for the patient's tissues. When too much implant is placed into too tight a pocket, the pocket pushes back, especially in the lower breast, and the implant is pushed upward. Under muscle, the pocket tends to be even tighter, especially if specific techniques aren't used to release pressure of the lower muscle on the implant. If you're thinking about a larger implant and have tight tissues, a binder or strap may make some sense, but . . .

Specific surgical techniques— accurate, precise pocket development and control—are more effective than binder devices at controlling implant position.

When you and your surgeon select an implant that is excessively large for your tissue characteristics, the risk of implant displacement increases.

How long are you willing to wear a binder device? What happens when you take it off? An excessively large implant exerts excessive pressure forever. Want to wear a binder device forever?

If the implant is in a good position for the first few weeks and then displaces upward, wound healing mechanisms beyond any surgeon's control may be the cause.

Special Bras

Some women love them; other women hate them! Some need them; some don't. If you ask women about bras following their augmentation, I promise you'll hear answers all over the map. Some will say you absolutely must wear a bra, even a certain type. Others will say no; it's not necessary. Surgical garment companies love bras and support garments because they boost the bottom line. But every different manufacturer will tell you that its design is better for several reasons. How many bras do you need? It depends on whom you ask. The companies will tell you several. You'll probably enjoy at least two, so you can wash one while using the other. The real bottom line?

If a bra or a certain type of bra were best, everyone would be using it. It just isn't so.

If special bras were really necessary at all, patients wouldn't do well without them. And believe me, a lot of patients do great without them every day!

If you or your surgeon feel that you need them or like them, use them. Just don't fool yourself into thinking they're really necessary from a medical standpoint, provided you make optimal decisions and apply certain surgical techniques.

Some surgeons feel that a bra holds the implant in place. My question is why do you need to hold the implant in place? If the pocket is created accurately in the right location, the pocket holds the implant in place. Other surgeons feel that the pressure of a bra decreases chances of bleeding and makes patients more comfortable. I can't envision depending on a bra to prevent bleeding. Surgical techniques prevent bleeding. And comfort? Just ask several women, and you'll get several answers. Some are more comfortable with a bra, and some without. It's a personal preference.

What do we tell our patients? "You'll go home with a single piece of tape over your incision. In the first few weeks after surgery, you can wear or not wear a bra. It's your choice. Wearing or not wearing a bra won't affect your final result at all. If you're more comfortable wearing a bra, or if you want to create a certain look, go for it, the sooner, the better. It's not necessary to worry about a bra harming your incision, even if it's an underwire bra and your incision is under your breast. On the other hand, if you're more comfortable not wearing a bra, don't wear one. You don't need it, especially in the first few weeks after surgery."

You need a bra, however, when you are engaging in any activity that causes your breasts to bounce, such as running, jogging, aerobics (even low-impact aerobics), horseback riding, etc. Why? Gravity alone, even with a bra, pulls breasts downward. Add the force of bouncing, and the migration will definitely start sooner. No way around it. If they're bouncing, they're sagging sooner and more! What type of bra will prevent this? Any tight bra that prevents bouncing. Sometimes two jog bras, one size too small. Whatever it takes, stop the bouncing! This rule applies from now on if you want to minimize tissue stretch and potential sagging.

RECOVERY TIMES AND LIMITATIONS

What is normal for recovery times? Which limitations are mandatory, and which are optional? Do all patients respond the same? What is a normal time to return to normal activities? To athletic activities? What does all this tell you about your upcoming surgery?

The shorter and easier a surgeon describes your recovery time, the less trauma that surgeon is causing to your tissues.

Patient Variations

All patients don't respond the same after surgery. Some have a higher tolerance for discomfort than others. Some don't have any tolerance at all—for any discomfort. Some follow instructions better than others. Some remember what they've learned better than others. Most are impatient for things to get back to normal regardless of how many times they've been told that tissue-healing takes time.

If you have a very low tolerance for discomfort, you will have a more difficult recovery. You're likely to request more pain medications and use them more frequently and longer. Pain medications make you sleepy while they make you comfortable; you won't get moving as well, and you may become constipated. It's always easier to take pain medications than to work through discomfort, but it's definitely not better. Optimal surgery lets you avoid strong, narcotic pain medicines, and most of all, makes your recovery a lot shorter and easier.

Pain medications are a very mixed blessing—the less the better, and the sooner you're off them, the better.

But despite patient variations, you can bank on the following:

The more you know what to expect, the easier your recovery.

The less trauma and bleeding during surgery, the faster and easier your recovery.

The better you follow instructions, the easier and less complicated your recovery.

The higher your discomfort tolerance, the more rapid your recovery.

The more rapidly you resume normal activities, the shorter your recovery.

Normal Activities

For the sake of discussion, let's define normal activities as

1. Lifting your arms above your head,

2. Lifting normal weight objects,

3. Driving your car,

4. Carrying out all normal (non-athletic) daily activities, and

5. Lying directly on your breasts.

Before your surgery, specifically ask when you can begin each of these activities. From the answers, you'll learn a lot about your upcoming surgery.

If you can't return to these normal activities within two weeks, something's not ideal. Tissue injury, low pain tolerance, too many pain medications, a complication—something!

If you can return to all normal activities in less than one week, you've probably made good choices of surgeon and techniques.

If you can return to all normal activities in less than four days, you and your surgeon are both doing well, but there's still room for improvement!

If you're able to return to normal activities within forty-eight hours or less, you and your surgeon are dynamite, and you just had a state-of-the-art surgical procedure!

Over 96 percent of our patients return to full, normal activities within twenty-four hours following their augmentations, even when placing the implant submuscular.[1,2]

If you're told that expecting to return to normal activities in less than four days is unreasonable and just won't happen, you might want to continue your surgeon search.

One of Our Typical Patients Describes Her Recovery . . .

The following letter was written by one of our patients to thank someone for providing information about us. It is reprinted with the patient's permission.

> _Jean:_
>
> _Here is a brief synopsis of my BA experience with Dr. Tebbetts. He was Fantastic. I flew in from the Midwest and arrived on a Thursday. I had my consultation with him that Thursday afternoon. I stayed with a friend of mine in Dallas, so we went out that evening, had dinner, and went home. The next morning, I went in at 7:45 for surgery. Even the waiting experience was pleasant. I waited in a comfortable recliner while I was being prepped for my surgery. I remember waking up immediately after surgery, and Dr. Tebbetts asked me to see if I_

could raise my arms above my head. I did it with no problem. That afternoon I went to the place where I was staying, with my friend, and I rested most of the day. However, I could change my own clothes (over my head) and do many other things with no problem. I took my prescribed medication that evening only. The next day (24 hours post-op) I took Advil and never took anything else beyond that. I showered, blow-dried my hair, went shopping, got dressed, all at 24 hours post-op. I remember that evening, I made myself a sandwich and had no problem reaching the bread, which was in a cabinet well above my head. When I flew home (48 hours post-op), my children were not feeling well, and I was able to squat down and pick up my 20-lb son with no problem. I'm now 4 days post-op and I have been sleeping on my side for the last two evenings. I must say that if I had to repeat this experience, I wouldn't change a thing. Dr. Tebbetts and his staff were very helpful and professional. I am extremely pleased with my choice. As for the look, the partial-submuscular, anatomical implants I received look great now, but I think that they will look even better when they drop in a few months. That's about it. Let me know if I can answer any other questions for you. Thanks again for helping me find Dr. Tebbetts!

Margaret

(Names are fictitious to protect patient privacy.)

This letter describes a typical experience for the vast majority of our patients. Because there is a normal variation in patients' tolerance to discomfort and their ability to follow our postoperative instructions, we can't guarantee this experience for every patient. But our commitment to patient education and the surgical techniques that we use in every case offer this type of experience to every augmentation patient.

Athletic Activities and Emotional Stress

Athletic activities and emotional stress increase your pulse rate. When your pulse rate rises, your blood pressure rises. A rise in blood pressure can cause internal bleeding in your breasts. Internal bleeding means another operation, tubes coming out of your body for a while, and a higher risk of capsular contracture. *It just isn't worth it!*

Athletic activities include any activity that causes your pulse rate to increase significantly (more than 20 percent above your resting pulse rate): running, fast walking, bicycling, aerobics of any kind, heavy or prolonged exercise of any sort.

Emotional stresses vary a lot, but the most likely involve personal relationships or severe job stresses. Believe it or not, these stresses can cause just as much pulse and blood pressure increase as athletic activities. Again, it's not worth it! Avoid emotional stress as much as possible.

Avoid athletic activities of any sort and severe emotional stress for at least two weeks following surgery.

You should be able to start a gradual return to normal exercise activities beginning two weeks after surgery. If it hurts, stop it and try again two days later. Your body is smarter than you. Listen to it!

If you aren't allowed to begin returning to athletic activities in less than four weeks, ask questions. Why not? What's going to happen? Ask other surgeons!

RECOVERY QUESTIONS . . . AND THE MESSAGE FROM THE ANSWERS

Before your surgery, ask questions about your recovery:

What will my recovery be like?

Will I have bruising?

Will I have drain tubes coming out of my body?

When can I return to normal activities, drive my car, lift normal objects, raise my arms above my head, etc.?

When can I bathe?

Do I need special bandages, bras, or binders?

When can I return to athletic activities?

The better the answers to these questions, the better you'll like your recovery and, likely, your result!

Ask Surgeons to Commit

If you get hedged answers to any of these questions from surgeons, persist. Ask the questions again. Ask for pinpoint answers. No surgeon can give absolute guarantees in any single case, but answers to these questions provide you with valuable information about what you can expect.

This subject isn't nuclear physics. Part of recovery is you, and part is your surgeon. What your surgeon does in the operating room can substantially affect your recovery. You can't see what the surgeon does in the operating room, but you can gain insight before surgery by asking about your recovery. Either way, once you choose your surgeon, the rest of recovery is up to you. *Your job will be easier if you make the right choice of a surgeon.*

THE NEXT STEP . . .

You've now done a major portion of your homework—learning information about every aspect of augmentation so that you'll have knowledge tools when you begin to consult surgeons. In the next chapters, we'll locate qualified surgeons and help you with the steps in consultation and decision-making.

References

1. Tebbetts, J. B. Achieving a predictable 24-hour return to normal activities after breast augmentation, part 1: refining practices using motion and time study principles. *Plast. Reconstr. Surg.* 109: 293-305, 2002.

2. Tebbetts, J. B. Achieving a predictable 24-hour return to normal activities after breast augmentation, part II: patient preparation, refined surgical techniques and instrumentation. *Plast. Reconstr. Surg.* 109: 293-305, 2002.

3. Tebbetts J. B., and Adams, W. P. Five critical decisions in breast augmentation using five measurements in five minutes: the high five system. *Plast. Reconstr. Surg.* 116(7): 2005-2016, 2005.

4. Tebbetts, J. B. Patient acceptance of adequately filled breast implants. *Plast. Reconstr. Surg.* 106(1): 139-147, 2000.

5. Tebbetts, J. B. A system for breast implant selection based on patient tissue characteristics and implant/soft-tissue dynamics. *Plast. Reconstr. Surg.* 109(4): 1396-1409, 2002.

6. Tebbetts, J. B. Dual plane (DP) breast augmentation: optimizing implant soft-tissue relationships in a wide range of breast types. *Plast. Reconstr. Surg.* 107: 1255, 2001.

PART III

USING YOUR INFORMATION:
CONSULTING SURGEONS AND MAKING DECISIONS

FINDING QUALIFIED SURGEONS:

WHO DO I CALL AND WHERE DO I GO?

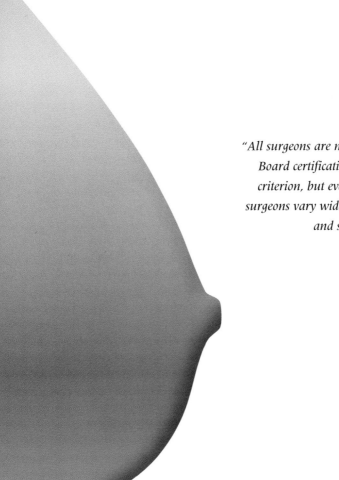

"All surgeons are not equally qualified. Board certification is an essential criterion, but even board certified surgeons vary widely in qualifications and skills."

The phone book is not the best resource! And in this new edition, we can tell you that the Internet is also not necessarily the best resource. Unfortunately, much of the "information" on the Internet by surgeons is purely advertisement that is often not backed by any track record that verifies their "expertise." You can certainly find names in both the phone book and on the Internet, but what you really need to know are 1) hard facts about a surgeon's credentials: education, training, and board certification and 2) documented evidence of a surgeon's experience—not just what the surgeon claims, but what the surgeon has published in respected scientific journals that document those claims.

Where did the surgeon train? How long? Is the surgeon board certified? By whom? What does board certification mean? What are the surgeon's other important credentials? Which credentials are important, and which are not? What are some important red flags? All of these questions involve surgeon credentials. Before you ever call a surgeon's office, you should check out the surgeon's basic credentials. Otherwise, you are more likely to waste valuable time and money or, worse yet, make poor decisions. Here are some things you need to know to check out a surgeon's credentials.

A SITUATION YOU'LL FIND DIFFICULT TO BELIEVE . . .

In most states in the United States, any physician who has completed four years of medical school and obtained an M.D. degree can legally advertise as a plastic surgeon or a neurosurgeon (brain surgeon) or any other type of surgeon without having obtained a single day of specialty training!

Any physician can call himself or herself a plastic surgeon! Legally!

Any licensed physician can advertise as a plastic surgeon without a day of specialty training in plastic surgery!

Any licensed physician can operate on you if you let them! Legally.

Can't happen, you say? It happens every day. Patients see an ad or hear a name, go to a surgeon, and submit to a procedure that changes their bodies forever. They do this without ever investigating the surgeon's credentials, without ever seeing more than one surgeon, without ever learning about the operation they're considering, and without confirming a surgeon's experience.

When a less-than-optimal outcome occurs (and _less-than-optimal_ covers everything from not so good to complete disasters), unbelievably, many patients allow the same surgeon to operate on them repeatedly—often without ever seeking another opinion or researching the surgeon's credentials! After the downhill slide (things often get worse with each reoperation), ultimately something or someone must get the blame. Incredibly, it's usually the breast implant or the last surgeon who operated trying to correct the problems! I've seen literally hundreds of such cases in my twenty-seven years of practice. Rarely have I seen a patient take responsibility for her lack of homework in selecting a surgeon.

Many patients spend more time shopping for a car than they spend selecting a plastic surgeon.

It's your body . . . you'll be looking at it for the rest of your life.

It's your job to select your surgeon. Don't complain later if you neglect your responsibilities.

Selecting your surgeon is the single most important thing you can do to assure an optimal result.

So, how do you go about it? The first step is to understand how a plastic surgeon is educated and what various credentials really mean. What is board certification? What does it mean? Board certified by whom? Some credentials are meaningful; many are less meaningful. Once you understand basic credentials, you can assemble a list of surgeons who have meaningful credentials. Then you'll need to shorten the list by looking past board certification to other useful information. After you shorten your list, you can begin calling surgeons' offices and requesting information. Your final decision and surgeon selection should be a combination of 1) credentials, 2) quality of information you receive (written and spoken), and 3) your experiences during your consultations. This chapter will introduce you to surgeon credentials and other useful tools to help you begin your search for a surgeon.

EDUCATING A PLASTIC SURGEON

After four years of college, most physicians complete four years of medical school to learn the basics of medicine. After medical school, most physicians who plan to specialize in a certain area then begin residency training. The length of residency training varies with the specialty. Plastic surgery and neurosurgery are among the longest residencies, requiring an additional six to eight years after medical school. Many board-certified plastic surgeons complete a five-year general surgery residency, then complete an additional two to three years of plastic surgery training.

Most plastic surgeons who are certified by the American Board of Plastic Surgery have completed six to eight years of specialty surgical residency training after medical school.

But remember! It is perfectly legal for a physician to set up a plastic surgery practice after four years of medical school without a single day of residency training in plastic surgery. Plastic surgery is an attractive specialty, and some physicians will shortcut the educational system any way possible. If a physician just skipped plastic surgery training (or some portion of it), the physician could begin doing plastic surgery six to eight years sooner—and could retire six to eight years sooner! It may be a great deal for the physician who may not even be aware of what he or she doesn't know, but it may not be a great deal for patients. Would you take your car for repair to a mechanic you knew started yesterday with no mechanic school or experience?

General practitioners perform plastic surgery. Dermatologists perform plastic surgery. Gynecologists perform plastic surgery. Ear, nose, and throat physicians (otolaryngologists) perform plastic surgery. Dentists perform plastic surgery. General surgeons perform plastic surgery. And the list goes on. Every specialty listed above has residency training, but none are as long or as comprehensive as plastic surgery residency. None focus on plastic surgery as much as a plastic surgery residency. Does that mean that none of these other specialists can do good plastic surgery? Not necessarily. But it's your job to decide how much training and experience you want your surgeon to have.

The following is my own perspective about surgical training. Many physicians who have completed medical school, with the help of a good book in the operating room (and some actually do this), can probably carry off a basic operation. If a physician has seen an operation performed several times or attended an instructional course of one or two days, so much the better. But neither compares with six to eight years of specialty training. Here's what I think:

A little plastic surgical training may be adequate for a basic operation when the patient expects only a basic result.

Do you really want only a basic result? You don't need in-depth surgical training until you need it!

A plastic surgeon with years of training has been there, seen that, done that, and, above all, doesn't panic when problems occur.

In surgery, the more you've seen, the more you know, and the better you deal with complex problems.

You don't see much in a weekend course or minimal residency training.

They don't put student pilots in the seat of the space shuttle for a reason. Training, training, training, experience, experience, experience. I can't imagine having too much!

If you're on the shuttle and it crashes, you don't have to worry about it. If lack of training and experience causes a problem with your plastic surgery, you'll get to look at it every day for the rest of your life!

Ask every surgeon specifically: How many years of residency training did you complete? In what specialty? In what location? Get the name of the residency program and the name of the surgeon who is in charge of that program.

Then check it out. Call the residency program and ask if the physician completed the program.

HOW NOT TO CHOOSE YOUR PLASTIC SURGEON

Just in case you don't want to read the rest of this chapter about sorting through surgeon credentials, you should at least know how not to pick a plastic surgeon. Here is a quick list:

- **The cost is much less with this surgeon.** You will largely get what you pay for, but even with higher prices, you should verify a lot more about the surgeon regarding matters that we will cover later in this chapter.

- **The surgeon was voted "Best in the City" by "The City" magazine.** Surgeons are provided space in magazines largely based on the amount of advertising dollars they spend with the magazine. Voting for "best physicians in a specialty" can be manipulated by surgeons and other physicians, health care organizations or corporations (to make their physicians look good), or by the magazine itself to make its advertiser surgeons happy. Unfortunately, the magazine never tells you how long it takes the surgeon to perform a breast augmentation (time in the operating room), how long it takes the surgeon's patients to recover (the best single question you can ask), how many reoperations the surgeon's patients require, how much experience the surgeon has, or whether the surgeon has published scientific articles in indexed, peer-reviewed medical journals. What is a simple solution? Ask your surgeon's hospital or surgical facility how long the surgeon usually requires to perform a breast augmentation. (That relates to your costs and the amount of drugs and anesthesia you'll receive and can significantly affect your recovery. The most skilled surgeons plan carefully before going to the operating room and execute the operation efficiently to optimize your safety and recovery.) Then ask your surgeon for confirmation of the surgeon's reoperation rates for breast augmentation. Those questions will quickly sort out self-proclaimed experts from true experts.

- **I was at a party and heard that the surgeon is good.** A large percentage of patients who think they have a great result may not realize how good a result they could have had if they had done more research and homework before having a breast augmentation. Ask them if they were able to go out to dinner the evening of surgery and resume full normal activities within twenty-four hours without taking any narcotic pain medications. (State-of-the-art decisions and surgical techniques routinely offer this type of recovery to patients.)

- **I had a friend who had surgery by the surgeon, and she thinks he's great.** You really don't know if you don't ask how long it took her to recover, how many reoperations she may have had, how long she's had her implants, or what her breasts look like without clothing or support.

- **I saw the surgeon on television.** Seeing a surgeon on television rarely proves anything, unless the surgeon is appearing on a credible educational channel where the surgeon cannot control the content of the program.

- **I went to a seminar and heard the surgeon speak.** Unless you have done considerable homework before attending the seminar, you have inadequate knowledge to judge what you hear from the surgeon. Continue reading this chapter.

BOARD CERTIFICATION—WHAT DOES IT MEAN?

Board certification can mean a lot, or it can mean nothing. A board can be nothing more than an individual or organization that will issue a certificate to anyone who pays a fee. Means absolutely nothing. Many different boards exist, but you need to sort out which mean something and which don't.

The key question to ask about board certification: Board certified by whom? By which board?

The American Medical Association's Board of Medical Specialties (ABMS) determines which boards are recognized as the most qualified boards to certify medical specialists in a specific specialty, including plastic surgery. You can access in-depth information about the ABMS at www.abms.org.

Currently, the AMA Board of Medical Specialties recognizes only one board to certify plastic surgeons— The American Board of Plastic Surgery (ABPS).

At the present time, the American Board of Plastic Surgery has the most stringent requirements for board certification in plastic surgery of any organization that certifies plastic surgeons. Other boards exist, but to my knowledge, none requires as much residency training, surgical experience, and rigorous examinations as the American Board of Plastic Surgery. Details of the requirements for certification can be found on the ABPS Web site at www.abplsurg.org.

How can I locate a plastic surgeon certified by the American Board of Plastic Surgery?

Plastic surgeons certified by the American Board of Plastic Surgery are listed in the directory published by Marquis Who's Who in cooperation with the American Board of Medical Specialties (ABMS). Instead of purchasing this expensive set of books, it's easier and cheaper to look up plastic surgeons in your area that are board certified by the American Board of Plastic Surgery on the following Web sites or at the following numbers:

- The American Society of Plastic and Reconstructive Surgeons at http://www.plasticsurgery.org/find_a_plastic_surgeon/ or call 1-888-4-PLASTIC (1-888-475-2784).

- American Society of Aesthetic Plastic Surgery at http://www.surgery.org/public/findasurgeon.php or call 1-888-ASAPS-11 (272-7711).

When you choose a surgeon who is a member of either of these organizations, the surgeon is certified by the American Board of Plastic Surgery. This means that the surgeon has graduated from an accredited medical school and completed at least five years of additional residency, usually three years of general surgery or its equivalent and two years of plastic surgery. (Many have completed six to eight years of residency training.) To be certified by the ABPS, a doctor must also practice plastic surgery for two years and pass comprehensive written and oral exams.

AFTER BOARD CERTIFICATION, THEN WHAT?

Board certification is not the only thing you should consider when selecting a surgeon.

Is board certification enough? What about experience?

Does board certification (even by the ABPS) guarantee you an expert in breast augmentation? Not necessarily. Board-certified plastic surgeons do a wide variety of procedures. Some focus on reconstructive surgery, some on cosmetic surgery, and others combine both in their practices. We mentioned earlier that experience is important, but there's no specific amount of experience that guarantees a good surgeon or a good result. A lot has to do with the personality of the surgeon, and you'll need to judge that during your consultation. In chapter 11, we'll give you more specific questions to ask your surgeon about experience, such as "What percentage of your practice is breast augmentation? How many augmentations do you average per year?" Based on what you've already learned about surgical options in chapter 6, you'll be able to quickly determine how much experience a surgeon has had with different augmentation options.

Subspecialization and the Surgeon's Curriculum Vitae

Some surgeons who perform only cosmetic surgery further specialize in specific types of cosmetic surgery. They will usually have more experience because that's what they do every day. They may have other credentials. Ask to see a copy of their curriculum vitae. It will list the surgeon's training in detail and all professional activities the surgeon has completed. Check out how many professional presentations the surgeon has given, courses taught to other surgeons, and professional papers published. Ask if they have a Web site, and check it out for content. (Almost all have a lot of fluff.)

Checking Out a Surgeon's Scientific Publications

A surgeon's curriculum vitae (and you should be able to easily obtain a copy from any surgeon's Web site), lists the surgeon's professional presentations and scientific publications. If a surgeon has not presented and published information that has been peer-reviewed and shared with other surgeons, does that necessarily mean that the surgeon isn't qualified? Absolutely not. But if a surgeon meets all of your other criteria *and* has presented and published extensively, it means that the quality of the surgeon's ideas has been recognized by colleagues who stringently review a surgeon's ideas and claims of experience.

First, two things you should understand: 1) What matters is not that a surgeon has published and presented, but *where* the surgeon published (what journals, and how respected the journals are), and 2) a surgeon's experience is nothing more than a claim until that experience is reviewed by peers (other specialized surgeons) and approved for publication.

A long printed list of scientific presentations and publications means absolutely *nothing* unless those presentations and publications have been to major groups of surgeons, subjected to very critical and thorough scientific review, and published in the most respected scientific journals.

How do you know which presentations and scientific publications are most significant? We're about to tell you.

The most respected scientific journals meet stringent criteria to assure the quality of what they publish. The most respected journal in plastic surgery with the largest circulation to surgeons worldwide is the *Plastic and Reconstructive Surgery* journal. This journal has the most demanding criteria and review processes of any journal that publishes information on plastic surgery. There are other journals that also focus on cosmetic surgery, but no other journal is as widely respected and no other journal has a track record of publishing the highest quality of peer-reviewed scientific articles as the Journal of *Plastic and Reconstructive Surgery.*

Index Medicus and its online counterpart, MEDLINE (the principal online bibliographic citation database of NLM's MEDLARS® system), are used internationally to provide access to the world's biomedical journal literature. The decision whether or not to index a journal for these services is an important one and is made by the director of the National Library of Medicine based on considerations of both scientific policy and scientific quality. The Board of Regents of the library sets policy for the library. The Literature Selection Technical Review Committee (LSTRC) has been established to review journal titles and assess the quality of their contents.

The most respected medical journals are indexed by Index Medicus and its online counterpart, MEDLINE. When a journal is indexed, a search of MEDLINE by medical professionals or by you will list scientific articles published in that journal. *If a journal is not indexed, the journal has not met the criteria for indexing that more respected journals have met.*

In order to become indexed, a journal must meet very tough criteria that assess the scientific quality of the information published in the journal. Details of the criteria and selection process for indexing can be found on the Internet at http://www.nlm.nih.gov/pubs/factsheets/jsel.html.

Some of the most respected medical journals in plastic surgery that have been approved for indexing include:

> *Plastic and Reconstructive Surgery*—by far the most respected source for information on cosmetic surgery and breast augmentation, in our opinion

> *Aesthetic Plastic Surgery*

> *Annals of Plastic Surgery*

> *British Journal of Plastic Surgery*

Although not peer-reviewed and indexed, one publication that has been widely respected by plastic surgeons for many years is *Clinics in Plastic Surgery*. This particular publication takes a specific topic, such as breast augmentation, and invites a wide range of specialists in that field to submit articles.

A comprehensive list of all currently indexed journals can be accessed on the Internet at

http://www.ncbi.nlm.nih.gov/entrez/linkout/journals/jourlists.cgi?typeid=1&type=journals&operation=Show

We are very proud that we have published more information and peer-reviewed scientific articles on the clinical aspects of breast augmentation than any surgeon in history. We are especially honored that we have produced more publications on clinical topics in clinical augmentation in *Plastic and Reconstructive Surgery* than has any other surgeon during the past decade.

Hospital Privileges

Another important way to assess a surgeon's credentials is to ask where the surgeon has hospital privileges. If a surgeon has hospital privileges at an accredited hospital in the community, it means that the surgeon's credentials have been reviewed by other surgeons and physicians before allowing the surgeon to operate in that hospital. Credentialing committees usually do much more homework than you can do. Many plastic surgeons operate in their own facilities, but to assure peer review of the surgeon, the surgeon should have hospital privileges. Call the hospital to be sure.

Professional Societies

There are many professional societies that use the name plastic surgery. But, like the various boards, some are more meaningful than others. The two major societies in plastic surgery that require members to be board certified by the American Board of Plastic Surgery are the American Society of Plastic and Reconstructive Surgeons (www.plasticsurgery.org or phone 1-888-4-PLASTIC [1-888-475-2784]) and the American Society of Aesthetic Plastic Surgery (www.surgery.org or phone 1-888-ASAPS-11 [272-7711]). Members of these societies also must adhere to a very stringent code of ethics and participate in continuing education. Other societies, including state and local societies, are less important when judging credentials.

Who's Who in America

Marquis Who's Who, in cooperation with the American Board of Medical Specialties (ABMS), publishes a directory of board-certified specialists with a summary of their credentials. This set of books is available at most libraries. *Who's Who in Medicine and Healthcare* is another publication that is available in libraries or on the Internet at **http://www.marquiswhoswho.com/products/HCprodinfo.asp.**

Best Doctors in America

The Best Doctors in America, published by Woodward/White, Inc., is also available at most libraries. Doctors are listed by specialty and by region. Combining *Who's Who* with *Best Doctors* gives you a good reference to locate experts in plastic surgery.

Recommendations from Friends

These recommendations can mean a lot or very little! Depends on the friend, how much she knows, and how much her surgeon educated her. If a friend is thrilled with her surgeon, ask why. Try to determine how much your friend really knows about augmentation. If you're impressed at the amount your friend learned from her surgeon, and even more importantly, if she returned to normal activities in less than forty-eight hours after her surgery, add the surgeon to your list.

CREDENTIALS AND SOURCES: A CHECKLIST

Credentials won't be the only thing you'll consider when selecting a surgeon. We'll cover a lot more in the coming chapters. But credentials are a start. Here's a useful checklist:

Essentials:

- Board certified by the American Board of Plastic Surgery

- Completed an approved residency training program in plastic surgery

- Member of ASPRS and ASAPS (see professional societies above)

- Has hospital privileges to do breast augmentation at an accredited hospital

- Curriculum vitae documents scientific presentations and publications

Cream on Top of the Essentials:

- Subspecializes in cosmetic surgery

- Subspecializes in breast augmentation

- Listed in *Who's Who*

- Listed in *Best Doctors in America*

- Recommended by a knowledgeable friend or physician

Not as Reliable:

- Advertisements

- Surgeon's Internet Web sites

- Web sites that market surgeons

- Media coverage

- General physician referral services (Most are paid by the surgeon to refer you.)

- Recommendations from anyone without in-depth knowledge about augmentation

Red Flags:

- Completed residency training in a specialty other than plastic surgery

- Certified in an unrelated specialty

- Not board certified by ABPS

- No hospital privileges

- Any false or misleading information—claims that aren't true

- Unwilling to answer questions about credentials

- Unwilling to provide access to curriculum vitae

You can check basic credentials without even calling a surgeon's office using the sources and references in this chapter. List the surgeons, check with the ASPRS and ASAPS, and check *Who's Who* for a summary of the surgeon's education and board certification. Use the checklist above to compare credentials. Shorten your list of surgeons based on credentials before you call their offices for information, and you'll save a lot of time.

What about surgeon "credentials" on the Internet?

In our opinion, the Internet has become more of a place for surgeons to market themselves than a source for credible information for patients. There is definitely some credible information on the Internet, but it is overwhelmed by self-serving, often paid advertisements by surgeons claiming to be "experts," a claim that is not backed up by a track record of peer-reviewed, scientific publications that truly measure their abilities against other surgeons.

If you seek a surgeon's name in your area through any Internet search engine or Web site, you should realize that the surgeon has almost certainly paid a fee to the entity sponsoring the Web site in order for the surgeon's name to be listed. In many cases, surgeons spend thousands of dollars to "purchase their way up the ladder of a Web site or search engine." None of those dollars necessarily correlate with a surgeon's skill or real expertise.

You should beware of all claims that you read on any Web site unless those claims are backed up by hard facts documenting the surgeon's credentials and experience, especially in peer-reviewed, scientific publications in indexed scientific journals, such as *Plastic and Reconstructive Surgery.*

What about Information on Internet "Bulletin Boards?"

Some of the best and the worst information can be found on bulletin boards.

The best information on bulletin boards? If you read of good patient experiences, especially when combined with a rapid (less than twenty-four hours) recovery, that information is usually meaningful.

The worst information on bulletin boards? If you read about a horror story, the best lesson you'll usually take away is that it's best to get it right the first time, and to do that, you've got to do your homework. Often the person telling the horror story didn't.

If you read about the "latest and greatest" implant or technique, you'd better dig deeper. There is a long list of latest and greatest that don't exist anymore, including peanut oil or soybean oil implants, Misti Gold implants, and great surgical techniques that were never published in an indexed scientific journal.

If you're looking at before-and-after pictures and anyone on a Web site tells you that you can make any type of good decision from a picture, they are insulting your intelligence. Just be sure you don't fall for it, or your intelligence may be speaking for itself! To better understand why, read our sections that tell you what pictures can and cannot tell you.

HAVING LOOKED AT CREDENTIALS, WHAT'S THE NEXT STEP?

Now you have a list of surgeons with good, basic credentials. The next step on the stairs is contacting the surgeon's office for information, not necessarily an appointment. In the next chapter, we'll supply guidelines of what to look for when you call for information and what to look for in the information you receive.

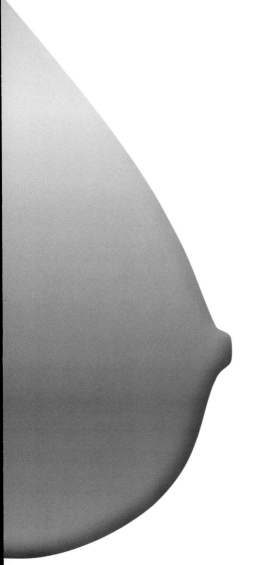

INFORMATION FROM SURGEONS' OFFICES:

GETTING AND EVALUATING IT

"A surgeon's habits are reflected in every aspect of the surgeon's practice. The quality and detail of a surgeon's information materials should tell you a lot about the surgeon."

You've obtained the names of several qualified surgeons, and you've checked their credentials. Now you're ready to call their offices and request information. Before you pick up the phone, do you know what to request? Do you know what questions to ask about breast augmentation? Do you want to simply request information, or would you like to spend some time on the phone talking with someone about breast augmentation? What do you hope to learn from your call? What would you like to get from the surgeon? To get the most from your time, you need answers to each of these questions—*before you call!* Other sources of information can also help: the Internet, the FDA, and implant manufacturers. Once you've gathered the information, what do you do with it? How do you evaluate information from surgeons? Before you visit a surgeon, gathering and evaluating information will make you better informed and better able to evaluate the surgeon during your consultation.

CALLING A SURGEON'S OFFICE

When a prospective augmentation patient calls our office, these are the three most commonly asked questions:

How much does it cost? Which way does the surgeon like to do it? Which type of implant does the surgeon use?

In our opinion, these three questions are not the most important things you should focus on during your first call to a surgeon's office. Yes, you may eventually want to know the answers to those questions. But initially, you might ask yourself, "Before I ask the price, is this a surgeon that I would even *consider*?" You can help answer this important question during your first phone call to a surgeon's office.

If you really want to start off asking questions that will tell you the most, ask: How long will it be after my surgery until I can do all my normal activities, such as lifting my arms above my head and lying with my full weight on my breasts?

When will I be able to drive my car and lift all normal-weight objects?

Will I have bandages, drains, or straps, and will I need narcotic pain medications?

Rather than asking questions on your first call to a surgeon's office, focus on listening.

Listen for three things in your first call to the office:

Courtesy, Service, and Knowledge.

Courtesy

How does the surgeon's office staff answer the telephone? If you select this surgeon, you'll be dealing with this staff before and after your surgery. Does the person who answers the phone have a name? What is it? Are you told? If not, I'd immediately hang up and try another surgeon!

Are you put on hold? For how long? Were you given a choice of a call back rather than holding? While wasting your time on hold (a discourtesy), is the surgeon trying to sell you additional operations with quasi-tasteful recorded commercials? Rather than listening to recorded commercials on hold, wouldn't it be nice to *get substance* and *information* without ever staying on hold? If your time is of no value to the surgeon now, how much more of your time will he or she waste in the course of caring for you?

Is the person on the other end of the line cheerful and enthusiastic, or is the attitude, "Yeah, what do you want?" Is the person appreciative that you chose to call this office? After all, you will be paying a substantial amount of money and could potentially refer more patients.

Is the person listening to you and your questions (a courtesy)? Or does the person immediately launch into something that sounds like a recorded answering machine, giving you answers to questions you didn't ask and don't need to know? What should you listen for?

> **We're glad you called us. We respect your time. I am listening to you. I want to give you information that will help you make the best decisions, whether you come to see us or not. I'm going to do everything I can to help you and make you want to come and see us.**

Service

Plastic surgery, especially cosmetic plastic surgery, is a service-oriented business. At least, it should be. You aren't sick. You don't require emergency care. You are choosing to have an operation that is not medically necessary, taking certain risks, and spending a considerable amount of money in the process. Why shouldn't you expect good service?

> **Service in plastic surgery means meeting your needs now, during your first call!**

To meet your needs, a surgeon's personnel must first show the courtesy of listening to your needs. What information are you seeking? What are you trying to achieve? If they don't listen or they immediately try to sell you two more operations or services you didn't ask for, beware!

Service means making things easy for you. Is every single word or question difficult? If you ask whether the surgeon does augmentation, does it take a while to receive the answer? Does every question seem to be an imposition or a problem? Does the person offer to send you information? Is it sent in a timely manner? Did someone call to be sure you received it? The only message you should hear is:

I want to make this easy for you. I want to help you whether you come to see us or not. Let's get started.

But what if you don't really know what you need?

One of the highest forms of service is helping you understand what you might need in a knowledgeable, friendly, no-pressure manner.

Another highest form of service is to provide information that can help you make the best decisions regardless of which surgeon you choose.

Which brings us to our next important point . . .

To help you understand your needs, a surgeon's staff must give you good information using terms that are easy to understand—and that requires knowledge!

Knowledge

One of the very best ways to judge a surgeon is to listen carefully to the surgeon's staff. The staff is a reflection of the surgeon.

I've never seen a highly knowledgeable staff that worked for an average-level surgeon.

It's difficult and time consuming for a surgeon to hire, train, and keep knowledgeable staff. If you find a knowledgeable, courteous, helpful staff, it probably didn't happen by accident. The kind of person who trained that staff is likely the kind of person you'd want doing your surgery!

You won't believe how easy it is to distinguish fact from fluff in plastic surgery. All you need to do is listen.

If it sounds too good to be true, it usually is. Is the surgeon trying to tell you there's only one best way to do augmentations? You already know that's not true. Is everything all roses with no thorns—all benefits with no trade-offs? You already know that no surgical option is without trade-offs. Does the surgeon tell you all augmentations are done a certain way? If so, you already know the surgeon is doing some of them wrong. Is the surgeon or staff willing to honestly and frankly discuss risks and trade-offs?

Are the surgeon and the surgeon's staff telling you things you need to know?

Are the surgeon and staff giving you information that will help you even if you choose another surgeon?

Does the answer sound reasonable? Pertinent?

When you ask a question, is there a huge void on the other end of the line when it comes to substance, or do you want to pick up a pen and take some notes? Do the minutes pass quickly on the phone? Do you feel you are really learning something useful?

Are the surgeon and the surgeon's staff willing to spend time with you?

Knowledge doesn't come quickly. Repetition is important if you really want to retain the most information and make the best decisions.

Are you getting the feeling that the person on the other end of the line would rather be doing anything rather than talking to you? Do you feel rushed? When you ask a question, do you hear a deep sigh that implies, "Are you really going to ask me another question?" Or does the person make you feel like you can ask all the questions you want—they'll be happy to spend any amount of time required to answer them. If the office is extremely busy, do they offer to call you back at a mutually agreeable time to spend more time answering your questions? No office is perfect at every one of these items, but some are definitely more nearly perfect than others.

Do the surgeon and the surgeon's staff help you even if you don't really need an operation or if this surgeon is not the best doctor to do your operation?

The ultimate in service and knowledge is not selling you an operation you don't need.

Am I dreaming, suggesting that any surgeon's office might, in good faith and with nothing to gain, refer you to another surgeon or help you with a nonsurgical service rather than suggesting an operation? It can happen. But don't hold your breath because it's rare. I've actually heard a well-known plastic surgeon say, "If they call my office, I assume they're looking for an operation, and I'm here to see that they get one!" That's not good service. That's greed.

Does the surgeon offer you an opportunity to come into the office and spend a considerable amount of time with a patient educator at no charge?

Surgeons who use patient educators almost always have better informed patients. No surgeon can spend as much time with every patient as a staff of patient educators. The best plastic surgery practices want to help you understand as much as possible. You'll often find that you are more comfortable with a patient educator than with the surgeon. If you're more comfortable, you'll listen better and learn more. If given the opportunity, take it!

Is the surgeon's staff willing to help guide you in the decision process?

Knowledgeable staff people are interested in helping you make the best decisions so that you and the surgeon can make the best team decisions. The more they know about the different options, the better they can help you understand which options are realistic for you, helping guide you in the decision-making process. The very best staff people also always know when to stop and never exceed the limits of their knowledge. There is always a point where the only correct answer is "You'll need to discuss that with the doctor. That's something that the two of you will decide after your consultation and examination."

Are you offered an opportunity to look at before-and-after pictures and speak with other patients if you desire?

We've already covered some of the pros and cons of before-and-after pictures. The most important thing to remember is that no other patient is just like you and that no picture (unless it has a ruler in the picture) can accurately estimate the three most important things when choosing implant size: 1) the base width of the breast, 2) tissue stretch, and 3) the amount of breast tissue present before the augmentation. Nevertheless, you want to be a bit skeptical if a surgeon can't or won't show you examples of results. Speaking with other patients can also be helpful. Not that you'll have the same experience, but hearing from another patient can sometimes make you more comfortable.

COSTS: HOW DO THEY EXPLAIN THEM?

When you ask about costs, are the costs broken down or all lumped together? Are there different costs for different procedures and different types of implants? Although a package price may seem attractive, you don't really know what you're paying for. Costs should be broken down by surgeon fees, implant costs, laboratory fees, mammogram fees, electrocardiogram fees, anesthesia fees, surgery facility costs, and any hidden costs such as preoperative and postoperative medications. Just ask about costs, and see how much detail you hear. Ask about each item separately. Is each item included in the price you were quoted?

WHAT TO ASK AND WHAT TO ASK FOR: A LIST OF QUESTIONS

When you first call a surgeon's office, the following questions will help you get what you need: 1) spoken answers that help you evaluate courtesy, service, and knowledge, and 2) written informational materials.

When you ask the following questions, listen carefully to the answers! Take notes, and keep the answers organized by surgeon. The answers are key to making good decisions when selecting a surgeon:

1. I'm interested in getting information about breast augmentation. Does Dr. X do breast augmentation?

2. How does Dr. X do breast augmentation?

3. Tell me what recovery is like for Dr. X's average patient? What about drains, bandages, straps, special bras, and pain medications, and when can I return to all my normal activities?

4. Could you send me some information about breast augmentation and about Dr. X and your practice?

5. What are the risks involved in having breast augmentation?

6. What are the costs of a consultation?

7. Do you have before-and-after photographs that I could see?

8. Would it be possible to speak with other patients of Dr. X who have had augmentations?

9. How long has Dr. X been in practice?

10. How many augmentations does Dr. X do every year?

11. Does Dr. X limit his practice to cosmetic surgery?

12. Where does Dr. X have hospital privileges?

13. Is Dr. X board certified? By which board?

14. How much will my augmentation cost?

After asking these questions, evaluate the answers. Did you get a little or a lot of information? Is the information quality or fluff?

EVALUATING WRITTEN INFORMATION YOU RECEIVE
FROM SURGEONS

When you receive written information from a surgeon, read it carefully. That's part of your job. At least 30 percent of patients never read information they receive. If you don't read it, you can't use the knowledge to make better decisions.

In later chapters, we will emphasize repeatedly that:

A surgeon's habits are reflected in everything a surgeon does. All you need to do is notice.

Informational materials reflect a surgeon's habits and commitment to educating patients.

What should you look for in written information and brochures? The following are some guidelines:

Is the information generic, or did the surgeon write the information personally?

If it's generic, you can tell. You'll probably see the same thing from other surgeons.

Is the information just the surgeon's opinion, or is it documented by scientific studies published by the surgeon that confirm the surgeon's opinions and support the surgeon's stated experience?

There is nothing wrong with just an opinion, but if it's not based on documented experience and has not been subjected to review by other surgeons, the opinions may not be as valid as the opinions of a surgeon who has met those stringent criteria.

Does it appear and sound distinctively different compared to other surgeons' information? If it doesn't sound different, it probably isn't much different. What might that say about your result?

What do the informational materials tell you about the surgeon's habits? Is the surgeon compulsive and different? Better? What might that say about your surgery?

Does the information contain substance or fluff? If you took away the fancy book, what does it SAY? Fluff with little substance? What might that say about the surgeon?

Does the information address most or all of your questions and concerns? How well?

If only 50 percent of the answers are there, what might that say about the percent of knowledge?

Is the information written in easy-to-understand language? And at the same time, is it informative? Can you study deeper and get more information if you'd like to?

If not, why not? Does the surgeon not know enough, or not care enough, or both?

THE INTERNET AS A SOURCE OF INFORMATION

Information from the Internet should be scrutinized using the same criteria as spoken and written information from surgeons. The questions listed earlier in this chapter apply to Internet information as well as spoken and written information.

Many individual plastic surgeons have Web sites. When visiting these sites, continually ask these questions:

How much is substance, and how much is fluff?

Is the surgeon a self-declared expert, or has the surgeon's expertise been supported by peer-reviewed scientific articles supporting the surgeon's opinions and confirming the surgeon's experience? The most respected professional journal in plastic surgery is **Plastic and Reconstructive Surgery.**

Have I seen and heard this before?

Is anything different?

Check all Internet information against surgeon credentials obtained from sources listed in this chapter and in chapter 9.

RED FLAGS IN INFORMATIONAL MATERIALS AND SPOKEN ANSWERS

If you read or hear any of the following, beware! Every statement listed here is an actual statement that a patient has told us she heard from a surgeon or a surgeon's staff.

Red Flag 1—Regarding Training

Oh, don't worry about formal plastic surgery residency training. Dr. X did special training in cosmetic surgery under Dr. Y and Dr. Z, world-famous cosmetic surgeons. Now he's the best in the world!

Dr. X is specially trained in cosmetic surgery, not plastic surgery.

I know that Dr. X is a dentist, but breasts are sometimes found in the mouth! Ha, Ha! That's why he does breast augmentations!

You don't need six years of training to do breast augmentations. It's a simple operation!

Red Flag 2—Regarding Credentials

Dr. X doesn't operate in any hospitals, so he doesn't need hospital privileges.

Dr. X is certified by the X!*$$$$ board of plastic surgery—the most famous board in the world! (Check to assure that the board certifying the surgeon is recognized by the American Board of Medical Specialties.)

Dr. X has only been in practice two months, but he's invented a completely new procedure for breast augmentation that is the most advanced in the world!

You don't need to worry about credentials. Dr. X has operated on five *Playboy* models and six famous actresses! Sorry, we can't give you their names! But you see his work in *Playboy* and *Penthouse* all the time!

Red Flag 3—Regarding Scientific Publications by a Surgeon

Scientific publications don't have anything to do with good surgery. Many good surgeons never publish scientific articles. (They may not, but if they don't, their opinions and experience have not been subjected to review and scrutiny by other expert surgeons in the field, so what you're getting is just one surgeon's opinion and statement of experience.)

Red Flag 4—Picking an Implant Size

Bring us a picture of the breasts you like, and Dr. X can make them for you!

Go buy a bra that's the size you'd like to be, and bring it with you to the office. We'll let you put implants in the bra and choose the size you'd like to be! (See chapters 4, 5, and 6.)

Fill your bra with panty hose. When it's full, take the panty hose out and soak them in water. Squeeze out the water and measure it. That's the size, we'll select for your implants!

Try on some breast enhancers in a bra size you'd like to be. Tell us the size, and we'll match your breast implant to it!

Fill plastic baggies with water (or peas, or anything else) and stuff them into a bra size you'd like to be. Bring them to the office with you, and we'll measure how much water is in the baggy and match your implant to that size!

Red Flag 5—Sending You Information

You won't need any written information. We'll tell you everything you need to know when you come in. It'll only take fifteen minutes.

Information? Sure we've got information we can send you! (Funny, it never arrives. Or if it does, it may only consist of a trifold from a generic source.)

You can get all the information you need on Dr. X's Web site (sure, at www.whatinfo, justfluff.com or believemeIamtheexpert.com).

We're just going to send you some brochures from the most prestigious plastic surgery society in the world.

You don't need any special information. Breast augmentations are pretty much all the same. Come on in, and we can get you taken care of!

Red Flag 6—Selling You What You Didn't Ask About

Breast augmentation? Sure, we do that! But you'll probably want to think about liposuction and a facelift, too!

You don't want to just do your breasts. You'll need some liposuction to perfectly balance your figure!

Your breasts will look so good that no man can look you in the face unless we get you on our special skin care program and do a facelift!

With those nice, tight breasts, you won't want to be seen with those loose facial wrinkles and frown lines. Why don't we get you on our program of collagen, hyaluronic acid, and/or botox injections for your frown lines and when those don't work very well, we can always sign you up for a facelift!

Red Flag 7—Discounts

Sure, we have discounts. How much can you pay?

If you choose two other operations at the same time as your breast augmentation, we can give you a huge discount!

We can offer you some nice, cheap implants. And by the way, we do charge for the operation when they need to be replaced.

(This list could go on forever, but you get the messages!)

THE NEXT STEP . . .

Having gathered and evaluated information from the list of surgeons with good credentials, now you're ready to decide which surgeons you want to see in consultation and prepare for the consultations well in advance.

CONSULTING WITH A PLASTIC SURGEON:

PREPARING AND DOING IT

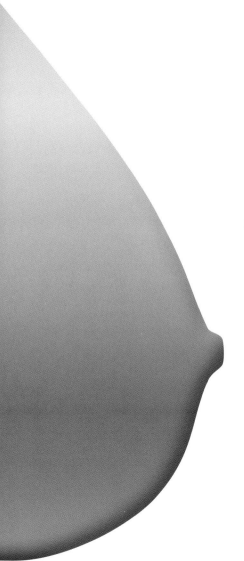

"A surgeon's habits are reflected in the surgeon's staff, information materials, office organization, and thoroughness, and in the logic of what the surgeon tells you. Look, listen, and ask yourself if these are the characteristics you want in your surgeon."

You've obtained names of surgeons (hopefully more than one), and you've checked their credentials (chapter 9). You narrowed the list based on credentials, then gathered and evaluated information from each of their offices (chapter 10). You narrowed the list again. Now it's time for the main event—your consultation with plastic surgeons. Notice I said plastic surgeons—plural. You're cheating yourself if you don't consult more than one. No matter how great you may think one is, you don't really know if you don't compare!

MAKING APPOINTMENTS

Complimentary Consultations with a Patient Educator

Most busy, experienced surgeons offer complimentary consultations with a nurse or patient educator prior to seeing the patient. A patient-educator consultation is a great opportunity for you for the following reasons:

- You have an opportunity to learn more before you see the surgeon.

- You'll be able to make better use of your time with the surgeon.

- You'll probably communicate better with most patient educators than with most surgeons.

- You have an opportunity to evaluate the surgeon, and, in general, the better the patient educator, the better the surgeon.

- You have an opportunity to save money on a surgeon consultation if anything is not right for you (the procedure, the information you hear or don't hear, what you hear about your recovery, how you're treated, and whether you're subjected to hard-sell techniques).

Most patient educators are willing to spend as much time with you as necessary, usually at least 30-45 minutes. The benefit is that you have that much additional time to gain information before you see the surgeon—regardless of how much time the surgeon spends with you!

If you have an opportunity to consult a patient educator before consulting the surgeon—do it! The best surgeons will almost always offer this service because they want you to know as much as possible.

Don't See the Surgeon Until You're Prepared

After visiting with patient educators in different surgeons' offices, you'll have a totally different perspective. There's a good chance you'll shorten your surgeon list, saving money and time in the process, based solely on your visit with the patient educators.

Don't make an appointment to see a surgeon until you're prepared. We'll give you a specific checklist later.

The more prepared you are before meeting with a surgeon, the better you'll understand the surgeon, and the better you can evaluate the surgeon.

Best Times for Appointments

Your best chance for a thorough consultation is at a time when the surgeon is least likely to be rushed. Many surgeons operate in the morning and see patients in the afternoons. Ask if appointments are available in the morning or any time on a day when the surgeon is not operating. You won't sit in the waiting room as long.

Be on Time

It's reasonable to expect a surgeon to respect your time. It's also reasonable to respect the surgeon's time. The surgeon has set aside time to see you. If you're late, your consultation will either be more rushed, which usually happens, or you totally disrupt the schedule for the surgeon and all of the other patients being seen that day.

Call If You Can't Make It

When you make an appointment with any professional and don't cancel if you can't make it, you are wasting that professional's time. Always call if you can't make it or need to change an appointment time. Most offices will appreciate your calling and be happy to make another appointment.

SEEING WHAT THEY DON'T TELL YOU—THINGS TO NOTICE

The Surroundings

A surgeon's office doesn't need to look like the Taj Mahal. If it does, you're paying for it.

You're not going to a museum or estate. You're going to see a surgeon. Statues, art, and expensive furniture don't tell you a thing about the quality of surgery you'll get, but guess who gets to pay for the décor? You!

A quiet, comfortable atmosphere that reflects good taste is all that's required. Anything more, and you're paying extra for the décor.

If the office looks like it may not belong to a plastic surgeon, there's a message. An overly "medical" appearing office is not typical of cosmetic surgery offices. Do you want someone operating on you that doesn't do those procedures very often?

The Organization

Watch the flow of the office and the flow of patients. Does it appear well organized, or does it look like feeding time at a zoo? The organization and function of a surgeon's office should tell you a lot. If it's a zoo, just ask yourself how organized the surgeon is.

The organization, function, and flow of every surgeon's office is a reflection of the surgeon's habits.

Ask yourself if you want someone with these habits operating on you.

Information versus Pressure Sales

Look around the office. Are you barraged at every turn with something trying to sell you another operation or service? Informational materials can be valuable, provided they aren't the same materials you see in other offices (generic materials personalized with a surgeon's name). As you look at materials and displays in an office, ask yourself:

Are they trying to inform me or trying to sell me? If you're sold by good information, that's fine. That's what you're looking for.

Does the Surgeon Respect Your Time?

If you're on time and the surgeon keeps you waiting excessively, ask why. Problems can occur in surgery, and patients before you want to talk about three more procedures than the one for which they made an appointment. But some surgeons are chronically late without a reasonable explanation.

> ### *If everything else about your experience with the surgeon is great, and the surgeon keeps you waiting, you may be satisfied by an apology.*

Our policy is that if we keep you waiting for a surgeon consultation longer than ten minutes, you will not be charged for your consultation regardless of the reason. You won't get excuses. You'll get a free consultation. If more surgeons adopted that policy, more patients would be treated more courteously.

Remember that with the best of intentions, if a patient before you needs to ask more questions or has a condition that demands more time that the surgeon didn't know about, your time with the surgeon may be delayed. Although we absolutely try to see that this doesn't happen, it sometimes even happens to us.

BEFORE-AND-AFTER PICTURES, COMPUTER IMAGING

In chapter 4, we discussed window shopping for breasts and the relative advantages and risks of using before-and-after pictures and computer imaging to make decisions. If you didn't read that section before, do it now! When you look at pictures or computer images, use the following checklist:

❏ Repeat the following sentence three times to yourself: "I cannot possibly make valid decisions by looking at any type of pictures of someone else." We know you would like to, but it's categorically impossible! If you or your surgeon fool yourself into thinking you can, you're both responsible for what may occur later.

❏ I must remember that if there's not a ruler in the picture, the picture cannot tell me anything about the three most important factors that affect appropriate size of breast implant: the base width of the breast, tissue stretch, and the amount of breast tissue present before the augmentation.

❏ Did the person in the picture look exactly like me before the operation? If not, I'm not going to look like her after my operation even if everything is done exactly the same. Even if she did, her tissue stretch is different, and my result won't match hers.

❏ Did the surgeon look at a magazine picture you brought and say, "Sure, we can make that breast! No problem!"? If so, consult other surgeons.

❏ Did the surgeon say, "I'll use the pictures to help me understand what you'd like, and then I'll try to help you understand our best options and trade-offs, given your tissues"? If so, GREAT!

❏ Were you given some excuse why there were no pictures for you to see? If so, consult other surgeons.

❏ Does every result look good? If so, you aren't seeing a range of results. Consult other surgeons.

❏ Did the book not contain a wide variety of breasts with some results better than others? If not, consult other surgeons.

❏ Did the surgeon or staff fully answer any question you asked about the pictures? If not, consult other surgeons.

❏ What about the quality of the pictures? Are they standardized? Good quality? Is the background consistent in all the pictures? A surgeon's habits are also reflected in the quality of the picture as well as the quality of the result.

❏ If you looked at computer images, remember that a technician can produce changes on a computer that no surgeon can produce with living tissue.

❏ If the surgeon uses the imager to help you understand some points, fine. If a technician or the surgeon uses the imager to try to sell you something that doesn't make sense or sell you other nonbreast operations, beware.

❏ If the surgeon morphs (changes the appearance of) your breasts on the computer and prints you a simulated before-and-after picture, don't look at it too much and try not to fix the image in your mind. Your result definitely won't match the image.

❏ Don't count on getting the result you've seen from imaging. Once you've seen a simulated result, you tend to expect that result even if the computer screen is covered with disclaimers informing you that this is only a simulation.

❏ If you used any type of software or a Web site to make choices of breast implant size or type, you are ignoring critical aspects of matching your implant to the stretch and dimensions of your tissues

PREPARING FOR MY VISIT—A CHECKLIST FOR MY CONSULTATION

Are You Ready for a Consultation?

If you can check all of the items on the following checklist, you're ready to consult with a plastic surgeon.

❏ I've read chapters 1 through 10.

❏ I made a list of surgeons and verified credentials.

❏ I called surgeons' offices and requested informational materials.

❏ I evaluated surgeons' staffs on the phone.

❏ I specifically asked in detail about what to expect while recovering from my augmentation and when I could return to normal activities.

❏ I've gathered information from at least three surgeons with solid credentials, good informational materials, and knowledgeable staffs.

❏ I took advantage of visits with patient educators.

❏ I've made a specific list of questions I want to ask the surgeon.

Questions to Ask Every Surgeon during the Consultation

If you don't already know the answers, review chapters 1–10. Ask the questions and take notes about the answers. You can review your notes and refer back to this book later.

❏ In what specialty was your residency training? How many years? Are you board certified? By whom?

❏   How long have you been in practice?

❏   Do you have hospital privileges? Where?

❏   How many breast augmentations have you done, and how many do you perform each year?

❏   What are the three most important things you'd advise me to think about with regard to breast augmentation?

❏   What is your preferred incision location? Why? How many of each location have you done? Can you show me pictures?

❏   Which do you prefer, over or under muscle? Why? When do you feel a dual-plane approach is appropriate? Do you perform over, under, and dual plane? How many of each have you done?

❏   What is your preferred implant? Why? Do you offer all different types of implants?

❏   Do you prefer round or anatomic implants? Why? Do you offer both? How many of each have you done?

❏   If you prefer round implants, how do you deal with the fill issue?

❏   Are round implants adequately filled with saline or silicone to prevent shell folding?

❏   Do you think shell folding can affect the life of the shell?

❏   If we overfill a round, saline-filled implant, are you willing to guarantee the implant if the manufacturer does not? What happens if my implant fails?

❏ What are the three worst things that can happen following my augmentation? What are the chances they will happen? Exactly what do we do in each case if they happen? What are the costs involved? Time off work, worst possible scenario?

❏ Would you ever recommend implant removal without replacement? If so, why? What affects how my breast will look if we had to remove implants?

❏ Does the size of the implant we choose affect my tissues as I get older? How?

❏ Do you charge me to replace my implant if it ruptures? Is there anything that can occur that you would charge me for in the future, including follow-up visits or surgery?

❏ Will anyone else perform any part of my surgery? Are they more qualified than you?

❏ When can I lift my arms above my head, drive my car, and lift my children or other objects?

❏ Will I have drains?

❏ Will I have bruising?

❏ Will I wear special bandages, bras, or binders? For how long?

❏ Why should I choose you to do my surgery?

Things to Notice during the Surgeon's Examination

❏ Is the surgeon organized?

❏ Did the surgeon or surgeon educator explain to you the key factors that neither the surgeon nor you can control following surgery (infection, capsular contracture, tissue stretch, etc.)? This important information is included later in this chapter.

❏ Does the surgeon explain what he or she is doing during the examination?

❏ Does the surgeon measure your breasts? Measurements demonstrate minor differences that even the most experienced surgeon cannot see by simply looking at the breasts, and remember, a surgeon cannot improve what a surgeon cannot see. Some of the basic measurements are illustrated in Figure 11-1, A–D.

❏ Does the surgeon use a precise record in your chart where measurements and details are recorded while you are being examined? An example of our clinical evaluation sheet used during the examination is illustrated in Figure 11-2.

❏ Does the surgeon demonstrate and discuss the specific characteristics of your tissues during the exam and how those tissue characteristics might affect your options and results?

❏ Does the surgeon explain during the exam how the width of the breast implant you choose might affect the result, depending on the width and amount of breast tissue that you have before surgery?

❏ Does the surgeon stretch your skin and measure the amount of stretch?

❏ Does the surgeon point out limitations of your tissues that might affect your choice of implant size or width?

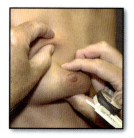 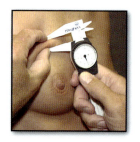

A. Thickness of tissue over implant

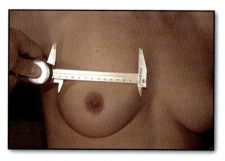

B. Base width of breast.

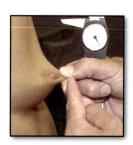 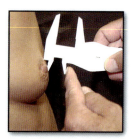

C. Skin stretch.

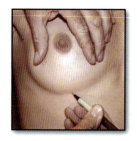 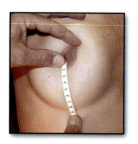

D. Nipple to inframammary fold distance.

FIGURE 11-1

Augmentation Mammaplasty Clinical Evaluation for _____

Patient Preferences, Objectives, Preparation, History, Limitations, Exam, Surgical Choices

Size: Pt. Desires: ❏ Natural appearing breast ❏ Unnatural, bulging upper breast ❏ Proportionate to protect tissues ❏ Very large Approximate Desired Cup _____ Requests specific cc's _____ ❏ Pt.Chooses Size ❏ Pt. Leaves Size Choice to Dr. Tebbetts
Implant: ❏ Round ❏ Anatomic ❏ Smooth ❏ Textured ❏ Saline ❏ Silicone ❏Pt. Leaves Type Choice to Dr. Tebbetts
Pocket Location: ❏PRP ❏RM ❏Dr. Tebbetts to decide
Incision Location: ❏IM ❏PA ❏AX ❏UMB
❏Pt. Leaves Incision Choice to Dr. Tebbetts Pts. Initials _____

Capsular Contracture and Tissue Stretch Factors:
❏ Implant choice may affect risk
❏Pt.accepts full responsibility for all costs for any surgery necessary to treat any capsule or tissue stretch deformities and costs exceed costs of original surgery Pts. Initials _____

Patient Has Completed, Read and Signed:
❏ Pt. Educator Consult ❏ Choice Documents
❏The Best Breast Book Pt. Ed. Initials: _____
Discussed/Patient Accepts That:
❏ Implants will be removed/not replaced if one infection or 2 capsular contracures occur
❏ The larger the implant , the more risks of sensory loss, tissue damage, and need for reoperations Pts. Initials _____

Age _____
Height _____ Wt._____lbs
Frame: ❏ Sm ❏ Med ❏ Lrg
Torso: ❏ NI ❏ Wide ❏ Nr
Gravida _____
Para _____
Bra **Band** Size: 32, 34, 36
Breast **Cup** Size (Approx.)
Prior to pregnancy_____
Largest with preg _____
Current Cup Size _____
Desired Cup Size _____
Previous Breast Disease:
❏ None
Biopsies: ❏ No ❏ Yes
_____
Family Hx. Breast Cancer
❏ No ❏ Yes
Mother Grandmother Aunt
❏ Maternal ❏ Paternal

Previous Mammograms:
❏ No ❏ Yes
Date: _____
Interpretation: ❏ Normal
❏ Other: _____
Pertinent Medical History:
❏ None

Smoker: ❏ No ❏ Yes _____
Allergies: ❏ NKA

Current Meds, Herbs, Vits:
_____
_____
_____
Companion: _____
Relation: _____

Specific Limitations Discussed with Patient:
❏ Your breasts will never match
❏ You may lose some or all sensation
❏You may see or feel edges of your implant due to thin tissues
❏ You may require reoperations and additional costs in the future due to implant size requested , your tissue stretch characteristics or capsule you form
❏ We give no guarantee of cup size
❏Any reoperation may require an inframammary incision
❏ Other: _____
_____
❏ Patient vocalizes under-standing and acceptance of all items checked above. Pt. Initials _____

Breast Masses
❏ None
❏ Size and Location:
_____
_____
Larger Breast:
❏ Left ❏ Right
Est. Vol. Diff. _____ cc TBD
Nipple Level
Discrepancy _____ cm N/A
IMF Level
Discrepancy _____ cm N/A
Envelope Compliance
❏ NI ❏ Inc ❏ Dec
❏ Constricted Lower Env.
❏ Short, fixed IMF
❏ Other:

Prioritized Decisions Based on Breast Measurements and Tissue Characteristics
The High Five™ System   Copyright 2005   John B. Tebbetts, M.D.

I. POCKET LOCATION SELECTED BASED ON THICKNESS OF TISSUE COVERAGE (Circle One)

| STPTUP | If <2.0 cm., consider dual plane (DP) or partial retropectoral (PRP), pectoralis origins intact across IMF) | DP |
| STPTIMF | If STPTIMF <0.5 cm, consider subpectoral pocket and leave pectoralis origins intact along IMF | PRP   RM |

II. IMPLANT VOLUME/WEIGHT BASED ON BREAST DIMENSIONS, TISSUE STRETCH, AND EXISTING PARENCHYMA

Base Width	B.W. Parenchyma (cm)	10.5	11.0	11.5	12.0	12.5	13.0	13.5	14.0	14.5	15.0	
	Initial Volume (cc)	200	250	275	300	300	325	350	375	375	400	
APSS$_{MaxStr}$	^{2}If APSS < 2.0, - 30cc; If APSS > 3.0, + 30cc; If APSS > 4.0, +60cc Place appropriate number in blank at right											cc
N:IMF$_{MaxSt}$	If N:IMF > 9.5, + 30cc Place appropriate number in blank at right											cc
PCSEF %	If PCSEF < 20%, +30cc; If PCSEF > 80%, - 30cc Place appropriate number in blank at right											cc
IDFDD cc	If Inamed Style 468, -30cc Place appropriate number in blank at right											cc
Pt. request												cc
NET ESTIMATED VOLUME TO FILL ENVELOPE BASED ON PATIENT TISSUE CHARACTERISTICS												cc
III. IMPLANT TYPE MFR:	STYLE/MODEL:					VOLUME:						cc

Volume: N:IMF Relationships		200	250	275	300	325	350	375	400	PreN:IMF
		7.0	7.0	7.5	8	8	8.5	9.0	9.5	cm
IV. NEW INFRAMAMMARY FOLD LEVEL	N:IMF$_{MaxSt}$ to set with preoperative markings and intraoperatively									cm
V. INCISION LOCATION (Circle One)				IM	AX	PA	UMB			

Breast Dimension Ranges (cm)				McGhan 468 Anatomic			Mentor Siltex Textured Round			Mentor Smooth Round			McGhan 410 FM		
Cup Size	A.D.	A:IMF	N:IMF	Base	Proj	Vol	Base	Proj	Vol	Base	Proj	Vol	Base	Proj	Wt.Gms.
B	3	3.5	5				9.5	3.0	125+25	9.5	3.0	125+25			
	4.5	5.5	8	10.0	4.0	195-205	10.0	3.1	150+25	10.0	3.1	150+25			
				10.5	4.2	230-240	10.6	3.3	175+25	10.6	3.3	175+25	10.5	3.8	195
C	4.5	5.5	8	11.0	4.3	270-285	11.0	3.4	200+25	11.0	3.4	200+25	11.0	4.0	235
	6.5	7.5	11	11.5	4.6	300-315	11.5	3.5	225+25	11.5	3.5	225+25	11.5	4.2	270
				12.0	4.8	350-370	11.9	3.6	250+25	11.9	3.6	250+25	12.0	4.4	310
D	5.5	7.0	8.0				12.3	3.7	275+25	12.3	3.7	275+25			
	7.5 >	9.0>	11.0	12.5	4.9	380-400	12.6	3.7	300+25	12.6	3.7	300+25	12.5	4.6	350
				13.0	5.3	450-475	13.0	3.8	325+50	13.0	3.8	325+50	13.0	4.8	395
DD	5.5	8.5	9.0	13.5	5.5	495-520	13.6	4.0	375+50	13.6	4.0	375+50	13.5	5.0	440
	7.5 >	9.5>	11.0>	14.0	5.7	560-590	14.2	4.1	425+50	14.2	4.1	425+50	14.0	5.2	500
				14.5	5.9	620-650	14.8	4.2	475+50	14.8	4.2	475+50			

FIGURE 11-2

❑ Does the surgeon demonstrate to you using your own tissues what might be achievable in terms of your result?

❑ Does the surgeon meticulously record the details of your examination during the examination? If not, how can the surgeon remember all the details of your exam later after examining several other patients?

❑ Does the surgeon review your pictures with you and explain in detail what would not change and what differences to expect in your breasts following surgery?

❑ Does the surgeon explain everything in terms that you clearly understand, and ask you if you have any other questions?

❑ Does the surgeon thank you for your coming for consultation?

FACTORS NEITHER YOU NOR YOUR SURGEON CAN CONTROL

Before you see a surgeon, just in case you don't hear it from the surgeon or the surgeon's staff, you should know the most common factors that neither you nor your surgeon can control that could cause problems or make additional reoperations necessary. The three most important are 1) infection, 2) capsular contracture, and 3) unpredictable tissue stretch. We've discussed these in greater detail in chapter 7 but will reemphasize a few important points.

Infection can occur in any operation. Every woman's breast tissue contains bacteria. Antibiotics may not eliminate the risk of infection regardless of the type of antibiotic, the dose, or when they are given. Infection is not totally preventable following augmentation. If you develop infection around your implant(s), our opinion is that the safest treatment with the least risk of additional future problems and increasing deformities is to remove the implants and not replace them.

Capsular contracture is affected by many factors, including your specific healing characteristics that genetically are factors you and your surgeon can't control. The degree of trauma and bleeding during surgery may affect risks of capsular contracture, and you can gain some insight into these factors by asking about your recovery. There is no type of implant currently available that prevents capsular contracture. If you develop capsular contracture and need a reoperation, that reoperation doesn't change your body's tendency to form capsules. Removing or opening a capsule does not prevent the formation of another capsule, and the tightness of the capsule that reforms is not predictable and could be worse than the original capsule.

How your tissues will respond to your implants depends on your tissue characteristics, your age, your pregnancy history, and the type and size of implant you choose. The larger the implant, the thinner your tissues, and the older you are, the more likely excessive stretch will occur. Excessive stretch can occur with any type of implant and any type of filler material. When excessive stretch occurs, the implants usually move down (bottoming, with the nipples pointing excessively upward) or out to the side (lateral displacement with widening of the space between the breasts). Additional surgery to attempt to correct excessive stretch is unpredictable at best because the tissues are the same tissues that stretched excessively in the first place.

What about Costs?

During your consultation visit, you need to inquire about costs. At this stage, you are gathering information. In chapter 13, we'll discuss costs,

costs analysis, and financing alternatives in more detail. From your surgeon or the staff, you'll need costs for each of the following items:

❏ Surgeon fees

❏ Laboratory fees (for lab work prior to surgery)

❏ Electrocardiogram fees (if needed)

❏ Mammogram fees (if surgeon requires mammogram)

❏ Surgery facility fees

❏ Costs of implants

❏ Anesthesia fees

❏ Medication fees or costs (for before and after surgery)

❏ Any other fees

If a surgeon offers a "package price," always insist that the price be broken down into the categories listed above.

If you don't, you won't be able to analyze what you're paying for to compare to other surgeons. See chapter 13.

Always ask for a written quote for costs signed by the surgeon or a staff member.

And ask how long the prices on the quote apply.

A Post-Consultation Checklist for Evaluation

In the next section, "Your Homework after the Consultation," is a checklist. Before your consultation, review the checklist thoroughly so that you'll notice all of the items listed.

YOUR HOMEWORK AFTER THE CONSULTATION

Doing your homework after the consultation is just as important as doing it before the consultation.

Record your impressions while they are fresh in your mind.

As soon as possible after your consultation, complete the following checklist, making brief notes beside each item. Don't procrastinate. Do it as soon as possible!

❏ Was the staff courteous, efficient, and knowledgeable?

❏ Were the surroundings pleasant, comfortable, and not excessive?

❏ Did anyone try to sell you operations or services that you weren't interested in?

❏ How thorough was the surgeon?

❏ Did the surgeon use a specific checklist during your exam or just rely on memory?

❏ How well did the surgeon explain the issues?

❏ Did the surgeon measure your breasts, especially the base width, tissue stretch, and distance from nipple to fold under stretch? Did the surgeon explain the importance of the measurements?

❏ What did the surgeon tell you specifically about your tissues?

❏ Did the surgeon present you several options and discuss the trade-offs of each?

❏ Did the surgeon discuss possible outcomes and trade-offs with respect to your specific tissues?

❏ How did you select an implant? Were your tissues a major consideration?

❏ Was the surgeon glad to see you?

❏ Was the surgeon's personal appearance neat, and did it reflect attention to detail?

❏ Did the surgeon seem to really care?

❏ Was the surgeon precise, with a lot of attention to detail?

❏ Did the surgeon thoroughly answer your questions?

❏ Did the surgeon say, "Thank you for coming to see me"?

Think about the Person You Just Met with and What You Heard!

It's your job to evaluate surgeons. Focus on substance instead of hype and fluff.

You'll recognize a great surgeon without the surgeon having to tell you. Substance usually shows. Fluff usually shows, too.

Gorgeous and charming don't contribute to what you'll get in the operating room.

Ask yourself how much substance is behind the appearance and charm.

Caring, thoroughness, attention to detail, and substance definitely contribute to what you'll get in the operating room.

How much of each did the surgeon have?

Remind yourself: "This person will be changing my body forever, and I'll look at it every day." Are you comfortable?

Were you offered options? A surgeon can't offer what the surgeon doesn't know how to do. There is definitely not one best way to do an augmentation if you know all the different ways.

Did you honestly and frankly discuss complications and what would be done? If the worst occurred, would you want this person to take care of you?

Did you discuss your tissues and how implant selection would affect them over time? If you didn't, you are very likely to make BAD TEAM DECISIONS!

Did you discuss what would likely NOT be accomplished by your augmentation? Did you discuss the specific factors that neither you or your surgeon could control, and if those factors caused a problem, who would be responsible for costs of reoperations?

Repeat this process for each surgeon that you consult. Make your notes, and file them with the information you obtained from each surgeon. When you're done, you will have all of the information that is reasonably necessary to make good decisions about surgeon selection. If you shortcut any of the steps, you may shortcut your quest for the best breast.

THE NEXT STEP . . .

Now that you've completed your surgeon consultations, it's time to finalize your choices.

PART IV

PUTTING IT ALL TOGETHER:
FINALIZING YOUR DECISIONS AND PREPARING FOR SURGERY

PUTTING IT ALL TOGETHER:

MAKING YOUR SELECTIONS

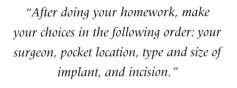

"After doing your homework, make your choices in the following order: your surgeon, pocket location, type and size of implant, and incision."

You've now completed all of your surgeon consultations and compiled your notes from those visits. It's time to select your surgeon.

WHAT TO DECIDE FIRST? DOES IT MATTER?

Yes, it matters. If you make the right choice of surgeon, the rest is easier. The best surgeon should always present you with options and should discuss the trade-offs of each option or set of options, as well as discussing factors that are not controllable and what an augmentation won't change about your breasts. Together, you'll make team decisions. You'll need to decide the following things, in order:

1. **Who is my surgeon?**
    - ❏ Dr. X
    - ❏ Dr. Y
    - ❏ Dr. Z

2. **What pocket location?**
    (This choice is critical because it determines how much tissue will cover your implant for your lifetime!)
    - ❏ Retromammary (behind breast tissue only)
    - ❏ Partial retropectoral (behind the pectoralis muscle)
    - ❏ Dual plane (behind muscle above, behind breast tissue below)
    - ❏ Total muscle coverage (behind pectoralis and serratus muscles)

3. **What type and size implant?**
    - ❏ Smooth
    - ❏ Textured
    - ❏ Round

Patient Decisions In Breast Augmentation

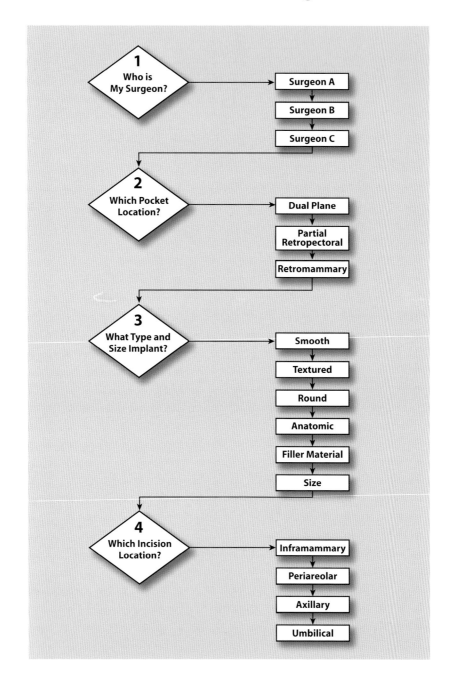

FIGURE 12-1

- ❏ Anatomic
- ❏ Filler material
- ❏ Size

4. **Which incision location?**

- ❏ Inframammary
- ❏ Periareolar
- ❏ Axillary
- ❏ Umbilical

PICKING YOUR SURGEON

If you've done your homework, picking your surgeon is usually easy.

Chances are good that you already know who you want to be your surgeon. One surgeon will often clearly stand out above the others, but if you are fortunate enough to have more than one surgeon who meets most of the guidelines we've given you, read on.

If you're making a choice of surgeon based primarily on price, you need not read any further.

In fact, you probably haven't even read this far, but if you have, you're likely to get exactly what you're paying for, and nothing you read is going to help you unless you prioritize quality over price. Amazingly but often predictably, you'll be the first to point fingers when something doesn't go right following surgery. Patients who prioritize price over quality rarely look in the mirror when pointing fingers.

How Do You Know Who's Right? The Comfort Level

First, review your checklists from chapter 11. If you evaluated each surgeon objectively using the criteria in the checklists, one surgeon will usually meet several criteria that other surgeons don't meet. If a surgeon clearly meets more criteria, go with that surgeon. But if you've found two or more surgeons who meet all of the objective criteria, it's time to go with your gut feeling.

Select your surgeon based on objective criteria from your homework.

Who makes you most comfortable? Never place comfort above qualifications!

Which surgeon listened to you best? Which do you feel best understands what you want? Which surgeon presented you the most options with the best explanation of trade-offs? Which surgeon emphasized reconciling your wishes with your tissues and demonstrated tissue limitations? Which surgeon seemed to care the most? Which was most thorough? We've mentioned all of these criteria before, but these are the ones that should weigh heavily on your gut feelings.

Which surgeon told you what you didn't want to hear? What are the factors you and the surgeon can't control? What characteristics of your breasts won't be changed following your augmentation? Truth based on knowledge and experience sometimes isn't pleasant, but it's still truth.

If you're still not sure, make a second visit to each surgeon you're still considering. Focus on which surgeon pays the most attention to detail. Look for distinguishing points to help with the final decision. Always focus on substance.

In the following sections, place a check mark beside your choices.

PICKING THE POCKET LOCATION

❏ **Retromammary** (behind breast tissue only or subfascial)

This choice is logical only if you have more than 2 cm. of pinch thickness of the tissues higher on your chest above your breast tissue. If your surgeon doesn't measure tissue pinch thickness, how do you know? A visual guess isn't as good as a measurement, and this has a lot to do with whether you'll see the edges of your implant. Fewer than one-fifth of patients we see have adequate tissue thickness to make this a logical, safe choice.

❏ **Subfascial coverage** (behind the breast tissue and behind a very thin, less than 1 mm thick layer of fascia)

This location has not been proved to add any significant coverage or have any benefits compared to a properly performed dual plane procedure and does not provide one-tenth of the coverage that dual plane allows. It is more of a surgeon gimmick than a pocket location that really adds tissue coverage.

❏ **Partial retropectoral** (behind the pectoralis muscle)

If you don't have more than 2 cm. of pinch thickness, put the implant partially behind the pectoral muscle regardless of the trade-offs. You may have some distortion of the breast when the muscle contracts (that's not often), and the distance between the breasts may widen slightly over time, but both of these trade-offs are better than putting an implant under tissues that are too thin!

❑ **Dual plane** (behind the pectoralis muscle in the upper breast, behind breast tissue in the lower breast)

If you don't have more than 2 cm. of pinch thickness, and you need muscle coverage in the upper breast but would like to reduce the trade-offs of traditional muscle coverage, the dual-plane location offers that option. The best of both worlds is a very good option for most, but not all, first-time augmentation patients. It is not necessarily the best approach if you are very, very thin (less than 0.5 cm pinch thickness immediately at the fold under your breast).

❑ **Total muscle coverage** (behind pectoralis and serratus muscles)

This is not usually a good choice for augmentation because it has too many trade-offs that affect the lower, outer shape of the breast and the shape and position of the fold beneath the breast. It is sometimes useful in reconstruction cases.

PICKING THE IMPLANT

What Type and Size Implant?

❑ **Size**

If your envelope has been stretched by pregnancy, you'll need enough to fill the envelope adequately for the best result. If you've not been pregnant, a good rule of thumb is to think about enlarging the breast the amount it would enlarge during pregnancy—about a cup size. If you want an especially large breast, you must accept the inevitable consequences of your decisions. The larger the implant (especially above 350 cc) and the thinner your tissues, the greater your risks of complications, additional surgery, visible implant edges, rippling, and possible shrinkage (atrophy) of your existing breast tissue. You need to consider what you want and balance that with what will happen to your tissues as you age, especially with a larger implant. Best choice? Ask your surgeon to enlarge your breast proportionate to your figure, filling the breast only enough to create an aesthetic result, not too large—and don't ever discuss ccs. You'll definitely be happier ten years or more later. Don't be too concerned when you hear many women say they want to be larger. They aren't thinking about the long-term consequences.

❏ **Smooth**

Do you prefer a smooth-surface implant? Why? Hopefully it isn't because smooth implants are cheaper. Don't make this choice believing that you'll be less able to feel the implant because it isn't so. Tissue coverage is the main issue that affects whether you can feel an implant. The fact that a smooth-wall implant can move around more than a textured is a positive and a negative. The main worry is whether smooth implants really are as good at preventing capsular contracture and how the smooth wall implant may affect tissues long term.

❏ **Textured**

Most surgeons believe that textured surface implants offer a decreased risk of capsular contracture (more so with silicone-gel filled implants compared to saline-filled implants). With anatomic or shaped implants, a textured surface helps maintain optimal position of the implant. If you choose a smooth wall implant and subsequently develop a capsular contracture, will you look back and wonder, "What if I had chosen a textured surface implant?"

❑ **Round**

Easier to use than an anatomic; hence, preferred by many surgeons. The main question is how to deal with the fill issues with current round, saline-filled implants. If you fill it to manufacturer's recommendations, the shell folds and risks visible rippling and shell failure. If you overfill, you currently are not assured in writing that the manufacturers will warranty the implant. If you're choosing a round implant because a surgeon has told you that "anatomic implants malposition," hopefully you asked exactly how many anatomic implants the surgeon had placed. The fact is that both round and anatomic implants can malposition, and published data[1-4] suggest that the incidence of reoperations with properly used anatomic implants is less than one-half of 1 percent.

❑ **Anatomic**

Looks more like a breast. More demanding of the surgeon. Offers better long-term control of upper-breast fill and breast shape. Best in first-time augmentations until a surgeon has plenty of experience, then okay for reoperations. Fill volumes are defined differently by the manufacturer, depending on the specific type of shaped or anatomic implant. (You must check.) Remember that all anatomic implants are not the same: some are full height and some are reduced height, and adequate fill to reduce risks of upper shell folding or collapse depends on the implant's passing the tilt test outside your body.

❏ Saline Filled

A better choice for any patient who, despite scientific evidence, has any concerns whatever about the safety or potentially higher capsular contracture rates with silicone gel filled implants. The primary tradeoff of all saline filled implants is that they are likely to have a shorter shell life compared to silicone gel implants, and therefore potentially require more replacements during a patient's lifetime. Saline implants are also currently less expensive compared to silicone gel filled implants.

❏ Silicone Filled

Silicone gel filled implants have been shown in FDA studies to have a longer shell life (lower failure rate) compared to saline implants. *Form stable silicone gel filled implants (the newest, anatomic implants that maintain their shape when upright, without shell collapse or folding) have a substantially lower shell failure rate compared to conventional silicone gel filled implants.* All silicone gel filled implants except form stable silicone gel implants have been shown in FDA PMA studies to have a higher rate of capsular contracture compared to saline implants. These rates also relate to how a surgeon performs your surgery—the less trauma and bleeding, the faster the recovery and the lower the capsular contracture rate. Silicone gel filled implants are more expensive compared to saline implants, and form stable silicone gel implants are more expensive compared to conventional silicone gel filled implants.

PICKING THE INCISION LOCATION

❏ **Inframammary** (in the fold under the breast)

The most commonly used incision in breast augmentation offers surgeons the greatest degree of control in the widest range of breast types and implant types and sizes: The standard by which all other incisions must be measured. The only reason not to have an inframammary incision is 1) you absolutely do not want a scar on the breast or 2) you have a documented history of hypertrophic (heavy) scarring from a surgical procedure (not from an accident where the cut was caused by trauma).

❏ **Periareolar** (around the areola)

A good selection if you have a history of hypertrophic scarring or if you just prefer this location. The implant has more exposure to bacteria in breast tissue by this approach, but no scientific studies prove a higher risk of infection or capsular contracture. Nipple sensation is an issue. Nursing should not be an issue if the procedure is performed properly.

❏ **Axillary** (in the armpit)

The ideal location if your main goal is to get the scar off the breast. Much better control during surgery compared to the umbilical approach. The entire pocket can be created under direct vision by the surgeon using endoscopic instruments. This scar is not visible in over 90 percent of patients even with the arms raised.

❑ **Umbilical** (around the belly button)

Attractive to some surgeons from a marketing standpoint. You'll find that the vast majority of highly experienced surgeons feel this approach offers much less control compared to other approaches, unnecessarily traumatizes abdominal tissues, and requires that most, if not all, dissection of the implant pocket be performed bluntly and blindly. The entire pocket is created by tearing tissue with an expander balloon and by forceful, manual movement of the inflated device or by using some other form of blunt dissector that tears tissues. You'll have injury with discomfort and bruising in the upper abdomen that rarely, if ever, occur with procedures that assure less tissue trauma and bleeding, and in a few cases, you may develop deformities of the upper abdomen. You can't judge by pictures because many of the irregularities under the breast or in the abdomen aren't visible in standard pictures. You get all of the benefits of the umbilical approach without the trade-offs and risks by selecting an axillary incision!

WHAT ABOUT COSTS?

We'll cover costs in the next chapter, and discuss options for dealing with costs.

THE NEXT STEP . . .

Congratulations! You've done your homework and made your choices. Now it's time to prepare for your surgery.

References

1. Tebbetts, J. B. Patient acceptance of adequately filled breast implants. *Plast. Reconstr. Surg.* 106(1): 139-147, 2000.

2. Tebbetts, J. B. Dual plan (DP) breast augmentation: Optimizing implant soft-tissue relationships in a wide range of breast types. *Plast. Reconstr. Surg.* 107: 1255, 2001.

3. Tebbetts, J. B. Achieving a predictable 24-hour return to normal activities after breast augmentation, part II: patient preparation, refined surgical techniques and instrumentation. *Plast. Reconstr. Surg.* 109: 293-305, 2002.

4. Tebbetts, J. B. Achieving a zero percent reoperation rate at 3 years in a 50 consecutive case augmentation mammaplasty PMA study. *Plast. Reconstr. Surg.* 108(6): 1453-1457, 2006.

PREPARING FOR SURGERY:

WHAT SHOULD YOU DO?

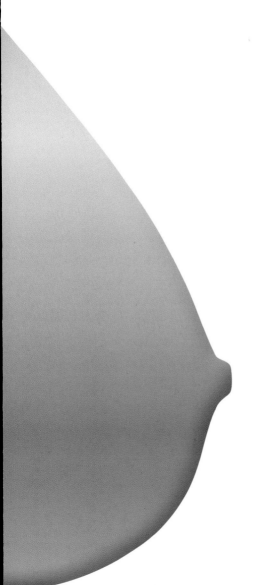

"You are ultimately responsible for thorough planning that assures optimally safe surroundings and the most pleasant experience."

Now that you've selected your surgeon, it's time to prepare for surgery. Preparations begin with money: what are the costs, which are justified, and where does the money come from? Next, you'll need to check into the surgery facility to be sure that you're not having surgery in someone's back room (Don't laugh; it happens every day in bargain basement situations.) Finally, it's important to clearly understand the scheduling policies and procedures of your surgeon and make all necessary arrangements in an organized manner. A lot of arrangements are required. Preparation and organization prevent glitches that can interfere with your surgery.

COSTS

Part of preparation is paying for your surgery. During your visits with surgeons, you collected a specific breakdown of costs from each surgeon. You've probably noticed that we didn't go into detail about analyzing costs while choosing a surgeon. The reasons?

If you want the best result, cost should not be the primary determining factor in choosing your surgeon. Choose based on qualifications, and then address the costs.

You can't pay enough later to undo problems from "bargain" surgery, but you will pay to correct them!

Are we saying that costs don't matter? No. Costs certainly *do* matter. But you're not going shopping for a dress. You're asking someone to permanently make changes in your body. If costs seem unreasonable or totally out of line with other quotes, investigate. Way too high or way too low is worth looking into. Ask questions! Why the high cost?

Or how can you get such a bargain? Look carefully at the breakdown list of costs we provided. Don't just accept a "package deal" if it seems out of line.

Bargain Surgery

Is there such a thing as "bargain surgery"? Undoubtedly, you can find low-cost plastic surgery. But a bargain? A bargain is *value* at a lower than expected price. The key word in this definition is *value*. If, in fact, you get top-quality surgery at a lower-than-expected price, then you're getting a real value. But it's not often that you get a *steal* when buying surgery. When bargain surgery seems attractive, ask yourself:

Am I getting top-quality surgery for this bargain price? How do you know? What might you be giving up?

How is the bargain surgeon able to offer such a good price?

Cheaper implants? "Back room" surgery, instead of an accredited surgical facility? Not many cases scheduled? Less qualified? Who pays for costs of reoperations if problems occur?

How many professionals (or anyone, for that matter) do you know who do more work for less money—at the same quality level?

Most of the better surgeons we know charge similar surgical fees. We don't know any top-quality surgeons who offer bargain basement prices. In fact, we don't even know any above-average surgeons who offer extremely low prices. If you encounter prices that are substantially lower than other surgeons you consult, beware. You may find some surgeons who do equivalent quality surgery at a lower price than other surgeons, but how do you really know until they've already operated on you? Once they've operated on you, you'll definitely have to live with the "bargain."

Our favorite answer when asked about surgeons and prices is:

If there is anyone who knows what a surgeon is really worth, it's the surgeon.

How Much Difference Is There, Really?

After all, this is just a breast augmentation, and breast augmentations are simple. Believe it or not, I've heard more than a few patients and surgeons make this statement. My response?

Anything seems simple if you don't know enough to understand why it's not simple.

If augmentations were really simple, all results would be outstanding, and you'd see very few reoperations.

If it's so simple, why the drains, bandages, special bras, pain pumps, narcotic pain medications, bruising, excessive pain, and prolonged recovery following surgery? Remember, with optimally performed surgery, there is a greater than 90 percent chance that you can return to full, normal activities within 24 hours of your surgery using techniques we have published in the most respected professional journal in plastic surgery[1] with no drains, bandages, special bras, straps, no bruising, and no narcotic pain medications!

Your best chance for a good result is at the first surgery.

After that, everything gets more difficult and risky, with more trade-offs and more costs.

Few patients appreciate the importance of getting a good result at the first operation. We can't overemphasize this important point. If you require a reoperation, even the best surgeon is working with previously operated tissues. Things are always more difficult, and every aspect of a reoperation is less predictable. Every reoperation involves even more factors that a surgeon cannot control. All augmentations and all surgeons are not the same. Reoperation and complication rates can vary significantly from one surgeon to another. In FDA studies where augmentations were performed by many surgeon investigators, an average of 17 percent of patients had a reoperation in just three years following their augmentation.[2,3] Using processes and techniques that we described in peer-reviewed and published journals, in 1,664 reported cases with up to seven-year follow-up, *instead of a 17 percent reoperation rate, we documented a 3 percent reoperation rate*[1,4,5] In a more recent study, we documented a zero percent reoperation rate in a 50-consecutive-case series supervised by an independent review organization in an FDA study.

Substantial differences in outcomes and reoperation rates can occur from one surgeon to another.

Many of the same techniques that speed recovery, combined with optimal decision processes, reduce complications and reoperations.

Costs by Category—The Details

It's easy to eliminate or reduce costs by eliminating tests and proce-dures prior to surgery. The key question is how much of your safety you may be sacrificing when you eliminate more thorough testing even if it seems to be overkill. What might an additional test or two be worth if it potentially prevented your having a cardiac arrest or other problem during or after surgery? If you didn't do the test and had a major problem during or after surgery, there's a good chance you'd question why you weren't as thorough as possible prior to your medi-cally unnecessary operation!

Fees for all cosmetic surgery are paid prior to surgery. We're not aware of a single quality cosmetic surgeon who does not follow this policy. To fully understand costs of your surgery, look at the breakdown of costs associated with first-time (primary) breast augmentation surgery:

Surgeon fees—These fees vary with the qualifications and experience of the surgeon. Cost range: $2,500–$5,500; average $3,500.

Laboratory fees (for lab work prior to surgery)—Some basic lab tests are usually required even if you're perfectly healthy. A routine blood count (to assure that you're not anemic and do not have an undiagnosed infection or other problem) and routine blood chemistry (to check fac-tors that could affect how you react to sedative drugs or anesthesia) are common. Some surgeons require HIV testing. Some surgeons don't feel that any lab tests are necessary in a healthy individual. We disagree. To make this surgery as completely safe as possible, leave no stones unturned. Check everything. It's not worth risking a problem. Costs of lab tests? Range: $150–$300; average $200.

Electrocardiogram fees (if needed)—If you are over 40 years old or have any history of any type of heart problem, your surgeon may require an electrocardiogram. Cost range: $150–$300 (including inter-pretation by a cardiologist); average $200.

Mammogram fees (if your surgeon requires mammogram)—Many surgeons require routine mammograms before a breast augmentation regardless of your age or family history of breast cancer. Some surgeons do not feel that routine mammograms are necessary. It's true that breast cancer is exceedingly rare in women below the age of 30-35 years, but it happens. We require mammograms on every patient over the age of 30 because operating in the area of an undiagnosed breast cancer may have significant effects on whether that cancer can be cured. We want to take no unnecessary risks with a totally elective operation even if a mammogram increases the costs. Have your mammogram at a breast center where they are familiar with breast augmentation patients. Cost range: $100–$350; average $150.

Surgery facility fees—This fee is the fee that a hospital or outpatient surgery facility charges for the costs of the facility and supplies required to do your surgery. If a surgeon operates in an office facility, this fee may be lumped with other fees. If this fee is excessively low, beware! The only way to substantially lower this fee is to use fewer or cheaper supplies, have fewer or less qualified personnel, or to have less equipment or cheaper equipment in the facility. Fully accreditied facilities with adequate, qualified staff and equipment must charge fees that allow them to remain in business. Cost range: $1,200–$2,000; average $1,500.

Costs of implants—Implant costs vary widely. In chapter 4, we discussed many of the factors affecting implant costs. Cheaper implants are usually cheaper. Enough said! If an implant fails sooner because it was cheaper with respect to quality, you didn't get a bargain. What you got was another operation with substantial costs and risks. Check carefully into implant costs and manufacturer before you implant this device. Cost range: $600–$1,600 per pair; average $1,200. Silicone-gel-filled implants, especially form-stable silicone-gel implants, cost more compared to saline-filled implants. These costs can vary widely, so check costs with your surgeon.

Anesthesia fees—Fees for anesthesia vary according to the type of anesthesia (general versus local) and increase with the level of person giving the anesthesia. Most state-of-the-art facilities require that CRNAs (certified registered nurse anesthetists) or anesthesiologists administer anesthesia—particularly general anesthesia. Cost range: $250–$750; average $350.

Medications fees or costs (for before and after surgery)—Costs of medications that are required before and after surgery vary significantly from surgeon to surgeon. The more medications a surgeon requires you to take, the more you'll spend! The most common medications required for breast augmentation surgery are antibiotics and pain medications. Other medications are optional, and the necessity varies with the surgeon. The less trauma a surgeon causes, the less medication you will need. Cost range: $15–$200; average, less than $40.

Any other fees—Always ask if there are any other fees. If other fees are charged, they are unusual, and you should carefully investigate the value of those charges. Special circumstances exist, but always check out any unusual fees.

The Totals

Adding individual costs listed above, you'll find that an augmentation at today's prices will cost between $4,965 and $11,000 with an average of $6,500. What a range! In our opinion, if you pay more than $8,000 for a top-quality augmentation, you are paying too much. If you pay less than $5,000 today, beware!

FINANCING FOR COSMETIC SURGERY

Financing options are available for patients desiring breast augmentation who cannot or don't wish to pay with cash or check. Common options include credit cards, bank financing, and finance companies specializing in cosmetic surgery. Let's examine these options.

Credit cards—A good option for those who 1) want to take advantage of payments over time or 2) want to take advantage of special perks associated with certain credit cards (free airline travel miles, for example). The downsides? Most credit cards charge high rates of interest compared to bank financing and other financing options. Spending limits may not be adequate to charge all surgical costs.

Bank financing—Banks usually offer better interest rates compared to credit cards, depending on your credit rating and banking relationships. Check with your bank or ask your surgeon about banks that finance cosmetic surgery.

Finance companies—Until recently, most finance companies that offered financing for cosmetic surgery charged exceedingly high interest rates and offered financing only when a patient selected a surgeon that had an agreement with the finance company. Needless to say, if a finance company is taking a portion of a surgeon's fee to refer you to the surgeon, you are hardly choosing a surgeon based on all of the information we've given you. Always choose your surgeon based on qualifications we've listed for you—then arrange financing. Today, there are better financing options for patients than before, but you must be very careful. Be sure that you understand the interest rates, payment options, and late or default penalties before arranging any financing. With better financing companies, the interest rate you'll be charged is directly related to your credit rating. The better your credit rating, the lower the rate of interest. Remember, the money you are borrowing is unsecured. If you don't pay, what can the finance company repossess? As a result, you'll pay higher interest rates compared to a secured loan.

The Realities of Financing

You can't afford what you can't afford.

Financing increases the costs for your surgery. Be sure your budget can support the increase.

For many women, the best financing option is to save until you can pay with cash or check for your breast augmentation. Meanwhile, you can learn more and better research your options, and the options only get better. If you choose financing, be absolutely sure that your income and budget will support the payments, and be sure that getting the operation a bit sooner is worth the increased cost of financing. If you find good financing and feel that's the best option for you—fine—but be sure to look at the total cost with and without financing, so you can place a dollar value on having the operation sooner.

SURGERY FACILITIES

For the greatest safety, you want to have your breast augmentation in an accredited surgical facility. What does that mean? How do you know? What difference does it make? What type of accreditation is adequate?

Facility Accreditation

Accredited means that a surgical facility has passed rigorous examination to assure that the equipment and procedures of the facility meet standards for optimal safety. To become accredited, a surgery facility must conform to a huge number of rigorous standards and requirements. Once the facility meets written standards, examiners perform an on-site inspection visit to assure full compliance with all standards, regulations, and requirements.

Who Accredits Surgery Facilities? How Do You Know?

The two most well-known and well-respected accrediting bodies are the Joint Commission on Accreditation of Hospitals (JCAH) and the American Association for Accreditation of Ambulatory Surgery Facilities (AAAASF). The regulations are as long as the names—a pain to those who must pass examination, but an asset to patients. The JCAH usually accredits hospital facilities and hospital-based outpatient surgery facilities. The AAAASF specializes in accrediting outpatient or ambulatory surgery facilities regardless of where they are based. How do you know if a facility is accredited? Ask to see the accreditation certificate of the facility where you'll have surgery. Often it's posted in the facility. Your surgeon should know.

What Accreditation Is Adequate?

If you want to assure that a surgical facility is properly equipped and staffed and follows procedures for optimal safety, we'd look for a facility accredited by the JCAH or AAAASF. Other accreditation bodies exist, but these two are most widely respected at this time. If a facility is not accredited, or if it is accredited by a less well-known organization, be very careful. How important is accreditation?

Would you climb aboard an airplane if you were not sure the equipment and check-out procedures met certain criteria?

An accredited surgical facility assures you that specific, high standards have been met.

One of the requirements of accreditation is to assure that personnel are trained and that procedures and equipment are in place to deal with any emergency from a power outage to cardiac arrest. Ask your surgeon for additional information about surgical facilities and emergency contingency plans. If you have doubts, ask other medical personnel you know or other surgeons about a facility.

If a facility is not accredited, ask to see the facility.

Then visit an accredited facility.

With no special expertise, you should notice a significant difference.

If you're not comfortable with a surgical facility, don't have surgery there. This is an important area that's often overlooked by patients, especially patients seeking bargain surgery. It's your job to ask and assure that you're having surgery under the best circumstances. If a problem occurs and you haven't done your homework to assure that you're in the best of surroundings, it's too late.

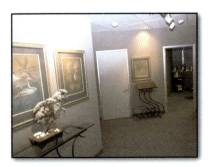

FIGURE 13-1

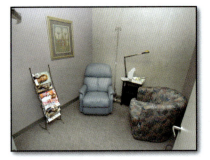

FIGURE 13-2

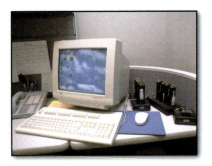

FIGURE 13-3

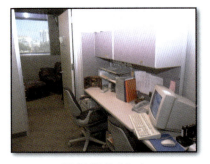

FIGURE 13-4

WHAT TO LOOK FOR IN A SURGERY FACILITY—THE THINGS WE THINK ARE IMPORTANT

When we designed our outpatient surgery facility, we tried to put ourselves in your place. What would we want if we were coming to this facility to have surgery? And how could we make it totally state-of-the-art medically, but make you feel less apprehensive compared to a hospital-type setting?

The surroundings and personnel in a surgery center can have a significant impact on your experience as a patient. If the surroundings and personnel are warm and personal (Figure 13-1), more like at home, you'll be more comfortable. The rooms where you will change and prepare for surgery need not be extravagant but should be comfortable (Figure 13-2) with reading material, television, and personnel immediately available. Computer information systems should be state-of-the-art (Figure 13-3), and the nursing station

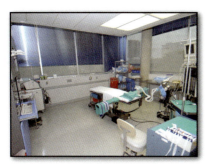

FIGURE 13-5 A

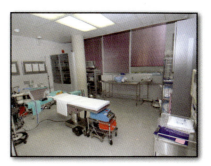

FIGURE 13-5 B.

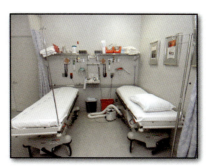

FIGURE 13-6

(Figure 13-4) should be immediately adjacent to your preparation and recovery rooms.

The operating rooms should appear state-of-the-art, spotlessly clean and equipped with the most up-to-date equipment (Figure Figure 13-5, A,B). Ideally, computer systems will also be present in the operating rooms that allow the surgeon access to your preoperative photographs and patient data. The recovery area should be immediately adjacent to the operating rooms (Figure 13-6) and should be state-of-the-art equipped.

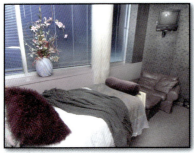

FIGURE 13-7 A

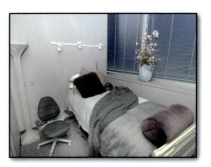

FIGURE 13-7 B

Some facilities may also provide overnight accommodations with immediately adjacent, one-on-one nursing care for patients who need overnight care after more extensive procedures (Figure 13-7 A,B).

SCHEDULING POLICIES AND PROCEDURES

When you are ready to schedule your surgery, the surgeon's staff will help with all the necessary arrangements. Specific scheduling policies and procedures are necessary to assure that arrangements are correct to the smallest detail. These procedures can vary among different surgeons, but each of the following activities should occur before arrangements are final.

A Surgical Arrangements Checklist . . .

- ❏ Select a date for surgery.

- ❏ Review surgeon's financial policies and policies for refunds.

- ❏ Pay scheduling deposit if surgeon requires.

- ❏ Sign informed consent documents and operative consent forms.

- ❏ Review and sign implant manufacturer's documents:

❏ Implant package insert

❏ Terms of implant guarantee

❏ Manufacturer's consent forms (if applicable)

❏ Verify that surgeon will register your implants with the national implant registry.

❏ Schedule lab tests and mammography.

❏ Review medications to avoid and medications to take before surgery.

❏ Review instructions for the night before surgery.

❏ Review instructions for the day of surgery.

Selecting a Date for Surgery

The type of recovery you expect (and it varies greatly from surgeon to surgeon) has a lot to do with selecting a date for surgery. The longer it takes for you to return to normal activity, the further ahead of any commitments you should schedule your surgery.

Check your schedule carefully before discussing dates with your surgeon's staff. Select a time at least one month in advance that allows you to have surgery without interfering with any other activities. Depending on the time required for recovery (you should already know this from information you've gathered from your surgeon), you'll need from three to ten or more days off work. Try to select at least two time periods when you could have surgery and recover, the first period being at least one month in advance. You need some flexibility to fit your surgeon's schedule.

Discuss available times with your surgeon's staff. The staff should be helpful and offer you alternative times, but you should also try to be helpful and flexible, if possible.

If you have a very specific time that you want to have surgery, the further in advance that you schedule, the more likely a busy surgeon can meet your needs.

If you are pressured to schedule, or if you hear "Why don't we just do this tomorrow?" RUN AWAY!

The best surgeons usually can't operate on you the next day!

Financial Policies and Conditions of Refunds

If you did not already receive written information from your surgeon detailing financial policies and procedures, ask for a written summary when you schedule. Every credible surgeon should provide you specific, written information that details all financial policies. Conditions for refunds vary from surgeon to surgeon, but you should know the details before you schedule. What if your child becomes ill the day before surgery? What if you just decide you'd rather have your hair done than have surgery on the day it's scheduled? Which fees are payable in advance of surgery, and when are they due? The answers to each of these questions should be spelled out in written financial policies. Read the information carefully. You'll be required to follow these policies!

Scheduling Deposits

Most busy, experienced, highly qualified surgeons require a scheduling deposit when you select a surgery date and schedule your surgery. An average scheduling deposit is 10–20 percent of the surgeon's fee, payable at the time of scheduling to reserve a surgery date. If a conflict occurs that prevents your having surgery on the date scheduled, most surgeons will reschedule your surgery once, but the scheduling deposit is usually nonrefundable if you cancel more than once. Scheduling deposits are necessary because you are reserving the surgeon's time and the time of many personnel. If you cancel, the surgical facility must pay these personnel, and the surgeon wastes time that could have been spent productively.

Signing Informed Consent Documents

Informed consent documents and operative consent forms are essential to document your understanding and acceptance of the potential benefits, trade-offs, and risks associated with your surgery. You will be required to sign these forms prior to surgery. The most thorough surgeons may require that you read and sign several documents at different times to try to assure that you thoroughly understand all of the information and the risks and trade-offs that you are accepting. Ideally, you should discuss the information contained in these forms with your surgeon and the surgeon's staff well in advance of surgery. Most surgeons provide you copies of all operative consent forms well in advance of surgery. Information on these documents should not be new! You should have heard all of it before during your patient educator visits and surgeon consultation.

Read all informed consent documents and operative permits carefully well in advance of your surgery.

Write down any questions, and be sure they are answered to your satisfaction before signing any documents.

You should never be put off or offended by requirements and procedures that are in place to try to assure that you thoroughly understand all of the important factors required for optimal decisions. Repetition should never insult your intelligence but should reinforce your comfort level that your surgeon is trying to do everything possible to ensure that you are optimally informed.

When you read about all of the risks and possible problems in the informed consent documents, don't be surprised if you feel a bit frightened. You should! These documents are designed to present you the very worst-case scenarios and risks regardless of how rarely they may occur. If you don't understand or feel that you can't accept any of the information in the informed consent documents, discuss your concerns with your surgeon, or don't have the surgery! The time for understanding is before your surgery.

Information from the Implant Manufacturer

At the very least, your surgeon should provide you 1) a copy of the package insert that comes with your implants, 2) terms of the implant guarantee, 3) any required manufacturer's consent forms, and 4) verification that your implants will be recorded in an implant registry program. The package insert contains a lot of information from the manufacturer that you should read and understand before having an implant device placed in your body. Terms of implant guarantees vary widely and are critically important. Read the guarantee carefully before you accept a surgeon's recommendation of implant. If the manufacturer requires additional consent forms, wonderful! That means the manufacturer cares about your being informed. Finally, ask your surgeon if your implant information will be recorded at surgery and the forms completed and submitted to assure that your implants are registered in the national implant registry program. If you have any questions about any of the information contained in these documents, ask your surgeon or contact the manufacturer before you sign or have surgery.

Scheduling Lab Tests and Mammography

Most surgeons require blood tests within two weeks of your scheduled surgery. Mammograms and electrocardiograms are usually acceptable if they have been performed within one year of your surgery date. Your surgeon's staff will assist with arranging for all necessary tests prior to surgery. Remember that these tests are important to assure your safety. Be absolutely certain to keep your appointments to have these tests done on schedule.

Medications to Avoid and Medications to Take

Every surgeon should provide a list of medications to avoid prior to surgery. The exact medications can vary from surgeon to surgeon, but some important basics:

Be sure that your surgeon is aware of all medications that you are taking.

Avoid all medications that contain aspirin for at least two weeks prior to surgery.

Read the labels carefully for all over-the-counter medications. Many contain aspirin.

Be very careful about herbs and herbal medicines. If you are using any herbal preparations, discuss them with your surgeon!

Many homeopathic and herbal medicines may be very effective in many ways, but if their specific interactions with medications used during anesthesia and surgery are not well known and documented, adverse interactions between the herbs and the surgical medications can cause serious problems. Be absolutely sure that you stop all herbal and homeopathic medications at least two weeks prior to surgery unless you have specifically discussed them with your surgeon and anesthesia personnel.

Aspirin and aspirin-containing products can interfere with your blood-clotting mechanisms and cause bleeding during and after surgery! Even one aspirin can cause problems within two weeks of surgery. Some herbs and herbal medicines can cause similar problems. Other medications can interfere with your anesthesia or produce undesirable effects if combined with anesthetic drugs. Your surgeon can't prevent these problems if you don't make the surgeon aware of medicines or herbs that you are taking before surgery.

Instructions for the Night Before

Normally, you'll be somewhat apprehensive the night before surgery. Generally, the better informed you are, the more comfortable you'll feel the night before surgery, but some apprehension is natural. Your surgeon will provide specific instructions for the night before surgery, but the most important basics are:

Never eat or drink anything after midnight the night before surgery.

If you do, material in your stomach can cause you to regurgitate, aspirate, and possibly die during surgery!

Sound drastic? It is drastic! Something as simple as having an empty stomach when you receive any sedative or anesthetic medicine is critically important to your safety. Don't cheat. Even if you think you're going into withdrawal without your coffee or cola in the morning!

Another tip that some surgeons forget to tell you. Stock your pantry before surgery. Pick up whatever you'd like to have after surgery, so you won't need to go get it the evening of surgery or the day after. Get some noncarbonated drinks as well as carbonated drinks. Stock some lighter foods you like, such as crackers, bagels, soups, etc., as well as your regular favorites. If you drink diet drinks, get one or two drinks that contain sugar for the night of surgery. You'll feel better quicker if you put a little sugar in your system immediately after surgery.

Ask your surgeon to give you any prescriptions you'll need after surgery, so that you can pick them up before surgery. Just one less thing you'll need to worry about!

Instructions for the Day of Surgery

You should receive specific instructions for the day of surgery, and these instructions can also vary among different surgeons. A few essentials:

Wear very comfortable clothing like a jogging suit that buttons or zips up the front.

**You won't enjoy tugging something on over your head.
Make arrangements for someone to drive you home
from the surgery facility and be with you overnight.
You'll receive medications that make driving
yourself unsafe.**

**Leave off your eye makeup; otherwise you'll wake up
with it in your eyes.
Protective eye lubricants during surgery make a total
mess of makeup.**

Also, leave off the body oils and lotions you might rub on or around your breasts. Your surgeon will need to make measurements and markings on you prior to your augmentation (if the surgeon is using state-of-the-art methods), and the markers sometimes don't perform optimally over oils or lotions.

Leave your jewelry and valuables at home!

Some surgical facilities prefer that you don't wear any type of makeup, nail polish, or belly button rings, but most facilities can work around these things that make you feel and look better. Just ask, or read the instructions you're given.

THE NEXT STEP . . .

Believe it or not, it's time to do it! You've gone through all the steps to get to the top of the stairs in the best possible manner, and now you're there. Try to relax as much as possible with the assurance that you've done your part toward getting the best breast. In the following chapters, we'll tell you what to expect during your recovery and offer suggestions for living with your new breasts.

References

1. Tebbetts, J. B. Achieving a predictable 24-hour return to normal activities after breast augmentation, part II: Patient preparation, refined surgical techniques and instrumentation. *Plast. Reconstr. Surg.* 109: 293-305, 2002.

2. U. S. Food and Drug Administration. General and Plastic Surgery Devices Panel Meeting Transcript. http://www.fda.gov/ohrms/dockets/ac/03/transcripts/3989T1.htm. Accessed January 13, 2004.

3. U. S. Food and Drug Administration. General and Plastic Surgery Devices Panel Meeting Transcript. Washington, DC. 1992 Feb 18.

4. Tebbetts, J. B. Patient acceptance of adequately filled breast implants. *Plast. Reconstr. Surg.* 106(1): 139-147, 2000.

5. Tebbetts, J. B. Dual plane (DP) breast augmentation: Optimizing implant soft-tissue relationships in a wide range of breast types. *Plast. Reconstr. Surg.* 107: 1255, 2001.

RECOVERY:

WHAT TO EXPECT

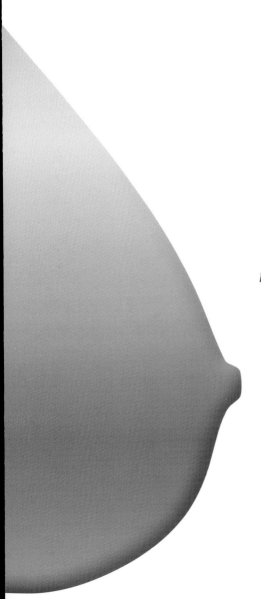

"The better your surgeon performs and the better you follow instructions, the more rapidly you will recover. Over 90 percent of our patients are able to be out to dinner the evening of their augmentation, and 96 percent return to full, normal activities within 24 hours.[1]"

Your recovery experience is the best indicator of the amount of tissue trauma and bleeding that occurred during your surgery.

Recovering from an augmentation is different from preparing for it. During preparation, there were many things that you could actively do to change the course of events. During recovery, your body does most of the work automatically, provided you don't expect everything to happen quickly and provided you don't tamper with the autopilot! If you understand what's normal, what to expect, and some of the reasons behind the dos and don'ts, the recovery process will be smoother.

Recovery is a team effort and depends on two key factors: what the surgeon does during the operation and how well you follow the surgeon's instructions postoperatively.

1. **The better your surgeon performs, the less the trauma to your tissues, and the less bleeding during surgery, and**

2. **The better you follow instructions following your augmentation, the more rapidly you should recover.**

RECOVERY IS VARIABLE

Is recovery similar from patient to patient? The answer varies from patient to patient and from surgeon to surgeon. If you understand some of the reasons for variations in recovery, the whole process should be easier.

Patient Variations

Your body and your breast tissues are different from other women's. The tighter your breast skin envelope and the more surgical manipulation required, the more tightness and tenderness you can expect following surgery. Everyone has some tightness and tenderness, but the amount varies according to what's required of your tissues. Generally, if you've had children prior to your augmentation, your tissues have been previously stretched, and you'll feel less tightness for a shorter time. If your skin is very tight and has never been stretched by pregnancy, you'll feel tighter longer.

Some patients are more tolerant of discomfort than others. Some patients are better able to get moving after surgery despite discomfort. Some patients follow instructions better than others.

Your individual pain tolerance, motivation, and ability to follow instructions will affect your recovery.

Adopt a positive attitude, follow instructions, get moving early and get well sooner!

Surgeon Variations

A surgeon can't change what you bring the surgeon to work with. But how the surgeon works with what you bring can significantly affect your recovery. The less surgical trauma the surgeon causes to your tissues, the easier and shorter your recovery.[1] The less bleeding the surgeon causes while creating the pocket for your implant, the easier and shorter your recovery. Hopefully, you learned from chapter 8 how to ask the right questions about recovery before surgery to help select a surgeon who minimizes surgical trauma.

In the previous edition of our book, we told you that if your tissues are thin and submuscular placement of the implant was necessary for adequate tissue coverage of your implant, you'll have more tenderness compared to patients whose implants are placed over the muscle. *With new, dual plane[2] and 24-hour recovery[1] techniques that we have published, you can experience the same 24-hour recovery whether your implant is over or under muscle.*

With optimal techniques and instruments, today there is no difference in pain or recovery if your implants are placed submuscular or submammary.[2]

Even if you choose a surgeon whose techniques still cause more post-operative discomfort if your implant is under muscle, this is a short-term inconvenience for long-term protection against seeing edges of your implant and possibly a greater risk of capsular contracture. If your surgeon used blunt dissection techniques, you can expect more tenderness and the possible inconvenience of drain tubes for a few days.

The easier your surgeon expects your recovery to be, the shorter the list of postoperative instructions.

The more the surgeon can do in the operating room, the less you'll be burdened with after surgery.

Surgeons' postoperative instructions vary a lot. The most important thing to remember is to follow your surgeon's instructions! A surgeon knows what is done in the operating room and because of that, what needs to be done or not done after surgery.

Don't try to outthink your surgeon! Follow your surgeon's instructions.

And don't follow your friend's postoperative instructions if she had a different surgeon.

If you personally know other patients who have had breast augmentations, especially subpectoral breast augmentations, one of your greatest difficulties will be in believing that 24-hour return to normal activities is even remotely possible. We assure you that this rapid return to normal activities is possible whether your implants are over or under the pectoralis muscle.

If you talk to several women who've had breast augmentation, you'll find a tremendous amount of variation in their recovery experiences. If your surgeon is giving you instructions that sound a lot simpler than what you've heard, be grateful! Your surgeon is probably doing a lot of things in the operating room that allow you to have an easier and shorter recovery. If you hear from another patient that you shouldn't lift your arms, lift your child, or drive your car, and your surgeon is telling you it's okay to do all these things immediately, go for it! Your surgeon just made your life easier. On the other hand, if your surgeon tells you not to do these things, the surgeon probably has reasons. Always follow instructions.

Your Surgeon's Staff

Your surgeon's staff is an extension of your surgeon. The goal is to help you get better sooner, so it's important to follow the staff's advice and instructions. When a person calls to check on you, listen carefully to that person's questions and instructions. The information you convey will help the staff make the best recommendations to speed your recovery. The more knowledgeable the surgeon's staff, the better they can help answer your questions and give you optimal advice. If you're in doubt about anything after speaking with staff, ask to speak directly with your surgeon or ask for an appointment to see your surgeon.

THE MOST IMPORTANT DO'S

The following is a checklist of the most important do's that apply to almost all postoperative augmentation patients:

- ❏ Follow your surgeon's instructions to the letter. Don't try to outthink your surgeon.

- ❏ Stay hydrated. Drink plenty of fluids for the first few days after surgery.

- ❏ Eat. And eat well. You need nutrition to heal.

- ❏ Never take any pain medication on an empty stomach.

- ❏ Resume normal activity as soon as possible, following your surgeon's instructions.

- ❏ Read your postoperative instruction sheets. They'll help you expect what's normal.

- ❏ Expect to be frustrated that your tissues don't change rapidly according to your schedule.

- ❏ Expect to be too big, too high, and too tight for a few weeks.

- ❏ Expect differences and constant changes in size and shape of your breasts for three to six weeks.

❏ Expect to feel bloated and heavier for a few days. You were given fluids during surgery that will increase your weight (sometimes by several pounds), make you feel tight and bloated in some instances, and may make you feel full in the lower ribs and upper abdomen areas. Don't worry. Within 24-72 hours, most of it all comes off as urine.

❏ Get out of the house and do something. Staring at your breasts does not reduce swelling and tightness.

❏ Don't expect shape changes to occur quickly. We don't make any judgments about shape for at least three months.

❏ Remember that two breasts *never match* and that no surgeon can make them match.

❏ If anything seems wrong, check your written instructions and information, then call your surgeon!

THE MOST IMPORTANT DON'TS

Your surgeon may give you a longer list of things to avoid, but the following is a basic checklist of don'ts that we use following augmentation:

❏ Avoid any type of aerobic or other activities or anything that causes a significant increase in your pulse for two weeks. Walking is okay; running is not. Sex is okay, but Olympic sex is not!

❏ Don't lift heavy objects (over 30–40 lbs) or strain hard for two weeks.

❏ Don't take too many pain pills. Pain pills can nauseate and constipate you.

❏ Avoid whatever else your surgeon tells you to avoid.

PAIN MEDICATIONS—RELIEF VERSUS RECOVERY

Pain medications are a two-edged sword. The less you need, the better.

They're necessary for relief, but they can interfere with recovery.

Pain medications may relieve discomfort, but all narcotic-strength pain medications have side effects that can interfere with recovery. The stronger the pain medication, the more side effects, such as drowsiness, nausea, and constipation. One of the most important things you can do to get better is to get moving. The trick is to use enough pain medications to dull the discomfort at first. As soon as you get moving, things get better, and you'll need less pain medication.

The three worst routine side effects of pain medications are drowsiness, nausea, and constipation.

If you're sleepy, nauseated, and constipated, nothing's going to get moving!

If you don't get moving in the first 6-8 hours after surgery, your recovery will definitely be longer and more difficult.

"Get moving" doesn't mean trying to be an Olympic woman. Just resume normal activities.

Any pain medication can cause nausea if you take it on an empty stomach. Nausea after taking pain medications is not an allergic reaction. It's a side effect. The stronger the pain medication, the more likely it will cause nausea, especially if taken on an empty stomach.

Always put something in your stomach before taking pain medications: Crackers, toast, bagel—just something.

Pain medications can be extremely habit forming quickly. If you insist on stronger narcotic pain medications, you're often creating a problem instead of solving one. Using 24-hour surgical techniques,[1] narcotic strength pain medications are totally and completely unnecessary. Even without 24-hour techniques, you should not need any pain medications that are stronger than codeine or a codeine-equivalent drug. Over 96 percent of our augmentation patients[1] receive nothing but 800 mg ibuprofen for pain, and the majority of them take it only for two or three days following surgery. At least 50 percent don't take any pain medication after 48 hours. More than 3000 patients now prove that being out to dinner the evening of surgery and returning to full, normal activities is routinely predictable without any narcotic-strength pain medications. Patients who take narcotic-strength pain medications rarely, if ever, experience this rapid recovery because they are drowsy, do not mobilize in the first eight hours after surgery, become stiff and more uncomfortable, and have much more difficult recoveries. We know because before we developed 24-hour recovery techniques, our patients required stronger pain medications and experienced three-to ten-day return to normal activities. There are countless examples of patients who have become addicted to stronger pain medications such as Demerol, Tylox, Percodan, or Valium after taking them for as little as seven days. Don't be one of them.

WHAT TO EXPECT THAT'S NORMAL

If you know what to expect that's normal, you'll be less frightened or concerned.

If you're more knowledgeable and less concerned, recovery is much easier.

When you get concerned about something, first consult the following checklist. Everything on this list is normal following augmentation, so expect it. And continue to expect it for at least six weeks after surgery. If it's gone before then, you'll be pleasantly surprised.

- ❏ They don't match! My breasts are a different size and shape! And they're different every day!

- ❏ They're too high!

- ❏ They're too big!

- ❏ They're too tight and shiny.

- ❏ They're too swollen!

- ❏ They're too firm!

- ❏ I hear sloshing inside my breasts.

- ❏ They don't move!

❏ They're numb or they're too sensitive or I have weird sensations.

❏ I can't lie on them because they feel like basketballs! (96 percent of 627 of our patients were lying on their breasts the evening of surgery![1])

❏ My waist has disappeared.

❏ The magic time when they'll feel like they belong to me is three months after surgery.

Remember, **breasts never match**. Your Creator didn't make them match, and neither can your surgeon. Early after your surgery, one will always swell more than the other, adding to the difference. All of that is normal! Your breasts are supposed to feel too big, too tight, too firm, too swollen, and weird. Remember, yesterday you didn't have this much inside your breast. Your skin envelope requires time to adapt and stretch, and until it does, you'll feel strange and variable sensations. After surgery, with or without drain tubes, you'll produce a little fluid inside the pocket around your implants. This fluid, combined with a small amount of air that stays in the pocket from surgery, can produce a sloshing sound that you may or may not hear for a week or two after surgery. Don't worry. Your body will absorb all of this in a few days. As long as your skin is tight from being filled, your breasts won't move normally. When the skin stretches, they will move.

The larger your implants or the tighter your skin envelope, the more stretch the implant will put on sensory nerves. When nerves are stretched, they usually do one of three things: go numb, get more sensitive, send weird sensations to your brain, or all three. Sensory changes are very variable and very unpredictable regardless of the surgical technique. Sensory changes can take a long time to resolve, as much as two years in rare cases. Most patients' sensory changes are resolved by one year, but some take even longer. Other patients experience virtually no problems with sensation. It's just very unpredictable.

There is something magic about three months. At about three months, most of our patients feel their implants are a normal part of their body. They stop referring to "them" and start talking about "my breasts." The reason that this time period is magic is because your tissues will require about three months to return to a more normal state that you don't constantly notice as "different."

Remember the two things that you and your surgeon can't control are capsular contracture and tissue stretch. Capsular formation and tightening of the capsule around the implant never occur the same in both breasts and neither does tissue stretch. Capsular tightening tends to tighten the lining around the implant, reducing the forces of the implant pushing downward that produce tissue stretch. A capsule forms around every breast implant, and the manner in which the capsule forms is always different from one breast to the other. Even if a capsule does not tighten excessively and cause a capsular contracture deformity, it will tighten slighty differently in one breast compared to the other, another reason why breasts never match on the two sides following augmentation. All of these factors happening differently in your two breasts over time assure that not only will your breasts never match, but how they don't match will constantly change over time, especially in the first three months following your augmentation.

WHAT'S NOT NORMAL . . . CONTACT YOUR SURGEON

If you develop any of the following, you should contact your surgeon:

❏ Fever higher than 102 degrees or fever with chills

❏ One breast that is much, much larger than the other

❏ One breast that appears much more bruised than the other

❏ Noticeable redness and tenderness in any area of the breast

❏ Any drainage from your incision area after three days

❏ Any unusual discomfort

❏ Any breathing problems

❏ Any other symptoms that your surgeon advises you to call about

A TYPICAL RECOVERY WITH OUR PATIENTS

The typical recovery of our augmentation patients has changed dramatically since we developed and published our methods that allow 24-hour return to normal activities[1] and allow most patients to be out to dinner the evening of surgery. If someone had told us seven years ago that this type of recovery is possible, we categorically wouldn't have believed them and probably would have questioned what substance might be producing their delusions. But the dramatic changes are real, are predictable, and are consistent. Dramatic improvement in our methods, techniques, and devices can truly impact the patient experience.

The following is a description of a routine recovery in our augmentation patients.

The Night of Surgery

You leave the surgery facility a bit drowsy but comfortable. You will already have raised your arms fully extended over your head several times before you leave the surgical facility. When you arrive home, make yourself comfortable on the couch or in bed but *no more than a two hour nap!* Get up, drink some liquids, and eat some crackers, a bagel, or something light. Take an ibuprofen pill, wait about twenty minutes, and get in a hot shower. Wash your breasts, and raise your arms and wash your hair. When you come out of the shower, you'll feel much less stiff. Lift your arms, fully extended, above your head and touch the backs of your hands together, like performing a "jumping jack." With your arms over your head, your upper arm biceps muscles should be touching your ears. Lower your arms and repeat four times for a set of five. Repeat this entire sequence, performing a set of five every hour before bedtime, and you'll be amazed at how much easier the rest of your recovery will be! If you are out to dinner, do your arm raises as soon as you return home.

After you return home, don't stay in bed or recumbent for more than two hours. Get up and perform normal activities or do minor house-work. Go out for a brief walk, shopping, or out to dinner the night of surgery. (More than 90 percent of our patients are now out of the house doing these activities the evening of surgery.)

When you feel really hungry, provided you didn't have nausea with lighter foods and drinks, eat whatever you'd like. Don't pig out, but feel free to eat anything that sounds good.

Before you go to bed for the night, we want you to lie totally flat on your breasts. Yes, we know you don't believe us, and yes, we know the thought frightens you, but *yes*, we want you to *do it!* Most patients report that when they first begin to put weight on the breasts, they are apprehensive, but as they apply more pressure to the breasts, apprehension and discomfort usually decrease significantly. Getting up is harder than getting down. Don't attempt a push up; that stresses your pectoralis muscles. Instead, just roll to the side and sit up. If you find it difficult the first time, you can have someone help by placing their hands under your shoulders, but most patients can sit up without assistance the first or second attempt.

When you're ready to go to sleep for the night, provided you've put food in your stomach, take one of your 800 mg ibuprofen tablets and enjoy your rest. If you awake during the night and have trouble going back to sleep, take one of your 50 mg Benedryl capsules, rearrange yourself to get comfortable, and try to go back to sleep without additional pain pills. Sometimes, hugging a pillow to your chest can make you feel more comfortable. If you want to slip into a soft bra or jog bra, feel free to try it. You can't harm anything! Most of our patients are more comfortable without a bra, but you can treat your breasts as normal breasts. Wear or do not wear a bra according to your comfort.

The Morning after Surgery

When you awaken in the morning, you'll feel stiff. That's normal. Roll to your side and sit up to get out of bed. Relax in a comfortable chair or on the couch, and have a light breakfast of whatever you like. As soon as you get something in your stomach, take one pain pill, and enjoy the rest of your breakfast. When you feel the pain pill taking effect (you'll feel less stiff with less discomfort), get into a very warm shower and let the water run over your shoulders, chest, and breasts for five to ten minutes. Then, gradually lift your arms above your head and you'll loosen up just as you did the night before. When you leave the shower, repeat your arm raising exercises. You won't believe how much better you'll feel after getting your arms moving. Expect to feel some tightness at first. That's normal.

If you're feeling good, it's fine to go out to shop, to a movie, or anything else you'd like to do. Don't plan a whole day of anything. You'll get tired easily for the first two or three days, so plan to do something, but then midafternoon, come home and relax. There's no reason you can't drive as soon as you feel like it. Most of our patients drive within the first 24 hours, the morning after their surgery. Never drive if you're taking any narcotic-type pain pills.

While we're on the subject of pain pills, you should be aware that some surgeons do not recommend Advil or other forms of ibuprofen because they feel that these medications can interfere with normal blood-clotting mechanisms. Over the past ten years, we have used Advil and other forms of ibuprofen in over 2,500 patients, have had no increased rates of bleeding, and find these medications invaluable in shortening recovery and avoiding the side effects and addiction potential of stronger medications. Although we have tried other types of medications that are chemically similar to ibuprofen with supposedly less risk of causing bleeding, none of these medications so far have been as effective as ibuprofen, and our studies confirm that the doses that we are using have not caused any excessive bleeding.[2,3,4]

As soon as you feel like picking up normal weight objects or your small children, do it! Most of our patients with small children are able to pick them up by the day following surgery. Again, you won't hurt anything by picking up normal weight objects. Just avoid heavy objects and straining.

Be sure to drink plenty of liquids to avoid constipation. Remember, we want everything moving.

The First Two Days Following Surgery

Don't be surprised if you feel bloated. You received fluids during surgery, and you'll accumulate some swelling around your breasts and chest. As this swelling gravitates downward, you'll begin to feel that your waist is getting bigger. Don't panic! All this will resolve, and you'll go to the bathroom more often over the next two to four days.

The first two days following surgery are filled with the most nuisances and discomfort.

Immediately try to get back into most of your normal activities. The sooner, the better! Just plan your days to allow for some rest if you get tired in the afternoons.

The First Three Weeks

Listen to your body when it comes to all activity. If something is too stressful, stop and try it again tomorrow.

Your body will tell you what you need to know if you'll just listen. That doesn't mean to stop everything at the least sign of discomfort. Go ahead and move. But if something hurts, back off! Try again tomorrow or the next day. Whenever you're comfortable, sex is fine. You probably won't be overly amorous if someone puts too much pressure on your breasts the first few days, but there are ways around too much pressure. Your significant other may require a bit of coaching and understanding at first. Be creative when you feel like it, but save Olympic-level sex for a week or two after surgery.

During the first three weeks, your breasts will feel very tight. For most patients, the worst tightness is in the first three days, but this begins to decrease a lot after the first week. If your skin was very tight before surgery, expect the tightness to take longer to resolve. You'll get used to it more after three or four days, and it won't constantly occupy your mind after the first week. By three weeks, you'll notice some tightness, but you won't think about it much.

If you heard some sloshing in your breasts, that will usually be gone in three weeks or less. Numbness, excessive sensitivity, and strange feelings (like pin pricks or electric shocks) are all normal. Most of these sensory changes won't disappear in the first three weeks. They take much longer to return to normal. Don't make any judgements about sensation for at least six months to one year because sensation will continue to change and improve.

Wearing a bra is totally up to you. If you're more comfortable in a bra (any type), wear it. If you want to create a certain look, wear it. If you're more comfortable out of a bra, don't wear one. Despite anything you might hear, a bra should not affect the results of your surgery using techniques we have published.[2] We've used this regimen in over 2,500 patients and have found that you know better about what makes you comfortable than anyone else.

By the end of three weeks, most of the worst nuisances are over, but your breasts still won't feel like they really belong to you.

After three weeks, start thinking three months.

The First Three Months

Most of the time during the first three months you'll refer to your breasts as "them." They simply won't feel like they belong to you. There are things inside your breasts. After the first three weeks, the skin begins to relax faster, but you don't notice day by day. As the skin relaxes, the excessive upper fullness begins to decrease, provided you haven't selected an excessively large implant for your tissue characteristics. The implants aren't really "dropping," but they appear to be. What's really happening? As the lower skin stretches, it's not pushing back against the implant as hard between the nipple and the fold under your breast. As pressure on the lower implant decreases, the filler inside the implant is not pushed upwards as much by pressure of the tight lower skin, and the filler redistributes into the lower part of the implant and the breast. As upper fullness decreases some, you may feel that your breasts are getting smaller. They're not, but you may think so because most of the time you're looking down at them. Check out a side view in the mirror. You'll see that you're gradually getting more fullness in the lower breast. This progression happens in every augmentation patient and more in some than others. Expect it, and don't worry that your breasts are getting smaller.

Suddenly shopping is a lot more fun! Although your breasts will continue to change during the first three months, it's a totally new experience to go shopping, wear anything you want, and look fabulous. Different patients feel comfortable shopping at different times, but when you feel like it, do it.

A patient gave us a great description of how augmented breasts feel during the first three months. She said that "they are like trying to dial a phone with false fingernails. They just feel weird until you get used to them." That's what over 90 percent of patients tell us. They're not painful. You just notice them. Toward the end of the three-month period, you'll begin to notice them less, and one day, all of a sudden, you don't notice them at all. They're just part of you.

The Years That Follow

Once you no longer notice your breast implants, you'll almost totally forget them . . . provided you don't develop capsular contracture and provided you have made wise choices about implant size.

Once your tissues heal and adapt to your implants, your breasts will no longer seem foreign to you. You incorporate the new you into your body image automatically. Your breasts are just your breasts. The implants are no longer an issue, and they usually don't even cross your mind.

If you escape the low risk of capsular contracture, and you'll usually know by the first six months to one year, your breasts won't change much, and they will seem totally normal. If you made good choices about implant size, your breasts will mature at about the same rate as a normal breast the same size. You may develop slightly more sagging over time, just as any normal, larger breast does with aging, but your breast looks a lot better while it is aging. The larger the implant you selected and the thinner your tissues, the more sagging and thinning of your tissues you can expect with time.

AND THE LAST STEP

After recovery, you'll enjoy living with your new breasts. In the next chapter, we'll discuss living with your breast implants and the care and maintenance of the best breast.

References

1. Tebbetts, J. B. Achieving a predictable 24-hour return to normal activities after breast augmentation. Part II: Patient preparation, refined surgical techniques and instrumentation. *Plast. Reconstr. Surg.* 109: 293-305, 2002.

2. Tebbetts, J. B. Dual plane (DP) breast augmentation: Optimizing implant-soft tissue relationships in a wide range of breast types. *Plast. Reconstr. Surg.* 107: 1255, 2001.

3. Tebbetts, J. B., and Adams, W. P. Five critical decisions in breast augmentation using 5 measurements in 5 minutes: The high five system. *Plast. Reconstr. Surg.* 116(7), 2005.

4. Tebbetts, J. B. Achieving a zero percent reoperation rate at 3 years in a 50 consecutive case augmentation mammaplasty PMA study. *Plast. Reconstr. Surg.* 108(6): 1452-1457, 2006.

FOLLOW-UP:

LIVING WITH YOUR NEW BREASTS

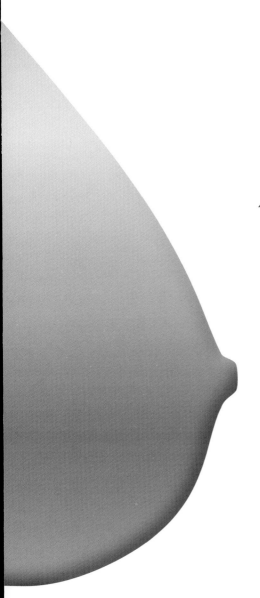

*"You don't need to baby your implants.
They should withstand any type of
normal, vigorous activity."*

Living with your new, augmented breasts is very similar to living with a normal breast, except that augmented breasts may require more maintenance.

More maintenance is the trade-off for feeling better about yourself.

ROUTINE MAINTENANCE

Follow-up Visits with Your Surgeon

Your surgeon can't give you optimal care if you don't show up for follow-up visits.

Routine follow-up visit schedules vary among surgeons. We like to check our patients within the first two days following surgery, then at three weeks, three months, one year, and every two years thereafter. We also instruct every patient to come in at any time they have any question or concern. One of the biggest problems with augmentation patients is failure to show up for follow-up visits. You think, "I'm doing great and don't have any problems, so I don't need to waste time and make a trip to see my surgeon." Wrong! Even if the visit is routine, your surgeon will be able to take better care of you and identify potential problems sooner if you do your part and show up. A surgeon should never charge you for follow-up visits following augmentation because they are part of the original costs. Take advantage of your surgeon's efforts to take the best possible care of you, no matter how well you think you're doing.

Supporting Your Breasts

Your breasts are supported primarily by your breast skin. As you get older, your breast skin usually becomes thinner and does not provide as much support. The larger your implants or the larger an unaugmented breast, the more weight in the breast and the more gravity will pull and stretch the skin over time, allowing your breast to sag.

Breasts that are supported some of the time sag less than breasts that are supported none of the time.

Sagging—how much and when—depends on your tissue characteristics, the size of your implants, your age, and how much you support your breasts.

Supporting your breasts, especially during activities that stress the skin and accelerate sagging, can decrease the amount of sagging and delay its onset. You can't totally escape the inevitable effects of gravity pulling on breast weight over time, but you can help. What happens if you never wear a bra? Check out pictures in _National Geographic_ of women who live in cultures where the breast is never supported. Aging is inevitable, but supporting the breast, at least some of the time, can delay the inevitable and reduce sagging.

If your breasts are bouncing, they are sagging faster than if they are not bouncing.

Support your breasts during any activity that causes bouncing.

Whenever you are doing any activity that causes your breasts to bounce, wear a bra or even two jog bras, if necessary, to immobilize the breasts as much as possible. Bouncing puts more stress on the skin in your lower breast and causes it to stretch more rapidly and to a greater degree. That stretch is what allows your breasts to sag. Bouncing is bad. Aside from activities that cause bouncing, wear a bra at least some of the time. At other times, enjoy your breasts. You don't need to wear a bra all the time.

Self-examination

Breast self-examination is an essential activity for every woman. One out of every ten or eleven women in the United States will develop breast cancer during her lifetime, and breast self-examination is one of the keys to early detection and cure.

Ask your gynecologist, family physician, or plastic surgeon to demonstrate optimal techniques. Perform breast self-examination every month about two weeks after the beginning of your menstrual period.

Your breast implants should not interfere with self-examination because the implants are behind, not within, the breast tissue. All of your breast tissue is in front of your implants and is totally accessible for examination by you or your physician. In fact, provided you don't have excessive firmness from capsular contracture, many physicians feel that breast examination is easier with implants in place.

Your breasts will feel different after you have implants. If you are thin and can feel your ribs with your fingers, you will probably be able to feel at least some part of your implants behind your breast regardless of the type of implants that you have. Wait until about three months after surgery to allow all swelling to resolve, and then ask your surgeon to demonstrate how to feel the edges of your implant in the lower or outer breast. Once you recognize the implant, you can distinguish it from anything else that is abnormal in either breast.

The larger your implants, the more you are likely to feel portions of the implant as you get older, because larger implants can cause more stretch and thinning that adds to the normal thinning most women experience as they age.

PHYSICIAN EXAMINATION

Every woman should have a thorough breast examination at least once every two years from age 20 to 35 and annually thereafter, by her family physician, gynecologist, or internal-medicine specialist.

Most women have breast exams at the time of routine gynecologic examinations. You will also have breast examinations at the times of your follow-up visits with your plastic surgeon. Most women who have breast augmentation have more frequent and more total breast examinations compared to the general population, provided they keep their follow-up appointments.

In addition to regular self-examination and physician examinations, you should immediately see your plastic surgeon, gynecologist, or family physician at any time that you notice anything substantially different in either breast or if you feel any mass or lump in either breast.

BREAST IMAGING: MAMMOGRAPHY AND MRI

Mammography recommendations differ among surgeons and other physicians. We require mammograms before any augmentation regardless of the patient's age. Following augmentation, we recommend waiting one year to allow all postoperative changes to resolve, then repeat a mammogram whenever it is convenient to establish a new baseline mammogram with your implant in place. Thereafter, you need mammograms annually or every other year after age 40, depending on the recommendations of your surgeon or gynecologist. If you have other risk factors, such as family history, that may increase your risks of breast cancer, more frequent mammograms will probably be necessary.

Mammograms for augmentation patients should be performed in a state-of-the-art breast center where all personnel are familiar with techniques of optimal imaging for breast augmentation patients.

If you ever hear any negative comments about augmentation during a visit to a mammogram facility, seek another facility because the personnel may not be familiar with optimal techniques.

Whenever you have a mammogram, ask the facility to fax a copy of the report to your plastic surgeon for your medical record.

Depending on the type of implant you choose and whether you may be enrolled in an FDA supervised study, check FDA recommendations and discuss with your surgeon the necessity and frequency of breast imaging studies following your augmentation.

Recreation and Athletics

Breast implants should not limit any type of recreational or athletic activities.

We have performed breast augmentation on several professional athletes in a wide range of sports: tennis, bodybuilding, race car driving, basketball, and others. Most of these have involved submuscular implant placement because most athletes have minimal body fat and thin tissues. Even with an implant under the pectoral muscle, these athletes don't miss a beat. Neither should you.

Theoretically, any high-impact blow can rupture an implant. A high-speed automobile accident or other severe trauma can rupture implants. But a lot of force is required, far more than you will encounter in any normal athletic activity.

DURABILITY, RUPTURE, DEFLATION

Today's state-of-the-art implants are much stronger and more durable than you might think. I've demonstrated the strength of Inamed-Allergan anatomic saline implants by filling an implant and standing with my full weight on the implant without rupturing it. Nevertheless, implant shells can fail, usually due to folding from underfill (see chapter 4), but also from rare manufacturing defects or valve failure. High-energy impact can also cause implant rupture, but even the most vigorous physical or sexual activity is unlikely to damage an implant without damaging you first. Allergan guarantees its implants for your lifetime, so any implant failure is more of a nuisance than a real problem.

You don't need to baby your implants. They should withstand any type of normal, vigorous activity.

However, your implants were not designed to withstand closed capsulotomy, the practice of forcefully squeezing your breast to correct capsular contracture.

We advise every augmentation patient that implant rupture is usually nothing more than a huge nuisance. I can replace any implant in less than 15 minutes in the operating room if implant replacement is all that's required, and you'll experience virtually no discomfort after surgery. The nuisance is filling out the necessary paperwork for the implant guarantee and doing the necessary preparations and laboratory tests prior to surgery. We never charge any patient on whom we performed an augmentation to replace the implant later if replacement becomes necessary. Amounts of coverage for anesthesia and operating room costs associated with replacement procedures vary among manufacturers, and you should read all of the fine print in manufacturers' warranties very closely.

Replacement of a ruptured silicone-gel implant, though slightly more involved than replacement of a saline-filled implant, is easy and routine for a qualified surgeon, provided you didn't have a previous closed capsulotomy performed on your breast. Closed capsulotomy is a forceful squeezing of the breast that some surgeons used (and some still use) to correct an excessively hard breast caused by excessive contraction or tightening of the capsule (lining) that forms around breast implants. Closed capsulotomy is attractive to patients who want to avoid surgery, but it can be very painful, cause bleeding and other complications, and does not predictably correct excessively firm breasts. In order to make a breast feel softer, closed capsulotomy produces tearing of the capsule (lining) surrounding the breast implant. Provided you didn't have a closed capsulotomy that disrupted the capsule around your implant, silicone gel that escapes from the implant is still surrounded by the capsule and is easy to remove. The only time that gel removal is complicated is following a closed capsulotomy when gel has been forced outside the capsule into the breast tissue. Never let anyone perform a closed capsulotomy on your breast!

With new, state-of-the-art, cohesive-gel anatomic implants from Allergan (the Inamed style 410, full-height anatomic implant), the implant was specifically designed to attempt to minimize or eliminate gel migration even if the implant shell disrupts (see chapter 4). The gel is so cohesive (sticky) that it is difficult to force it out of the shell even if the shell is cut.

If you ever have any type of problem with implant deflation or rupture, insist on a qualified surgeon.

Implant deflation or rupture is no big deal if your surgeon knows how to deal with it.

Anything can be difficult if you don't know how to do it, and the last thing you need is someone who doesn't know how to easily manage problems!

The Three Ss—Sex, Scuba Diving, and Skydiving

For some reason, we get more questions about these three activities than all others combined. Implants can withstand almost any sexual activities. The pressure changes that occur with scuba diving, skydiving, or airline travel are of virtually no consequence to state-of-the-art breast implants. Go for it! You shouldn't need to worry about your implants.

IF PROBLEMS OCCUR . . .

We can't comprehensively address every problem that can potentially happen with a breast implant, but chapter 7 covers most problems in detail. The following is a summary overview of some problems for your review.

Excessive Firmness

Capsular contracture usually occurs in the first six months to one year following augmentation. Although the development and tightening of the capsules always vary slightly on the two sides, if you notice one breast becoming noticeably firmer than the other, contact your surgeon. The best treatment is to completely remove the capsule and replace the implant and hope that your body won't do it again. If it does, we recommend removing both implants rather than increasing risks with repeated surgeries.

Displacement

If implants significantly displace from their desired position, the deformity is often difficult to treat. To reposition implants, the surgeon must close a portion of the pocket. That's relatively easy. Keeping it closed to prevent recurrent displacement is not easy because the surgeon is working with the same tissues that allowed excessive stretching in the first place. The larger the implant and the thinner your tissues, the less likely you'll get a long-term correction. Don't cause the problem with excessively large implants to begin with, and hope that your tissues are not genetically prone to excessive stretch.

Change in Size or Shape

Remember that your breasts will never match. Small changes in shape often may seem to be changes in size and are normal in every patient. However, a dramatic change in size usually means an implant leak or rupture. Treatment? Replace the implant.

A dramatic change in shape usually indicates that an area of the pocket has closed or the capsule is squeezing on the implant affecting its shape and its position. The best treatment is to partially or completely remove the capsule and replace the implant.

Tenderness

Tenderness in the breast is usually a response to hormonal changes that occur with aging or with changes in hormone or birth-control medications. Tenderness can also occur in response to caffeine, chocolate, and other medications.

During the first three months following augmentation, tenderness can be due to the implant stretching nerves, usually at the sides of the breasts. After three months, nerve stretch tenderness is unusual. If you develop severe capsular contracture that causes excessive firmness of the breasts, the breasts can become tender.

More than three months after augmentation, if you don't have capsular contracture or an excessively large implant stretching breast nerves, tenderness is usually not due to your implants.

If you develop tenderness, pay close attention to whether it changes during your hormonal cycle. If it does, it's usually due to hormonal changes. If it is constant and persists, contact your surgeon or gynecologist.

Breast cancer almost never causes tenderness.

"I've Lost Sensation"

Read more about sensation and sensory changes in chapter 7. Most patients lose some sensation immediately after augmentation, and most get significant return of that sensation six to twelve months following surgery. Many patients lose no sensation what so ever, and some patients actually develop hypersensitivity. Sensation just isn't very predictable.

Sensory changes are common regardless of the incision location, type of implant, or whether the implant is above or below muscle. Sensory changes are very unpredictable and depend on several factors, many of which you and your surgeon can't control.

Generally, the larger the implant, the larger the pocket the surgeon must create, the more stretch on nerves, and the more sensation you'll lose.

If you don't get the sensation back in two years, don't expect it to return.

Many patients want larger implants after their tissues have stretched and adapted to their current implants.

Very few patients think about the consequences of placing larger implants.

Every surgeon has heard this request from patients following augmentation. Perhaps it's due to the "if a little is good, a lot is better" rationale. Perhaps it's due to women feeling that their breasts are getting smaller as the excessive upper fill in the breast redistributes more into the lower breast. Placing larger implants doesn't solve either problem. This move just creates new questions and problems. How much is enough? How will we know? Are you willing to accept all the risks of your first surgery again, plus some new risks? Remember:

You can't keep a lot of fill in the upper breast by placing larger implants.

Over time and with aging, your lower-breast skin will stretch, and you'll always lose some upper fullness unless you have capsular contracture.

With larger implants, sagging will occur sooner and more, and you face added risks of implant-edge visibility, visible traction rippling of the breast, thinning of your breast envelope tissues, shrinkage of your existing breast tissue, and other surgical complications.

Is it really worth it? Past a proportionate amount of enlargement, bigger is definitely not better if you want to minimize risks, reoperations, and uncorrectable tissue deformities.

One Is Different from the Other

One breast is always different from the other. No surgeon can make two breasts match exactly. Don't expect your breasts to match. If they are close, wonderful! That means you're like every other woman who has a normal amount of variation between the size and shape of her breasts.

Don't fall into the trap of thinking that if one is smaller than the other, the solution is simple. Just put more implant or more filler in the current implant in the smaller breast. It's not that simple. The smaller breast has less skin. If you try to put more filler into less skin, you'll often get permanent, excessive bulging in the upper breast. A difference in shape with more upper bulging on one side is much more noticeable than a difference in size.

Remember, a difference in size is normal. Every woman has it.

Don't chase small differences in size and shape. You could end up looking worse!

Complications—When to Quit

Although we've mentioned this before, it's important to mention again. A huge majority of patients have absolutely no problems whatsoever with their implants. But a few patients have a lot of problems— sometimes because of factors neither surgeon nor patient can control and sometimes the result of bad team decisions by the patient and the surgeon.

There are worse things than removing and not replacing breast implants. You may not like your breasts as well, but if you seem to have persistent or severe problems, there's a very logical solution. Get rid of your implants. Over 90 percent of the implant "horror cases" we've reviewed could have been averted if someone, either patient or surgeon, had said, "Enough! Let's get them out!" If you used good judgement in your initial selection of implant, your breasts should not look any worse than they would look after a pregnancy.

THE LAST WORD

We'll stop where we started.

The BEST BREAST is the natural female breast until nature misses a beat or takes a toll, or a woman decides that it's not.

It's normal to want to feel normal. It's also normal to want to be the best that you can be. Breast augmentation can help with those normal goals.

Whether breast augmentation is right for you is a personal decision. Whether you get the best breast depends on how much you know, how well you do your homework, how well you make decisions, how qualified and skilled your surgeon is, and Mother Nature factors that neither you nor your surgeon can control. One thing is for sure. You're better prepared now than when you started, and you have a better chance of getting the Best Breast!

BREAST AUGMENTATION:

ELEVEN IMPORTANT VISUAL

LESSONS

"Perfection or change to a different breast is never an option. Improvement in the existing breast is the only realistic alternative. When looking at pictures, look for breasts that look like your breasts BEFORE surgery."

Pictures best illustrate some of the most important principles in augmentation. Pictures can also be misleading and confusing. What you see depends on what you know. The more you know, the more thoroughly and systematically you can evaluate pictures. Many of the terms and concepts used in this chapter have been explained in earlier chapters, so this chapter will be most meaningful and useful if you have read the previous chapters.

These visual lessons in augmentation focus on important concepts that every augmentation patient should know.

Every woman's augmentation result is determined by two factors:

1) What the woman WANTS, and

2) What the woman's body (her tissues) will ALLOW HER TO HAVE (what the surgeon has to work with).

As you look at any pictures of augmentation results, remember:

This woman's breasts are unique in shape and appearance, different from any other woman's. This woman's tissues are different from any other woman's.

This woman's wishes are different from any other woman's.

It's impossible to look at a catalog of breast pictures and pick out what you'd like to have, unless your breasts are exactly the same as the woman's in the picture before surgery—and they are never the same! Remember, the three most critically important factors in determining optimal implant size can never be accurately assessed in any two-dimensional picture (without special equipment for scaling): 1) the base width of the breast, 2) the amount of stretch, and 3) the amount of existing breast tissue. It's also impossible to know exactly what the woman in the picture requested. What she wanted might be very different from what you want. And, most importantly, the characteristics of her breast tissues are not exactly like yours.

We have chosen each set of images to make a point. Each breast is not the most beautiful breast or the most "perfect" breast. Any experienced surgeon can select a large number of "best" results, but if education is the goal, you need to see a full range of breast types, results, and common problems. As you study the lessons, focus on the message of each image. Don't necessarily ask yourself whether you particularly like the breast. Remember, what you see in a before image is all the surgeon had to work with. Perfection or a change to a different breast is never an option. Improvement in the existing breast is the only realistic alternative.

LESSON I:

Each woman's breasts have unique tissue characteristics. The skin envelope and breast tissue are different in every woman. A surgeon can work only with what the patient brings (her unique tissue characteristics). Ideal choices are different for each woman, depending on her wishes and her tissues.

This important principle is illustrated by the following before-and-after case studies. Compare each case to the other cases. Focus on the substantial differences among patients' tissues before augmentation and how those differences affected the results. Concentrate on the two major components of the breast: the skin envelope and the breast tissue (parenchyma) that fills the skin envelope. For each different combination of skin envelope and breast tissue, we will emphasize principles that affect the choices of implant and technique in each different type of breast.

Skin Envelope: Tight, Unstretched
Breast Tissue: Minimal

(Figure 16-1 A,B)

Before   **After**

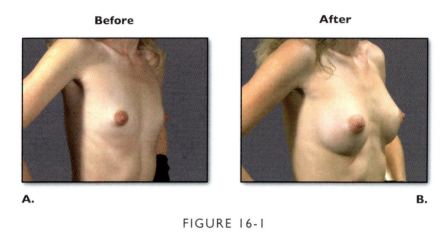

A.   B.

FIGURE 16-1

When the skin is tight and thin with minimal breast tissue to cover a breast implant, the most important considerations are these:

1. Avoid an excessively large implant. The skin will stretch only a moderate amount without permanently damaging or thinning the skin. Choose an implant that will not cause excessive skin stretch.

2. When tissues are thin and a patient can feel and see her ribs, she will also be able to feel the edges and possibly the shell of her implant regardless of the type of implant chosen.

3. Positioning the upper portion of the implant partially under the pectoralis muscle (in a dual-plane or submuscular pocket location) reduces the risk of the upper edge of the implants being visible.

4. Thin tissues will not support the weight of an excessively large implant as a patient ages. With an excessively large implant, the breast will sag more, the skin will become thinner, implant edges can become visible, visible rippling can occur, and shrinkage of existing breast tissue can occur from the weight of the implant pulling on the thin overlying tissues.

Skin Envelope: Stretched, Looser
Breast Tissue: Minimal

(Figure 16-2, A–C)

Before   **After**

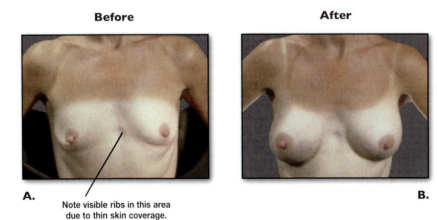

A.

Note visible ribs in this area
due to thin skin coverage.

B.

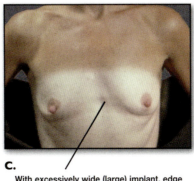

C.

With excessively wide (large) implant, edge
would be visible here.

FIGURE 16-2

Breast enlargement with pregnancy usually stretches the skin, leaving the skin envelope looser. The breast tissue inside the envelope often shrinks following pregnancy. The result is less filler in a larger, looser skin envelope. The most important considerations with loose skin and minimal breast tissue are these:

1. Adequately fill the loose envelope for the best result, but avoid overfilling. An excessively small implant will fill the lower breast, but leaves the upper breast empty (the rock-in-a-sock look). When the loose envelope skin is thin (note the patient's visible ribs), the goal should be to provide just enough fill (implant size) to expand the envelope for a natural upper-breast profile. Any implant larger than that required for adequate fill will cause excessive stretching and further thinning of the envelope as this patient ages, and risks all of the same long-term problems described previously.

2. A thin skin envelope with minimal breast tissue covering the implant almost guarantees that the patient may feel some portion of the implant, just as she could feel her ribs beneath the thin tissues.

3. Notice the extremely thin skin in the cleavage area between the breasts. If the implants selected were wider than the existing breast tissue (Figure 16-2, C) in an attempt to narrow the gap between the breasts, the edge of the implant would be visible beneath the thin skin between the breasts. To avoid a visible implant edge between the breasts, an implant was selected that was slightly narrower than the patient's breast tissue. The patient had to choose between a) narrowing the gap between the breasts more and risking a visible implant edge or b) accepting a slightly wider gap between the breasts and avoiding a visible implant edge. She chose option b.

Skin Envelope: Stretched, Looser
Breast Tissue: Moderate

(Figure 16-3 A,B)

Before   **After**

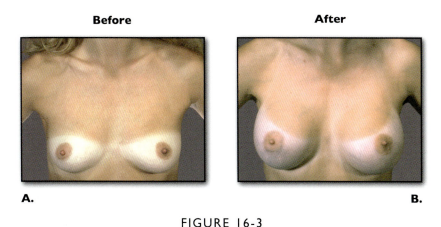

A.   **B.**

FIGURE 16-3

1. When more breast tissue is present in a stretched envelope, the breast tissue provides more cover for the implant, and the patient is less likely to feel portions of the implant.

2. The combination of skin already stretched by pregnancy with adequate breast tissue to cover an implant is ideal for augmentation.

3. The patient and surgeon can select from a wider range of implant sizes or widths without risking implant edge visibility when more breast tissue is present (a wider base width of the breast mound in front view).

Skin Envelope: Very Loose
Breast Tissue: Moderate

(Figure 16-4 A,B)

Before **After**

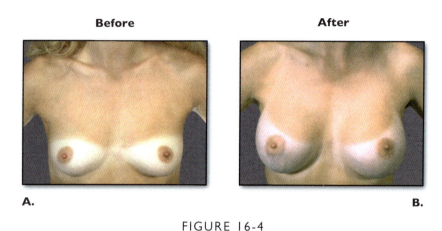

A. B.

FIGURE 16-4

1. The larger a breast, whether normally or during pregnancy or nursing, the more the skin envelope stretches. This patient's stretched skin envelope could be the result of gravity pulling on a moderately large breast as she aged or could have resulted from breast enlargement during pregnancy or nursing. In either case, the appearance could be exactly the same.

2. Although it's important to adequately fill a stretched envelope for an optimal result, when we see sagging of the breast before surgery, the skin envelope tissues are sending a message. The skin envelope did not support the weight of the patient's own tissue, or it wouldn't have stretched and allowed the breast to sag!

3. Although this stretched envelope could accommodate a very large implant and maintain a natural appearance, what will the excessively large implant cause when placed in an envelope that has already proved that it cannot support the weight of the patient's own tissues? More sagging and more tissue thinning!

4. The key to a good long-term result in this type of breast is to select an implant that will provide adaquate fill but avoid selecting the largest implant that the envelope could accommodate. The largest implant might look good, but only for a while. It would rapidly cause more stretch, more sagging with loss of fill in the upper breast, thinning of the skin envelope, increased risks of visible rippling in the upper breast, and increased risks of shrinkage of existing breast tissue. Excessive sagging could necessitate a breast-lift procedure (mastopexy) with additional trade-offs of more scars on the breast and possible increased loss of sensation. Making the right choices is important at the first operation.

LESSON 2:

A woman's breasts are never the same on both sides, and no two women have breasts that are exactly the same. No surgeon can make both breasts exactly the same; differences will always exist after surgery. Each type of breast presents unique problems, and every correction involves limitations and trade-offs.

In each of the following cases, we will point out the unique characteristics of the patient's tissues, the different problems that each patient's tissues present, and the corrections that were achieved by augmentation. In each case, we will also emphasize the *limitations* that each patient's tissues imposed and the *trade-offs* that were present during the decision-making process.

These different patients prior to augmentation emphasize the extreme variations in breast characteristics from one woman to another (Figure 16-5, A–J). To further appreciate the differences, select one characteristic from the following list. Then scan up and down the left and right columns on these pages. Notice how each characteristic varies from breast to breast.

Breasts differ tremendously from woman to woman.

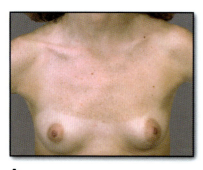 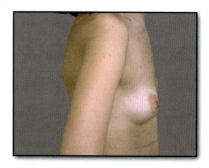

A.   **B.**

FIGURE 16-5

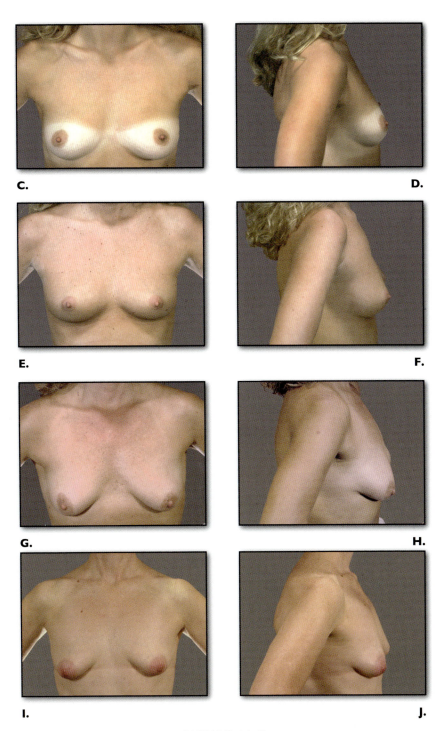

C.

D.

E.

F.

G.

H.

I.

J.

FIGURE 16-5

- Breast size

- Gap between the breasts in front view

- Breast shape

- Nipple location on one side compared to the other (one higher or lower)

- Sag of breast in side view compared to the other (one higher than lower)

- Upper breast fullness inside view

- Nipple tilt (pointing up or down)

- Ribs or breastbone visible, indicating thin overlying tissues

- Nipple orientation (pointing inward or outward)

- Breast size variation from side to side in each patient in front view

- Width of the breast in front view

All breasts look different after augmentation because all breasts look different before augmentation. A surgeon can improve only what the patient brings. A surgeon cannot exchange a patient's tissues for a different set of tissues. In the before-and-after illustrations that follow, notice that each result is only an improvement over what the patient has before surgery. The appearance of the breast before surgery is a major factor affecting the appearance of the result. Breast augmentation surgery offers improvement, not perfection.

FIGURE 16-6

Tissues:

No pregnancies, skin envelope not stretched, minimal breast tissue, thin tissues.

Problems:

Breasts too small for torso, left smaller than right, left higher than right, left nipple higher than right, wide gap between the breasts, inadequate upper fullness.

Corrections, Limitations, Trade-offs:

Size and proportion improved, left nipple higher than right (patient declined lifting the right nipple to avoid more scars and possible loss of sensation), gap between breasts narrowed some. Patient elected to acccpt a slightly wider gap following surgery rather than risk a visible implant edge in the cleavage area if we had selected a wider implant to further narrow the gap.

Before

After

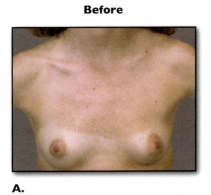

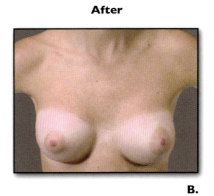

A.

B.

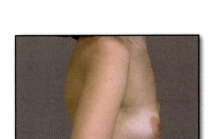

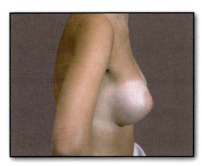

C.

D.

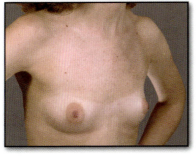

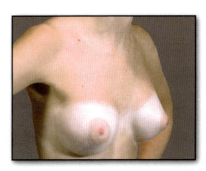

E.

F.

FIGURE 16-6

FIGURE 16-7

Tissues:

Two pregnancies, skin envelope moderately stretched, moderate breast tissue, tissues thin. (Note visible ribs beneath breasts.)

Problems:

Loss of upper fullness, loss of forward projection, excessively wide gap between the breasts or not enough cleavage.

Corrections, Limitations, Trade-offs:

Improved upper fullness, cleavage, and projection. Better overall proportion with torso by widening breasts at the sides. In front view, widening the breasts at the sides improves the balance of breast width with hip width and makes the waist appear smaller.

Before

After

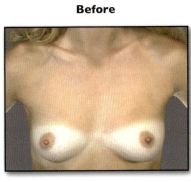

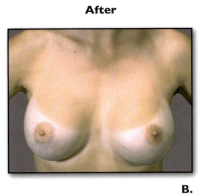

A.

B.

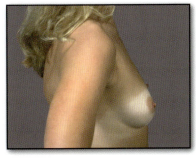

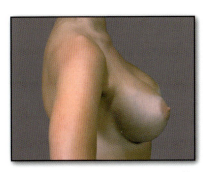

C.

D.

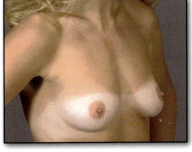

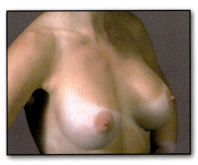

E.

F.

FIGURE 16-7

FIGURE 16-8

Tissues:

Two pregnancies, stretched envelope, minimal breast tissue.

Problems:

Very narrow breasts in front view with wide gap between breasts, thin skin in gap between breasts, thin skin envelope with ribs visible, breasts too triangular or "pointy" rather than round in front view, no upper breast fullness, down-pointing nipples.

Corrections, Limitations, Trade-offs:

Overall improved appearance, with a rounder, fuller, lifted appearance. Gap between breasts narrowed some, but limited because of thin skin between breasts and risk of visible implant edge if wider implant were used to narrow the gap more. Dramatic improvement in upper fullness and overall breast shape while preserving a natural breast appearance after augmentation. Nipples remain slightly down pointing.

Before

After

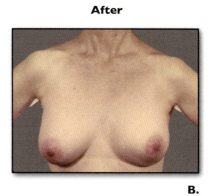

A.

B.

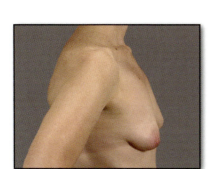

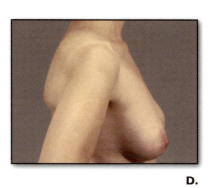

C.

D.

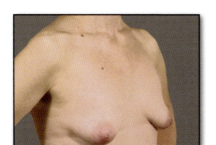

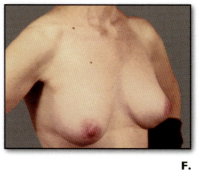

E.

F.

FIGURE 16-8

FIGURE 16-9

Tissues:

Two pregnancies, but minimal stretch of the skin envelope, moderate amount of breast tissue, envelope already relatively full. (Note upper breast is relatively full in side view before surgery.)

Problems:

Patient desires more cleavage, larger, fuller breasts to improve balance with hips and torso, overall figure balance.

Corrections, Limitations, Trade-offs:

Dramatic improvement in cleavage was possible because the gap between the breasts was narrower prior to surgery, the breast tissue was wider (to cover the edges of the implant), and the patient's skin was thicker in the gap between the breasts. All of these factors reduce the risk of seeing an implant edge between the breasts and allowed use of a wider implant to maximally improve the cleavage. Overall breast fullness improved, overall balance with figure improved.

Before

After

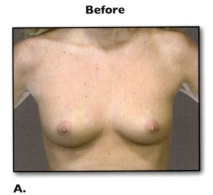

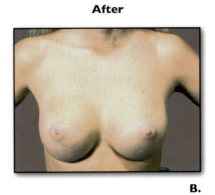

A.

B.

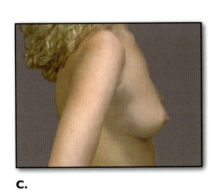

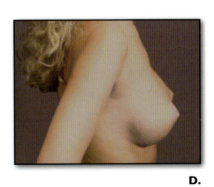

C.

D.

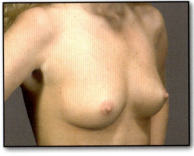

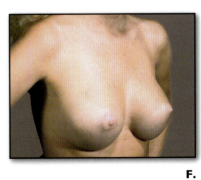

E.

F.

FIGURE 16-9

FIGURE 16-10

Tissues:

No pregnancies, skin envelope not stretched by pregnancy, but stretched by gravity pulling downward on breasts over time. Moderate amount of breast tissue, located primarily in the lower portion of the skin envelope. Breast shape determined by developmental factors during puberty and by gravity over time.

Problems:

Extreme down-pointing breasts, nipple-areola located low on breast mound and down-pointing, sagging appearance, inadequate fullness upper breast, inadequate cleavage or fullness in the middle area of each breast. Nipples located toward the outside of each breast mound rather than more centrally.

Corrections, Limitations, Trade-offs:

Patient declined nipple repositioning due to trade-offs of scar around nipple-areola and possible sensory loss. Overall appearance improved but with limitations. Nipples lifted, but still somewhat down-pointing. Nipples still located toward the outside of each breast mound. Upper fullness improved, overall breast shape improved, cleavage improved. Narrowing of the gap between the breasts limited due to risk of visible implant edge under the thin skin between the breasts if a wider implant were placed.

Before

After

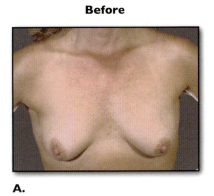

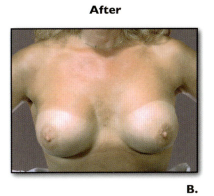

A.

B.

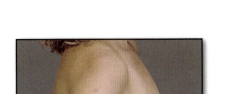

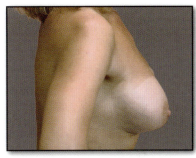

C.

D.

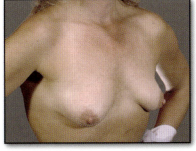

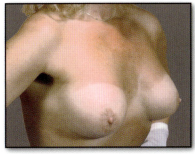

E.

F.

FIGURE 16-10

FIGURE 16-11

Tissues:

Envelope thin, not stretched, virtually no breast tissue present.

Problems:

Very little skin to work with, very difficult to achieve a normal appearing breast without the implant being obvious; lack of fullness in all areas of the breast, figure imbalance between breasts and torso and hips, lack of cleavage with wide gap between the breasts.

Corrections, Limitations, Trade-offs:

Improved overall breast shape and fullness, natural appearing breast, implant not obvious, improved cleavage and narrowing of gap between breasts but limited due to thin skin between breasts and risk of implant edge visibility. Note the visible ribs and breast bone between the breasts. Using any larger implant would produce visible implant edges in this area.

Before

After

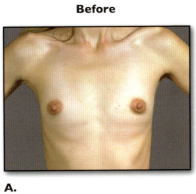

A.

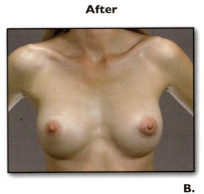

B.

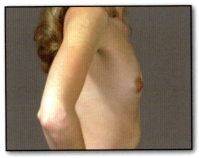

C.

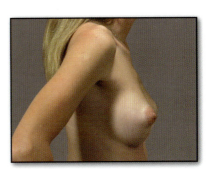

D.

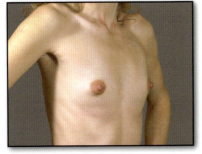

E.

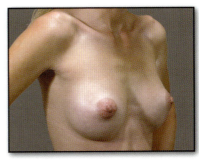

F.

FIGURE 16-11

LESSON 3:

What is enough, and what is too much?

The ideal size of implant is different from one woman to another, depending on the size of the woman's skin envelope before augmentation. If we could insert a funnel into the top of the breast, as we pour fluid into the funnel, the bottom of the breast would fill first, but the top would not be adequately filled (Figure 16-12, A). As we continue to add fluid, at some point, the upper breast would be full but still have a natural appearance (Figure 16-12, B). If we continued to add fluid, the upper breast would begin to bulge outwardly, with an excessively full and somewhat unnatural appearance (Figure 16-12, C).

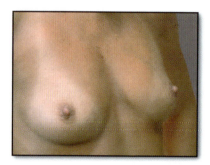

A.

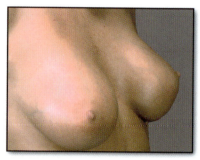

B.

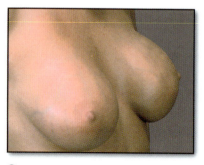

C.

FIGURE 16-12

VERY IMPORTANT TO REMEMBER!

The ideal size implant for any breast is the implant that will adequately fill the breast, but not overfill it. A surgeon can always put a larger-than-ideal implant in a breast, and many patients request implants that are too large for their tissues. Many patients actually prefer the appearance of an excessively full upper breast with outward bulging—the too-much look *without* a bra. When any implant that is larger than ideal for a specific patient's tissues is placed in a breast, the patient will pay a price in the future. The skin envelope will stretch and thin, the breast will sag, and all of the following risks increase: feeling the implant, seeing an implant edge, loss of upper fullness, visible rippling at the top or sides of the breast from the large implant pulling downward on thin tissues, compression and shrinkage of existing breast tissue, and likely a necessity of additional surgery to correct problems.

LESSON 4:

You won't look like your friend.

Let's assume that two friends (we'll call them Sharon and Janet, but the names are fictitious) decide to have breast augmentation. Sharon (Figure 16-13, A-B) has her augmentation first (Figure 16-13, C–D).

Janet sees Sharon's result, and says, "I want my result to look just like Sharon's." When we examined Janet, we found that her breasts were very different than Sharon's (Figure 16-14, A–B). Can we produce the same breast that we produced for Sharon? Of course not, because the breasts were so different before augmentation. Janet's result is shown in Figure 16-14, C–D.

Sharon

Before

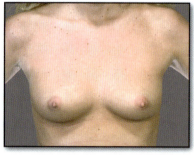

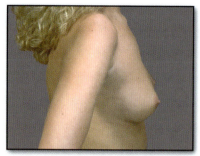

A.

B.

After

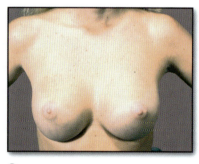

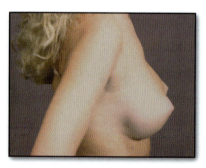

C.

D.

FIGURE 16-13

Wide breast in front view

Narrow gap between breasts

More breast tissue in skin envelope

Thicker skin envelope

Skin envelope not very stretched

Janet wants to achieve the same result that Sharon achieved. Can any surgeon match Janet's breasts to Sharon's?

Janet

Before

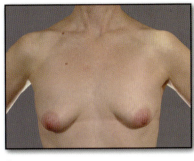

A.

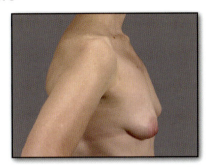

B.

After

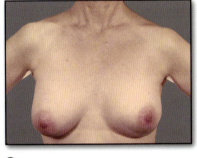

C.

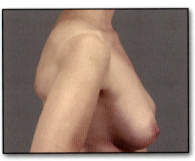

D.

FIGURE 16-14

Narrow breast in front view

Wide gap between breasts

Less breast tissue in skin envelope

Thin skin envelope

Skin envelope very stretched

Note the differences in Sharon and Janet *before* surgery:

A surgeon cannot change the *differences in these two patients' tissues before surgery*. Different tissues before surgery guarantee that their breasts will be different after surgery.

You can't select a certain breast from a picture and realistically expect to achieve that result.

Optimal implant size depends on base width of the breast, degree of skin stretch, amount of existing breast tissue (parenchyma)

LESSON 5:

A certain size implant does not produce a certain size breast.

Let's look again at our two hypothetical friends from Lesson 4 (see figures 16-13, A–D and 16-14, A–D). These friends, Sharon and Janet, requested and received exactly the same size implant. Are their breasts the same size after surgery? No. A certain size implant does not produce a certain size breast. Remember our formula from chapter 4?

Augmentation Result = Envelope + Parenchyma (breast tissue) + Implant

Sharon had more breast tissue *before* surgery than Janet, so with the *same size* implant, Sharon's breasts will be larger than Janet's breasts *after* surgery. The size of implant required to achieve the breast size you want after surgery depends on how much breast tissue you have *before* surgery.

We frequently see patients who have a certain size implant in mind based on what a friend had or what they may have heard, read in magazines, or learned from a chat group on the Internet.

Many women believe that a certain size implant (in ccs) is required to achieve a certain cup-size breast. This lesson clearly illustrates that a certain size implant does not produce a certain cup-size breast.

You should know that when you request a certain size implant, the easiest thing for a surgeon to do is fulfill your request rather than try to explain to you why that size implant may not be the best for you long-term. If you want the best result and the least risk of problems and additional operations as you age, discuss your wishes with your surgeon, but ask your surgeon to help you make the best decisions about implant size. Remember that "excessively large" carries a price as you get older.

LESSON 6:

Cleavage—what makes it and how much can I get?

Normal breasts don't cleave. Bras make breasts cleave. If breasts were intended to look like buttocks, they would be touching in most patients, and they are not! As breasts develop during puberty, the breast tissue develops on a curved surface, the chest wall. Gravity pulls the breasts outward slightly, so most breasts point slightly outward. Very few women's breasts point straight ahead. The width of the gap between the breasts depends on two factors: 1) the width of the woman's breast in front view, and 2) the total width of the torso. For a specific width torso, the wider the breast, the narrower the gap between the breasts. Stated another way, for a specific width breast, the wider the torso, the wider the gap between the breasts.

When the gap between the breasts is wide (Figure 16–17, A), two factors determine how much the gap can be narrowed: 1) the width, amount, and consistency of the patient's own breast tissue, and 2) the width and size of the breast implant. The wider the implant (Figure 16-17, B), the more the gap narrows, but distinct trade-offs and risks exist. If the implant is wider than the patient's breast tissue (Figure 16-17,C), the breast tissue no longer covers the edge of the implant, and the edge rests beneath only the thin skin in the gap between the breasts. When thin tissues cover an implant edge, the patient must accept a higher risk of the implant being visible in the cleavage area. What is the message to remember? If you request narrowing of the gap between your breasts, ask your surgeon to demonstrate how much the gap can be narrowed without risking edge visibility of your implant. If you want more narrowing than the surgeon demonstrates, be prepared to sign an

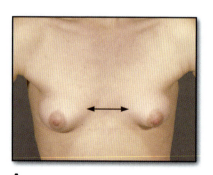

A.

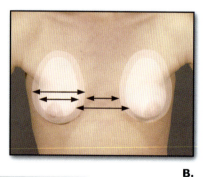

B.

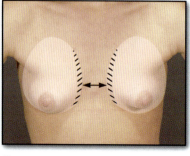

C.

FIGURE 16-17

informed-consent document that confirms your acceptance of the risk of implant-edge visibility and traction rippling developing with time as you get older and the implants pull on the thin, overlying tissues.

The patient below (see Figure 16–18, A) has extremely narrow breasts and a wide gap between the breasts. Following augmentation (see Figure 16-18, B), the gap between the breasts is narrower but not extremely narrow. Notice in the picture after augmentation that the sternum (the central chest bone) is visible under the thin skin between the breasts. If a wider implant had been used to narrow the gap further, the edge of the implant would be just as visible as the breastbone and ribs. More fullness in the middle would further emphasize the already outwordly pointing nipples.

Before   **After**

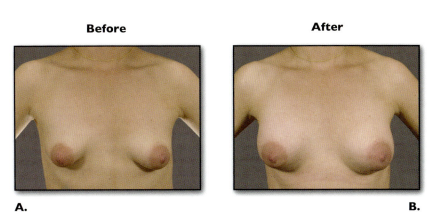

A.   **B.**

FIGURE 16-18

LESSON 7:

A certain incision location or pocket location (beneath breast or beneath muscle) does not produce a specific appearance in the result. Put another way, you absolutely can't reliably tell from looking at a picture whether an implant is over or under muscle nor through which incision the implants were placed.

An experienced augmentation surgeon can produce almost exactly the same result above or below muscle provided the surgeon has adequate experience with both locations and can produce exactly the same result through multiple incision approaches.

Look at the following results following augmentation (Figure 16–19). Which are over muscle and which are under muscle?

The implants are under muscle (A), over muscle (B), over muscle (C), and under muscle (D). Incision locations are under the breast (A), in the armpit (B), in the armpit (C), under the breast and around the areola (D). Each incision location and pocket location have advantages and trade-offs that are described in detail in chapter 6.

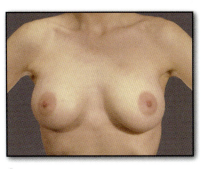

A.

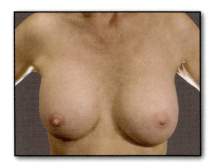

B.

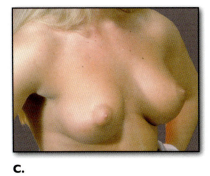

C.

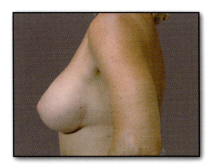

D.

FIGURE 16-19

LESSON 8:

Nipples point where they point. Surgically repositioning nipples involves substantial trade-offs.

Ideally, the nipple, surrounded by the pigmented skin called the areola, is located slightly outside the middle of the breast mound when viewing the breast from the front. In reality, nipple-areola position is extremely variable from woman to woman. In the pictures that follow (Figure 16–20, A–D), notice the wide variation in the position of the nipples from patient to patient as well as the differences in nipple position from side to side in the same patient.

Following augmentation, notice that the nipples basically point in the same direction as before surgery. Although the implant can be positioned to change nipple tilt and position slightly, any major correction of nipple position requires surgical repositioning. When the nipple-areola complex is repositioned surgically, the patient must accept the following trade-offs: increased risk of sensory loss, possible interference with ability to nurse, and visible scar around the areola. Every woman has differences in nipple position, but surgical repositioning should be reserved for very significant differences and for patients willing to accept the trade-offs.

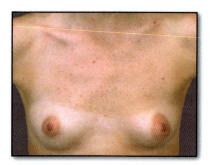 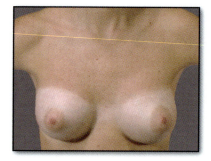

A.   **Left nipple-areola larger and more outwardly pointing.**

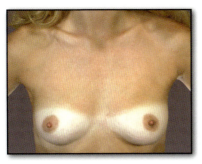 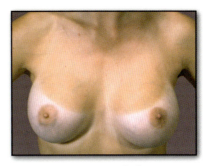

B. **Nipple-areola point outwardly right more than left,
both tilt upward.**

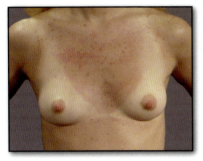 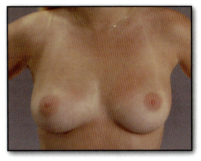

C. **Right nipple-areola smaller than left, left higher than right.**

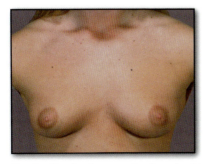 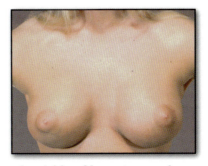

D. **Both nipple-areolas located toward outside of breast mound,
left higher than right.**

FIGURE 16-20

LESSON 9:

A round implant can produce a breast that looks good but may have a folded implant shell that can fail earlier. An anatomic-shaped implant can be filled adequately to protect the shell and still achieve a natural appearing upper breast.

If a breast looks natural following augmentation using a round implant (Figure 16-21, A–B), chances are that the shell of the round implant has collapsed vertically and the upper shell is folded (Figure 16–21, C). A folded shell risks early shell failure and implant rupture and requires additional surgery to replace the implant. If the round implant were filled enough to protect the shell and prevent collapse with the implant in the upright position (Figure 16–21, D) in the breast, the implant would usually cause excessive upper bulging or an excessively globular appearance (Figure 16–21, E).

An anatomically shaped implant (Figure 16–22, A) can be filled adequately to prevent upper-shell folding (Figure 16–22, B, C) with the implant upright, protecting the shell against shell collapse, shell folding, and early shell failure. When an adequately filled anatomic implant is placed in the breast (Figure 16-23), the tapered shape of the upper portion of the anatomic implant does not cause excessive upper-breast bulging. The result is a natural appearing breast and an implant without a folded shell that could fail sooner.

Before

After

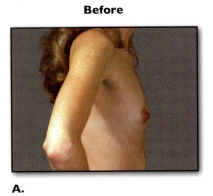

A.

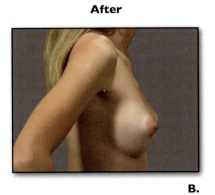

B.

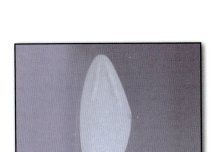

C.

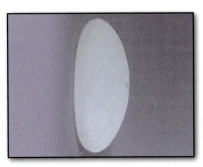

D.

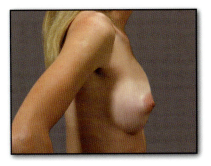

E.

FIGURE 16-21

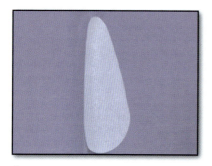

A.

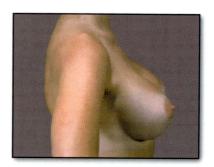

B.

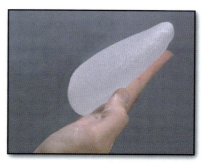

C.

FIGURE 16-22

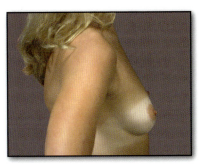

A.

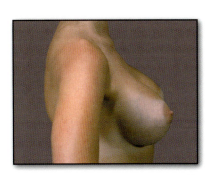

B.

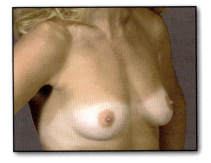

C.

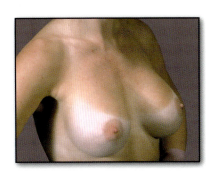

D.

FIGURE 16-23

LESSON 10:

The prices you can pay for selecting an excessively large implant

The skin envelope of the breast stretches to accommodate the enlargement of the breast during pregnancy and nursing, but this enlargement is a natural, physiologic process that occurs over several months and is usually limited to a moderate amount of enlargement. Breast augmentation enlarges the breast very rapidly, and the amount of enlargement depends on the patient's wishes and her tissues.

When a woman selects excessively large implants, she may enjoy the result for a while, but she is choosing long-term risks that she may not like. The skin envelope of the breast does not improve as a woman ages. Visualize your grandmother's breasts. Skin usually gets thinner and stretches as gravity pulls on the breast over time, with or without an implant. The larger the implant, the heavier the implant, the more stretch and thinning of tissues occurs, and the more rapidly it occurs. Excessively large implants can cause any or all of the following problems:

- Excessive skin stretching

- Sagging of the breast

- Loss of upper-breast fullness as the lower breast stretches

- Thinning of the skin envelope

- Shrinkage of the patient's own breast tissue from pressure by the implant

- Visible implant edges

- Visible rippling caused by the heavy implant pulling downward on the skin envelope (Figure 16-24, A–D)

- Distortion of breast shape

What implant size is safe and what is excessive? In part, the answer depends on a patient's tissues. *The thinner the tissues, the more a large implant can affect those tissues.* The rule of thumb that we follow is that any breast implant larger than 350 cc to 400 cc can produce the problems listed under lesson 10. Special circumstances may require larger breast implants, but whenever a patient needs or selects an implant larger than 350 cc, we advise the patient of the increased risks of the problems listed above.

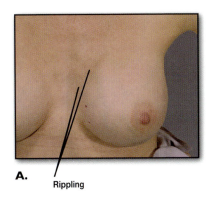

A.
Rippling

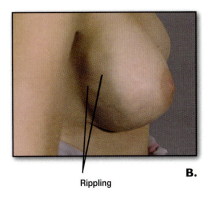

Rippling
B.

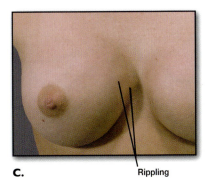

C.
Rippling

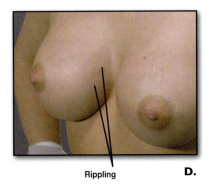

Rippling
D.

FIGURE 16-24

The following patients (see Figures 16-25 A–F, 16-26 A–F) had larger breasts that had been significantly stretched by pregnancy and nursing, requiring larger implants to adequately fill the envelope. The trade-offs of breast lift (mastopexy) were unacceptable to both patients, and both accepted the trade-offs of placing large implants. Both were fully aware that they might well require breast lifts in the future with removal of the large implants, and either no implant replacement or replacement with a much smaller implant. Remember, as you age, your tissues won't support weight as well.

Patient with markedly stretched tissues who refused breast lift (mastopexy) and requested very large implants.

Before

After

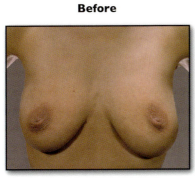

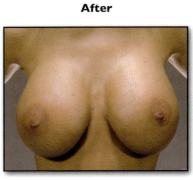

A.

B.

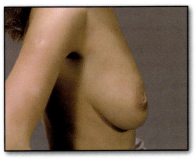

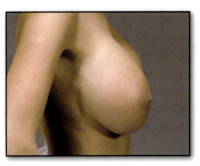

C.

D.

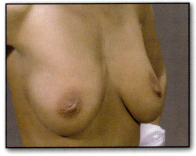

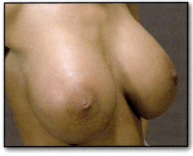

E.

F.

FIGURE 16-25

Patient with stretched envelope and sagging following pregnancy who required a large implant to adequately fill her envelope.

Before · **After**

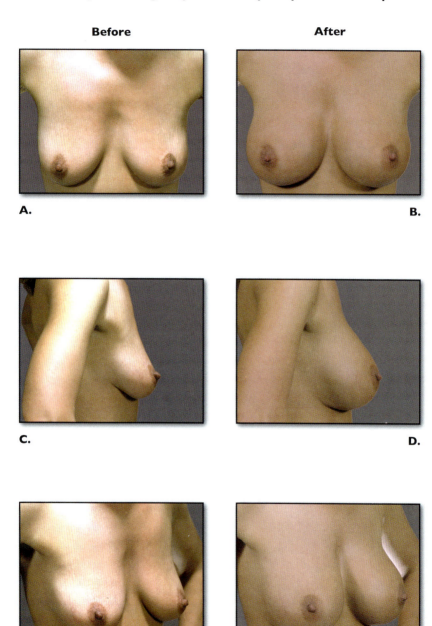

A. · B.

C. · D.

E. · F.

FIGURE 16-26

LESSON II:

What is capsular contracture?

When a medical device is placed in the body, the body forms a tissue lining around the device. This lining, called a capsule, forms around every breast implant in every patient. In most patients, the lining surrounds the implant but does not cause any problem. In a small percentage of patients, the capsule contracts or tightens excessively squeezing on the implant, making the implant feel too hard, and often pushing the implant out of position and distorting breast shape.

The risk of capsular contracture varies with the type of implant, implant shell characteristics, and type of filler material, but the average risk is 2–5 percent for textured-shell, saline-filled implants. This means that from two to five of every hundred patients will develop a capsular contracture on one or both sides.

Figure 16-27, A–F illustrates a patient who developed a capsular contracture of the right breast. As the capsule tightens excessively around the implant, it often displaces the implant upward (A) making one breast appear higher than the other. In side view (B), as the implant is pushed upward by the contracting capsule, the upper breast bulges, and the breast feels very firm compared to the left breast. After correction (D, E, F), the breasts appear more symmetrical (D), the excessive upper bulging is corrected (E), and both breasts have a very natural appearance (F).

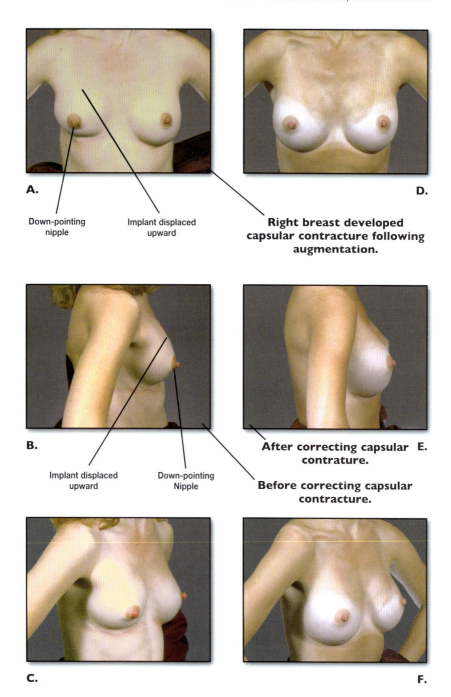

A.

Down-pointing nipple

Implant displaced upward

D.

Right breast developed capsular contracture following augmentation.

B.

Implant displaced upward

Down-pointing Nipple

After correcting capsular contrature. **E.**

Before correcting capsular contracture.

C.

F.

FIGURE 16-27

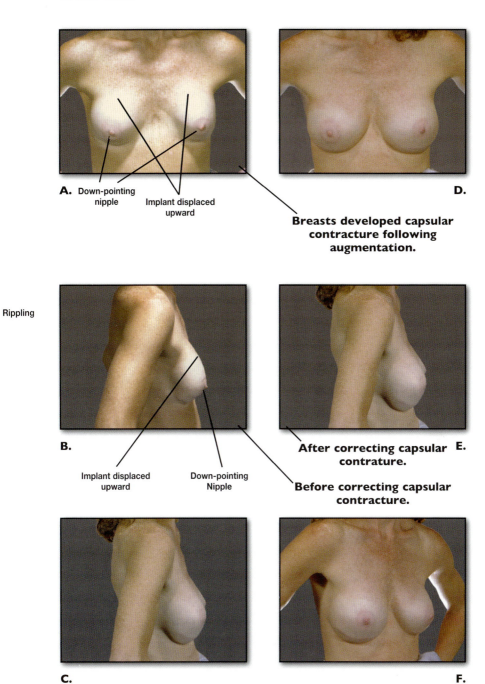

A. Down-pointing nipple   Implant displaced upward

D.

Rippling

B.   Implant displaced upward   Down-pointing Nipple

Breasts developed capsular contracture following augmentation.

After correcting capsular contrature. **E.**

Before correcting capsular contracture.

C.   **F.**

FIGURE 16-28

Another patient who has severe capsular contractures on both sides is illustrated in Figure 16-28, A–F. Both breasts are displaced upward (A) producing excessive upward bulging and down-pointing nipples (B,C). The middle portion of the left breast is flattened and distorted (A), and both breasts feel extremely hard. After removal of the capsules and implant replacement (D, E, F), the breasts appear much more symmetrical and natural with normal contours, a natural slope to the upper breast, and a softer feel.

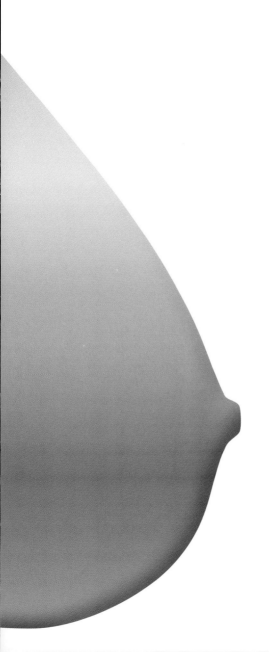

PATIENT SELF-ASSESSMENT
AND MEASURING TECHNIQUES

Are measurements really necessary, and are patient outcomes better with defined decision processes?

While plastic surgery is partially art, optimal results with minimal risks, rapid recovery, and minimal reoperations require that surgeons use art after they apply science, not in lieu of science. The scientific method is based on using objective, measurable data to test a theory or hypothesis. Absent objective data, methods are not scientific; instead, the methods are simply opinions. To determine whether results based on opinions are better compared to results based on scientifically tested and valid methods, it is important for you as a patient to consider data on results that have been scientifically peer reviewed and published in indexed medical journals.

Optimal results and outcomes with minimal reoperations require that you and your surgeon make optimal decisions before your augmentation. For the past three decades, surgeons and patients have based most of their decisions on subjective parameters, such as cup size (which no surgeon or patient can define), terms such as *thin* (How thin is thin?), and terms such as *tight skin* (How tight is tight?). To determine implant size, many surgeons allow patients to judge size by pictures (inaccurate unless the picture measures breast width and skin stretch). Other surgeons allow patients to purchase a bra of the size they desire and place test implants into the bra to determine the size implant to place during the augmentation (ignoring a basic fact that the width and stretch of the bra never match the width and stretch characteristics of the patient's breast). Many of these methods allow patients to define their wishes and then force their desires on their tissues whether or not the desires consider the dimensions and characteristics of their tissues. When patient and surgeon force tissues to a desired result instead of defining realistic limits of what each individual patient's tissues will safely allow, irreversible tissue compromises and uncorrectable deformities can result. These compromises can include skin thinning, shrinkage and loss of breast tissue, visible implant edges, visible traction rippling, excessive sagging of the breasts, implant malpositions, and even chest wall deformities.

Traditionally, many surgeons have resisted using measurements, instead preferring to rely on their "aesthetic eyes" to make decisions. Decisions based on subjective parameters without objective measurements contributed to an unenviable track record of an average 17 percent reoperation rate within just three years following augmentation in FDA studies.[1,2]

During the past seven years, we have developed more objective methods of assessing the dimensions and tissues of the breast. Instead of using terms like *small, big, tight, loose, proportional, cup size* and other terms that are subject to wide differences in interpretation and cannot be studied scientifically, we now rely on a few very specific, objective measurements and defined decision processes to make critical decisions before augmentation.[3,4] A key question is whether these more objective methods using simple measurements and defined decision processes actually improve patients' outcomes and reduce reoperation rates.

Instead of a 17 percent reoperation rate in just three years following augmentation,[1,2] these new methods[3,4] have enabled us to reduce reoperation rates to only 3 percent up to seven years after augmentation in 1,664 patients,[5–7] and for the first time in history, to document a zero percent reoperation rate in fifty consecutive breast augmentation patients at three years following augmentation in an FDA study.[8] Combined with redefined surgical techniques, these processes have enabled more than 80 percent of our patients to be out to dinner the evening of surgery, and 96 percent to return to full, normal activities within twenty-four hours following their breast augmentation.[7]

Decisions based on subjective terms and methods cannot be tested scientifically.

Decisions based on subjective terms and methods had a 17 percent reoperation rate in just three years.

Decisions based on objective measurements and defined decision processes CAN and HAVE BEEN tested scientifically.[3-8]

Decisions based on objective measurements and defined decision processes produced a 3 percent overall reoperation rate at up to seven years, and a zero percent reoperation rate at three years postop.

CAN AND SHOULD PATIENTS MEASURE THEMSELVES?

Patient measurements should never replace measurements and decision-support by an expert, board-certified plastic surgeon. Based on our experience and testing self-measurement techniques in many of our patients, we are convinced that interested, motivated, intelligent patients are completely capable of performing basic measurements on their breasts and applying basic decision-making processes to help establish safe, realistic expectations.

Every patient who performs self-measurements should thoroughly understand that her measurements will likely never exactly match her surgeon's measurements, and that fact should not disturb any patient. Measurements vary even among surgeons, but each individual surgeon's or patient's measurements become very consistent with repetition. Your surgeon will likely make more measurements than you make and will likely interpret the measurements differently and with more depth due to training and experience.

Our experience with patients measuring themselves has been overwhelmingly positive provided the patient understands the principles described above and provided the patient understands that patient measurements are always less comprehensive and somewhat less accurate compared to surgeon measurements. When surgeons and patients formerly e-mailed us with questions, we relied on photographs to try to help with answers or advice. Today, we rely totally on measurements, because we know how misleading photographs can be and realize that photographs convey very little or no information about the actual dimensions and tissue stretch of a breast—critical factors in every breast augmentation.

An obvious question is "How accurate and useful are patient measurements and decisions compared to surgeon measurements and decisions?" We tested a series of patients by combining our thorough and repetitive patient education processes described earlier in the book[9] with basic measurement techniques and decision methods and found that in 90 percent of cases, the patients' measurements and preliminary choices required absolutely no change in basic preoperative decisions by the surgeon. While the patient's measurements varied slightly in every case from the surgeon's measurements, the variations did not significantly affect the ultimate decisions of the surgeon. These findings surprised us and convinced us that many patients, adequately informed and motivated, are capable of performing basic self-measurements and making preliminary assessment decisions with remarkable accuracy.

BASIC MEASURING TOOLS

In order to perform basic measurements on your breast, you will need a flexible cloth or plastic tape measure that is marked in both inches and centimeters. Most sewing, fabric, or crafts stores and some hardware stores stock these types of tape measures, and many are very inexpensive. If you happen to have access to a set of calipers, they can be helpful but are not essential. In addition, you will need a ballpoint pen or washable marker to place dots on your breast at key measuring points.

A measuring kit that we assembled for our out-of-town patients (Figure A1-1) includes a caliper, measuring tape, and DVD with instructions for measuring. This kit is available on www.amazon.com or by calling our office. (Search for breast measurement kit and DVD.)

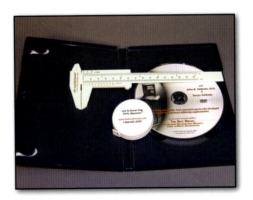

FIGURE A1-1

KEY MEASUREMENTS AND MEASUREMENT TECHNIQUES

Measuring the Thickness of Your Upper Breast Tissues

One of the most important priorities in breast augmentation is choosing an implant pocket location that assures optimal soft-tissue coverage over your implant for your entire lifetime. Your tissues are likely to become thinner with age, and thin tissues overlying any portion of a breast implant can allow visible implant edges, visible rippling, and excessive stretch that may be uncorrectable. Subjectively assessing whether you appear thin is inaccurate and inadequate. Making optimal decisions about implant pocket location requires objective measurements of tissue thickness.

The most accurate and effective method for determining the thickness of tissues that will lie over the upper portion of your breast implant is to measure tissue thickness in the upper breast using a simple pinch test and measuring with your caliper.

With one hand, gently grasp the mass or your breast tissue and pull it downward toward your feet to assure that you are not grasping breast tissue when you perform the pinch tissue measurement in the upper breast (Figure A1-2, A). With the opposite hand, open your thumb and index finger about an inch-and-a-half apart, then grasp the skin and underlying fat above the breast tissue, pinch firmly, and measure the thickness of the pinched tissue with the caliper (Fgure A1-2, B). It is important to avoid starting with your fingers extremely wide apart and pushing hard against the chest wall as you pick up tissues because you may tend to include the underlying pectoralis muscle in your measurement.

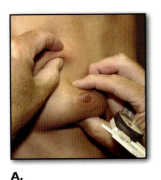

A.

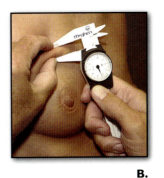

B.

FIGURE A1-2

Measuring the Base Width of Your Breast

The most accurate method for measuring the base width of your breast is to use a caliper, but if you do not have a caliper available, you will be able to make an approximate measurement with your tape measure.

While standing in front of the mirror, look at the cleavage area between your breasts. You'll notice a flat area between the breasts. Try to locate a point where this flat area first begins to slope upward onto your breast mound, and place a dot at the beginning of the upslope of the breast mound.

While looking in the mirror, visualize the line that forms the outside curve of your breast directly across the breast from the dot you placed in the cleavage area. You will be measuring from the dot in the cleavage area straight across to the outside border of the breast mound to determine the base width of the breast mound (Figure A1-3). The measurement should be a straight-line measurement, not a measurement over the curve of the breast.

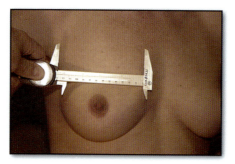

FIGURE A1-3

If you are using a tape measure in order to get a straight line measurement, you'll need to hold the tip of the tape measure in front of your chest locating the tip directly over the dot you placed in the cleavage area. Stretch the tape directly across in front of your breast, not touching your breast, and note the number on the tape where the outer profile line of your breast crosses behind the tape. This measurement from the beginning of the upslope of the breast in your cleavage area to the visible outer boundary of the breast is the base width of the breast mound.

Perform this measurement three times and record the three measurements, then average the measurements.

Measurement #1 (base width)	Measurement #2 (base width)	Measurement #3 (base width)	Average (base width)

Measuring the Nipple-to-Inframammary Fold Distance

While standing in front of a mirror, gently lift your breast, and locate the crease or fold beneath the breast. This is the inframammary fold. Using a ballpoint pen or marker, place a small dot exactly in the fold beneath your breast on a line directly beneath your nipple, near the six o'clock position of the fold (Figure A1-4, A).

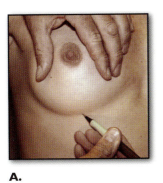

A.

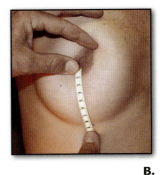

B.

FIGURE A1-4

Release your breast, and place a second dot exactly beside the midpoint of your nipple on the skin of the areola (the pigmented skin surrounding the nipple).

Place the tip of a flexible tape measure on the dot you just placed beside the nipple. With one hand, push the tip of the tape measure toward your back to hold it in place, and use the same hand (pushing backward and upward) to lift your breast upward toward your collar bone. This puts the skin between the nipple and the fold beneath your breast under maximum stretch. Pull the tape measure straight downward past the dot you placed in the fold under your breast, and read the nipple-to-fold distance on the tape at a point immediately beside the dot you placed in the fold (Figure A1-4, B). If you have someone who can help you, you can lift the breast and stretch the skin while they make the measurement.

Perform this measurement three times and record the three measurements, then average the measurements.

Measurement #1 (nipple to fold)	Measurement #2 (nipple to fold)	Measurement #3 (nipple to fold)	Average (nipple to fold)

Measuring Skin Stretch

Measuring skin stretch is somewhat more difficult compared to the previous measurements, and your surgeon will be able to more accurately repeat this measurement during your consultation. Nevertheless, you should be able to perform a very basic measurement that can provide useful information. A caliper is almost essential to perform this measurement accurately.

Pick up your caliper in your right hand (or in your left hand if you are left handed) and hold it in the palm of your hand leaving your thumb and index finger of the same hand free to grasp the skin of your areola.

Grasp the skin of your areola immediately adjacent to the nipple and pull if straight forward away from your chest as far as you can possibly force it to go (see figure A1-5, A). Use the fingernail of your opposite hand to mark the maximum point of skin stretch forward, and while holding the fingernail in the air to mark the point, release the skin and measure from the fingernail marker back to the relaxed skin of the areola on the chest (see figure A1-5, B). This distance represents the maximum forward (anterior) pull—skin stretch of your breast.

Perform this measurement three times and record the three measurements, then average the measurements.

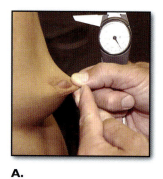
A.

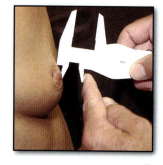
B.

FIGURE A1-5

Measurement #1 (skin stretch)	Measurement #2 (skin stretch)	Measurement #3 (skin stretch)	Average (skin stretch)

USING YOUR MEASUREMENTS TO MAKE PRELIMINARY DECISIONS

The measurements you have made can help you better understand options for implant size and implant pocket location that minimize your risk of reoperations, tissue compromises, and uncorrectable deformities in the future. If you understand that the caliper and tape measure are impersonal and totally objective, understanding the limitations that measurements can point out to you can be invaluable as you and your surgeon make critical decisions for your augmentation.

Before we discuss how to use measurements to help make decisions, you should clearly understand that the final decisions you and your surgeon make will depend on additional measurements and other factors that are individual to each patient. The information we will provide is general and is not intended to be definitive, but to provide a framework for you to better understand tissue limitations based on tissue measurements. The principles of using measurements to make important decisions in augmentation are derived from peer-reviewed scientific studies that we have published.[3,4] These are the same principles used by surgeons who are delivering 24-hour return[4,7] to normal activity and 3 percent or lower reoperation rates at up to seven years following augmentation.[5-8]

CHOOSING A POCKET LOCATION TO OPTIMIZE TISSUE COVERAGE OF YOUR IMPLANTS

The highest priority decision in breast augmentation is choosing a pocket location and using surgical techniques to provide optimal, maximal soft-tissue coverage over your implants for your entire lifetime. This is the highest priority decision in the high five priority decisions that surgeons use in the High Five Decision System[4] to minimize risks of uncorrectable deformities, such as implant edge visibility, visible rippling or wrinkling, and irreversible tissue thinning. These uncorrectable deformities and tissue compromises are almost totally avoidable by making simple decisions about pocket location that are based on objective measurements instead of subjective opinions and by making choices that maximize tissue coverage over your implants instead of choosing options that may or may not be adequate as you age and your tissues become thinner.

Table A1-1 is a flowchart that uses your measurement of the tissue thickness above your breast tissue (soft tissue pinch thickness of the upper pole or STPTUP) to help you select the best option for implant pocket location to assure optimal long-term coverage over your implant.

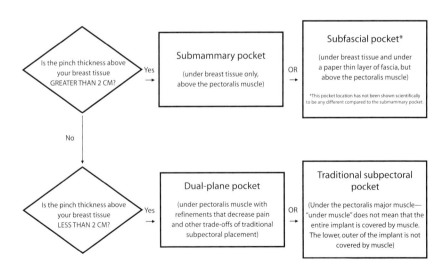

TABLE AI-I

If the soft-tissue pinch thickness you measured above your breast tissue was less than 2 cm thick, to minimize risks of reoperations and uncorrectable deformities, you should choose an implant pocket location that provides additional muscle coverage over the upper and middle portions of your implant.

Two options for pocket location that add muscle coverage include a traditional retropectoral pocket, and the newer, dual-plane pocket that provides muscle cover in the upper breast while minimizing trade-offs associated with the traditional submuscular pocket. (For more detailed information on pocket locations, see chapter 6.)

If your pinch thickness measurement above your breast tissue was greater than 2 cm, placing the implant behind breast tissue (submammary) or behind breast tissue and a thin layer of fascia (subfascial) are also reasonable options. With the development of the dual-plane pocket option that minimizes trade-offs of the traditional submuscular pocket location, more and more patients are asking, "Why not just be as safe as possible and provide muscle cover over the upper and middle portions of the implant?" More and more, we agree with them. Our peer-reviewed and published scientific studies indicate the dual-plane pocket location has the lowest reoperation rate and a zero rate of uncorrectable compromises. No other published studies currently match the track record of the dual-plane pocket location.[3–8]

Implant size (volume) options-Using base width, stretch, and nipple-to fold measurements

Table A-2 is a simplified version of the decision process table from our peer-reviewed and published TEPID™ and High Five systems. To use the table to estimate an approximate implant volume based on the width and stretch of your tissues, perform the following steps:

Base Width	Base Width (cm)	10.5	11.0	11.5	12.0	12.5	13.0	13.5	14.0	14.5	15.0
	Estimated Volume (cc)	200	250	275	300	300	325	350	375	375	400

TABLE A-2

a) In the far left column of the table, enter the measurements you performed in the following spaces: pinch thickness in the STPTUP space, base width in the BW space, skin stretch in the APSS (anterior pull skin stretch) space, and nipple-to-fold measurement in the N:IMF space.

b) In the top row of the table, locate the base width average measurement of your breast.

c) Immediately beneath the base width measurement, the table lists an approximate starting implant volume for your base width. This volume is a starting volume that will be adjusted depending on the correlation of your other measurements with your surgeon's measurements.

d) The suggested volume from c) above also depends on the degree of skin stretch in your breast. If your skin stretch is less than 2 cm, subtract 30cc from the volume suggested by your base width. If your skin stretch is greater than 3 cm, add 30cc to the suggested volume, and if your skin stretch is 40cc, add 60cc to the suggested volume. These volumes are all approximate and will depend on you and your surgeon's assessments and discussion.

References

1. U. S. Food and Drug Administration. Product labeling for Mentor and Allergen/Inamed core studies of saline implants. http://www.fda.gov/cdrh/breastimplants/labeling/mentor_patient_labeling_5900.html. Accessed: January 1, 2007, FDA web site updated November 17, 2006..

2. U. S. Food and Drug Administration. Product labeling for mentor and Allergan/Inamed core studies of conventional silicone gel implants. http:///www.fda.gov/cdrh/breastimplants/labeling.html. Accessed: December 5, 2006, FDA web site updated Nov 17, 2006.

3. Tebbetts, J. B. A system for breast implant selection based on patient tissue characteristics and implant-soft tissue dynamics. *Plast. Reconstr. Surg.* 109(4): 1396-1409, 2002.

4. Tebbetts, J. B., and Adams, W. P. Five critical decisions in breast augmentation using 5 measurements in 5 minutes: The high five system. *Plast. Reconstr. Surg.* 116(7): 2005.

5. Tebbetts, J. B. Patient acceptance of adequately filled breast implants. *Plast. Reconstr. Surg.* 106(1): 139-147, 2000.

6. Tebbetts, J. B. Dual-plane (DP) breast augmentation: Optimizing implant-soft tissue relationships in a wide range of breast types. *Plast. Reconstr. Surg.* 107: 1255, 2001.

7. Tebbetts, J. B. Achieving a predictable 24-hour return to normal activities after breast augmentation, part II: Patient preparation, refined surgical techniques and instrumentation. *Plast. Reconstr. Surg.* 109: 293-305, 2002.

8. Tebbetts, J. B. Achieving a zero percent reoperation rate at 3 years in a 50 consecutive case augmentation mammaplasty PMA study. *Plast. Reconstr. Surg.* 108(6): 1453-1457, 2006.

9. Tebbetts, J. B. An approach that integrates patient education and informed consent in breast augmentation. *Plast. Reconstr. Surg.* 110(3): 971-978, 2002.

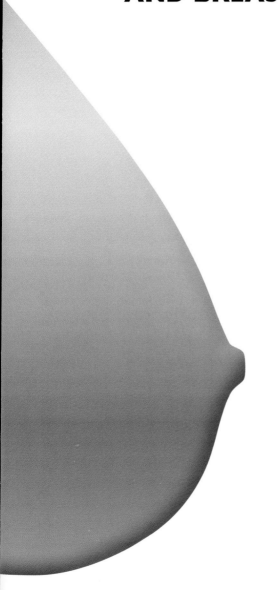

U.S. AND INTERNATIONAL STUDIES OF BREAST IMPLANTS AND BREAST CANCER

The following is a summary of the epidemiology studies of breast implants and breast cancer conducted by prominent researchers at prestigious institutions. Unlike the reports of individual women (often called case reports or case series), these studies were designed to make comparisons between groups of women with and without breast implants. These more rigorous epidemiology studies provide the opportunity to determine whether breast cancer among women with implants is occurring more frequently than might be expected.

International Epidemiology Institute, Karolinska Institute, and the U. S. National Cancer Institute, McLaughlin, PhD; Nyren, MD; Blot, PhD; et al; Rockville, MD. 1998

Breast Implants/Breast Cancer

This nationwide Swedish study included 3,473 women who had cosmetic breast implant procedures from 1965 through 1993. Followed for an average of 10.3 years, eighteen women developed breast cancer compared to twenty-five expected cases. The authors concluded, *"Our study showed a statistically nonsignificant reduction in the incidence of breast cancer that may be due to concomitant risk factors (e.g., lower age at first pregnancy and decreased glandular density)."*

In an earlier publication (1995), McLaughlin and colleagues reported similar findings based on 1,756 women with cosmetic breast implants in Sweden.

University of Southern California School of Medicine, Deapen, DrPh; Bernstein, PhD; Brody, MD; Los Angeles, CA. 1997

Breast Implants/Breast Cancer

This study reports continued follow-up of more than 3,100 women in Los Angeles County who received cosmetic breast implants between 1953 and 1980. Followed for a median of 14.4 years, thirty-one women with implants subsequently developed breast cancer compared to 49.2 expected cases of breast cancer. The authors concluded, *"In Los Angeles County, augmentation mammaplasty patients experience a significantly lower than expected risk of breast cancer and no delay in breast cancer detection . . ."*

In two earlier publications (1986, 1992), Deapen and colleagues reported similar conclusions based on following these same women for a median of 6.2 and 10.6 years, respectively.

Directly funded by Dow Corning Corporation.

Danish Cancer Society, International Epidemiology Institute, and the U. S. National Cancer Institute, Friis, MD McLaughlin, PhD; Mellemkjaer, MS; et al; Copenhagen, Denmark. 1997

Breast Implants/ Breast Cancer

This nationwide Danish study included 1,135 women who had cosmetic breast implant procedures between 1977 and 1992. Followed for an average of 8.4 years, eight women developed breast cancer versus 7.8 expected cases. The authors stated, *"In summary, breast implants were not related to an excess risk of breast or other cancers in our population-based cohort study."*

In an earlier publication (1994), McLaughlin and colleagues reported similar conclusions based on 824 women with cosmetic breast implants in Denmark.

Hartford Hospital, Kern, MD; Flannery; Kuehn, MD; Hartford, CT. 1997

Breast Implants/Breast Cancer

These authors reported on subsequent cancers in 680 Connecticut women who had breast implant surgery compared to 1,022 women who had tubal ligation surgery and no breast implants. No woman had a prior history of cancer. Women were followed for an average of 4.6 years after implant surgery and 5.4 years after tubal ligation surgery. Women with breast implants had a nonsignificantly lower rate of breast cancer compared to women without implants. The authors stated, *"Based on these data, it was concluded that silicone breast implants are not carcinogenic, because they are not associated with increased rates of either breast or nonbreast cancers."*

U. S. National Cancer Institute, Brinton, PhD; Malone, PhD; Coates, PhD; et al; Bethesda, MD. 1996

Breast Implants/Breast Cancer

This study included 2,174 women who had breast cancer and 2,009 women without breast cancer. Breast implants were reported by 36 women with cancer versus 44 women without cancer. This study found that the risk for breast cancer was lower among women who had breast implants. Furthermore, the decreased risk for breast cancer persisted as the time since implantation increased. The authors stated, *"In this study, we found that women who had received breast implants were not at an excess risk for developing breast cancer. This finding agrees with all the other analytical studies that have examined the relationship."*

Alberta Cancer Board, Bryant, MD; Brasher, PhD; Alberta, Canada. 1995

Breast Implants/Breast Cancer

This study was a reanalysis of data presented by Berkel, Birdsell, and Jenkins (1992), who reported a lower risk for breast cancer among women with breast implants in Alberta, Canada. Among the 10,835 women included in this reanalysis who had undergone breast augmentation surgery, 45 women subsequently developed breast cancer compared to 59 expected cases of breast cancer. Although the number of cancer cases was lower than expected and consistent with other research studies, since the results were not statistically significant, the authors concluded, *". . . the apparent risk of breast cancer cannot be said to be either higher or significantly lower than that of the general population."*

Birdsell and colleagues (1993), in an earlier study of this general group of women, investigated the survival experience of women with breast cancer diagnosed after breast augmentation. Among the 11,670 women with cosmetic breast implants included in this report, 41 developed breast cancer after augmentation. The survival experience for these 41 women was compared to the survival of all women diagnosed with breast cancer during the same time period (1973-1990 inclusive). The researchers concluded, *"In summary, our study shows that women with a breast tumor diagnosed after having had an implant survive as long as women with breast cancer without implants. We did not find that the tumors in women with implants were diagnosed at a later stage and in fact, these tumors were smaller at diagnosis. This . . . allows in our opinion the conclusion that cosmetic breast augmentation is not a cause of concern in regard to breast cancer."*

Institut Gustave Roussy, Petit, MD; Le, MD; Mouriesse, MS; et al; Villejuif, France. 1994

Breast Implants/Breast Cancer

The researchers studied 146 patients with breast cancer treated by mastectomy who received a gel-filled silicone implant between 1976 and 1984 for reconstruction compared to 146 matched controls with breast cancer who were treated in the same center without reconstruction. The risks of distant metastasis and death due to breast cancer were significantly lower in the breast reconstruction group than in the control group. The risk for second breast cancer did not differ between the two groups of women. The researchers stated, *"In conclusion, our results do not support the hypothesis of a detrimental effect of gel-filled silicone implants either in the course of breast cancer or in the risk of death due to other diseases."*

Fred Hutchinson Cancer Research Center, Malone; Stanford; Daling, PhD; et al; Seattle, WA. 1992

Breast Implants/Breast Cancer

The authors compared the incidence of breast implants among women with breast cancer to the incidence of implants among women without cancer. For their two study groups of women with cancer (women aged 21-44 years and women aged 50-64 years), compared to women without breast cancer, there was no apparent risk for breast cancer due to silicone breast implants.

Centers for Disease Control and Prevention, Glasser, PhD; Lee; Wingo; Atlanta, GA. 1989

Breast Augmentation/ Breast Cancer

Researchers compared 4,742 women with breast cancer (12 of whom had breast augmentation prior to their disease) to 4,754 women without breast cancer (8 of whom had breast augmentation). They found no association between breast augmentation and breast cancer.

BIBLIOGRAPHY FOR U.S. AND INTERNATIONAL STUDIES OF BREAST IMPLANTS AND BREAST CANCER

Berkel H, Birdsell DC, Jenkins H. Breast augmentation: a risk factor for breast cancer? *N Engl J Med.* 1992;326:1649-1653.

Birdsell DC, Jenkins H, Berkel H. Breast cancer diagnosis and survival in women with and without breast implants. *Plast. Reconstr. Surg.* 1993;92:795-800.

Brinton LA, Malone KE, Coates RJ, et al. Breast enlargement and reduction: Results from a breast cancer case-control study. *Plast. Reconstr. Surg.* 1996;97:269-275.

Bryant H, Brasher P. Breast implants and breast cancer-reanalysis of a linkage study. *N Engl J Med.* 1995;332:1535-1539.

Deapen DM, Bernstein L, Brody GS. Are breast implants anticarcinogenic? A 14-year follow-up of the Los Angeles study. *Plast. Reconstr. Surg.* 1997;99:1346-1353.

Deapen DM, Brody GS. Augmentation mammaplasty and breast cancer: A 5-year update of the Los Angeles study. *Plast. Reconstr. Surg.* 1992;89:660-665.

Deapen DM, Pike MC, Casagrande JT, Brody GS. The relationship between breast cancer and augmentation mammaplasty: an epidemiologic study. *Plast. Reconstr. Surg.* 1986;77:361-367.

Friis S, McLaughlin JK, Mellemkjaer L, et al. Breast implants and cancer risk in Denmark. *Int J Cancer.* 1997;714:956-958.

Glassner JW, Lee NC, Wingo PA. Does breast augmentation increase the risk of breast cancer? The Epidemic Intelligence Service Conference, April, 1989.

Kern KA, Flannery JT, Kuehn PG. Carcinogenic potential of silicone breast implants: a Connecticuit statewide study. *Plast. Reconstr. Surg.* 1997;100:737-749.

Malone KE, Stanford JL, Daling JR, Voigt LF. Implants and breast cancer. *The Lancet.* 1992;339:1365.

McLaughlin JK, Nyren O, Blot WJ, et al. Cancer risk among women with cosmetic breast implants: a population-based cohort study in Sweden. *J Natl Cancer Inst.* 1998;90:156-158.

McLaughlin JK, Fraumeni JF, Nyren O, Adami HO. Silicone breast implants and the risk of cancer? *JAMA.* 1995;273:116.

McLaughlin JK, Fraumeni JF, Olsen J, Mellemkjaer L. Re: breast implants, cancer, and systemic sclerosis. *J Natl Cancer Inst.* 1994;86:1424.

Petit JY, Le MG, Mouriesse H, Rietjens M, Gill P, Contesso G, Lehmann A. Can breast reconstruction with gel-filled silicone implants increase the risk of death and second primary cancer in patients treated by mastectomy for breast cancer? *Plast. Reconstr. Surg.* 1994;94:115-119.

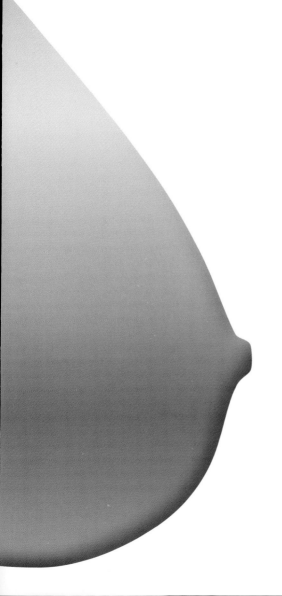

U.S. AND INTERNATIONAL EPIDEMIOLOGY STUDIES OF BREAST IMPLANTS AND CONNECTIVE TISSUE DISEASE

The following is a summary of the epidemiology studies of connective tissue disease (CTD) and breast implants conducted by prominent researchers at prestigious institutions. Unlike the reports of individual women (often called case reports or case series), the following studies were designed to make comparisons between groups of women with and without implants. In contrast to case reports, these more rigorous epidemiology studies provide the opportunity to determine whether CTD among women with implants is occurring more frequently than might be expected.

University of Michigan, School of Public Health, Lacey, MPH; Laing, MD; Gillespie, PhD; et al.; Ann Arbor, MI. 1997

Breast Implants, Environmental Exposures/Scleroderma

This large-scale, population-based study looked at all women in the state of Ohio diagnosed with scleroderma between 1985 and 1992. The analyses compared the 189 women diagnosed with scleroderma to the 1,043 women in a control group who did not have scleroderma. The authors stated, *"There was no association between SSc and silicone gel breast implants [adjusted odds ratio (aOR) 1.01, 95% confidence interval (CI) 0.13 to 8.15], any breast implants (aOR 1.48, 95% CI 0.34 to 6.39), or all silicone breast and facial implants (aOR 1.44, 95% CI 0.33 to 6.22)."*

These investigators conducted a comparable study in Michigan and found similar results (see Burns et al. 1994 in this summary).

Directly funded by Dow Corning Corporation.

University of Maryland, School of Medicine; University of Pittsburgh, School of Medicine; University of California San Diego, School of Medicine, Hochberg, MD; Perlmutter, MS; Medsger MD; et al.; Baltimore, MD. 1996

Breast Implants/Scleroderma

This multicenter study compared the frequency of augmentation mammaplasty among 837 women with scleroderma to 2,507 women without scleroderma. The authors concluded, *"These results fail to demonstrate a significant association between augmentation mammaplasty and SSc, and are consistent with those reported from other epidemiologic studies."*

Funded in part by the Plastic Surgery Educational Foundation. Dow Corning has contributed money to this foundation but has no control over what research the foundation chooses to fund.

Brigham & Women's Hospital, The Women's Health Cohort Study, Harvard Medical School, Hennekens, MD, DrPH; Lee, MBBS, ScD; Cook, ScD; et al.; Boston, MA. 1996

Breast Implants/Reports of Connective Tissue Disease

This study of female health professionals assessed self-reported data on six connective tissue diseases and breast implants. It included 10,830 women with breast implants and 384,713 women without breast implants. The authors concluded that, based on the self-reported data, the study's major contribution was to exclude large risks of connective tissue disease following breast implant surgery. Although the research raised the possibility of a small increased risk for women with implants, the investigators said the study could not reliably distinguish between this possibility and no risk. The study also found no difference in risk according to how long an implant was in place. According to Dr. Charles Hennekens, the lead investigator, *"Considering all available evidence, women with breast implants should be reassured that there is no large risk of connective tissue disease."* The authors stated that the next phase of this study will attempt to validate the self-reported diagnoses of connective tissue diseases by independent medical record review.

Funded by the National Institutes of Health and Dow Corning Corporation.

University of Michigan, School of Public Health, Laing, MD; Gillespie, PhD; Lacey; et al.; Ann Arbor, MI. 1996

Breast Implants, Medical Devices/UCTD

This study identified 206 women in Michigan and Ohio with undifferentiated connective tissue disease (UCTD) and compared them with 2,239 women without the condition. No association was found with silicone breast implants. When considering medical devices in general (both those containing silicone and those not containing silicone, including breast implants), however, the authors found a statistically significant association with this condition. UCTD is a condition with signs and symptoms that may evolve over time to a recognizable connective tissue disease, may never progress, or may disappear.

Directly funded by Dow Corning Corporation.

Brigham and Women's Hospital, Nurses' Health Study, Harvard Medical School, Sanchez-Guerrero, MD; Colditz, DrPH; Karlson, MD; et al.; Boston, MA. 1995

Breast Implants/Connective Tissue Disease, Signs, Symptoms, and Laboratory Tests

This study examined the incidence of connective tissue disease and 41 signs, symptoms, or laboratory findings of connective tissue disease among registered nurses followed from 1976 to 1990. Funded by the National Institutes of Health, the study compared the findings in 1,183 women with implants to the findings in 86,318 women without implants. The authors concluded, *"In a large cohort study, we did not find an association between silicone breast implants and connective-tissue diseases, defined according to a variety of standardized criteria, or signs and symptoms of these diseases."*

Emory University, Goldman, MD; Greenblatt, MD; Joines, MD; et al.; Atlanta, GA. 1995

Silicone Breast Implants/Connective Tissue Disease

A study of 4,229 women with and without breast implants from a rheumatology clinic found *"no evidence that women with breast implants are at an increased risk for having rheumatoid arthritis or other diffuse connective tissue disease."*

Directly funded by Dow Corning Corporation.

University of Kansas, Arthritis Center, Wolfe, MD; Wichita, KS. 1995

Silicone Breast Implants/Rheumatoid Arthritis

This study compared 637 women with rheumatoid arthritis to 1,134 controls (479 women with osteoarthritis and 655 women selected at random from the general population). The author stated, *"No associations between SBI [silicone breast implants] and RA [rheumatoid arthritis] were identified."*

Mayo Clinic, Gabriel, MD; O'Fallon, PhD; Kurland, MD; et al.; Rochester, MN. 1994

Breast Implants/Connective Tissue Diseases and Other Disorders

This study looked at medical records for all women in Olmsted County, Minnesota, who received breast implants between 1964 and 1991, identified 749 women who had received breast implants and compared them with 1,498 women who had not received implants. The investigators stated, *"We found no association between breast implants and the connective-tissue diseases and other disorders that were studied."*

Funded in part by the Plastic Surgery Educational Foundation. Dow Corning has contributed money to this foundation but has no control over what research the foundation chooses to fund.

Mayo Clinic, Duffy, MD; Woods, MD; Rochester, MN. 1994

Breast Implants/Connective Tissue Diseases and Other Disorders

This study looked at the medical records for 200 women who had 681 implants replaced or removed between 1970 and 1992. These women may be included in the Gabriel Mayo Clinic study noted previously. They found 85 percent of the implants were intact. The investigators stated, *"In our 30-year experience with silicone-gel breast implants for augmentation mammaplasty or breast reconstruction, the data from this study suggest that no clinically evident adverse health problems were incurred by those women who subsequently experienced a silicone gel-implant failure."*

University of Michigan, School of Public Health, Burns, PhD; Schottenfeld, MD; et al.; Ann Arbor, MI. 1994

Breast Implants, Environmental Exposures, and Family History/ Scleroderma

This large-scale, population-based study looked at all women in the state of Michigan diagnosed with scleroderma between 1980 and 1991. Most of the analyses compared the 274 women diagnosed with scleroderma between 1985 and 1991 with the 1,184 women in a control group who did not have scleroderma. The 1994 dissertation by Burns stated, *"'There was no association between any contact with silicone and scleroderma.' Their subsequent 1996 publication of this work concluded, 'Consistent with other studies, we found no increased risk of [scleroderma] among women with silicone breast implants.'"*

Directly funded by Dow Corning Corporation.

University of South Florida, College of Medicine and College of Public Health, Wells, MD; Cruse, MD; Baker, MD; et al.; Tampa, FL. 1994

Breast Implants/Symptoms and Diseases

The authors examined the incidence of 23 symptoms and four connective tissue diseases among 222 women with breast implant surgery compared to 80 women with other cosmetic surgery procedures. While the symptoms of tender and swollen glands under the arms were more frequent among the women with breast implants, the symptom of change in skin color was more frequent among those with non-breast implant cosmetic surgery. The study reported, *"No cases of scleroderma or lupus were found, and the incidence of arthritis was not significantly different between the implant and control groups."*

University of Pennsylvania, School of Medicine, Strom, MD; Reidenberg, MD; Freundlich, MD; et al.; Philadelphia, PA. 1994

Breast Implants/Systemic Lupus Erythematosus

The researchers interviewed 133 women with systemic lupus erythematosus (SLE) and 100 age-matched friend controls who did not have SLE. From this study, the authors concluded, "No association was seen between silicone breast implants and the subsequent development of SLE."

University of Texas M. D. Anderson Cancer Center, Schusterman, MD; Kroll, MD; Reece, MD; et al.; Houston, TX. 1993

Breast Implants/Autoimmune Disease

Results from this study of 603 patients (250 with breast implants and 353 with reconstruction from their own tissue) showed, *"The incidence of autoimmune disease in mastectomy patients receiving silicone-gel implants is not different than in patients who had reconstruction with autogenous tissue."*

The Johns Hopkins Medical Institutions, Wigley, MD; Miller; Hochberg, MD; et al.; Baltimore, MD. 1992

Breast Implants/Scleroderma

This is part of the Hochberg study conducted at the University of Maryland School of Medicine noted previously. Among 210 Baltimore respondents and 531 from Pittsburgh with scleroderma (SSc), the frequency of breast implants was about the same as that estimated for the U.S. adult female population. The investigators concluded, *"These data fail to support the hypothesis that augmentation mammaplasty with silicone-gel-filled prostheses is a risk factor for the development of SSc."*

University of Washington, Fred Hutchinson Cancer Research Center, Dugowson, MD; Daling, PhD; Koepsell, MD; et al.; Seattle, WA. 1992

Silicone Breast Implants/Rheumatoid Arthritis

A population-based study of 300 women with rheumatoid arthritis and 1,456 similarly aged control women showed, *"These data do not support an increased risk for rheumatoid arthritis among women with silicone breast implants."*

University of California, Weisman, MD; Vecchione, MD; Albert, MD; et al.; San Diego, CA. 1988

Breast Implants/Connective Tissue Disease

The authors followed a group of 125 women from a plastic and cosmetic surgical practice in San Diego and stated, *"Our survey did not reveal a single subject with an inflammatory rheumatic disease or condition following breast augmentation."* They added, *"It does not appear likely that augmentation mammaplasty is a significant or major inducer of inflammatory connective-tissue diseases in general."*

INDEX

IT'S IN THE CARDS

. . . forty cards with essential information for every woman considering breast augmentation . . . excerpted from

The Best Breast
By John B. Tebbetts, MD, & Terrye Tebbetts

John B. Tebbetts, MD
2801 Lemmon Avenue West
Suite 300
Dallas, Texas 75204
(214) 220-2712 office
(214) 969-0933 fax

www.thebestbreast.com
email: email@thebestbreast.com

1

STEPS IN THE QUEST FOR THE BEST BREAST

I—PREPARATION
Whether to even consider augmentation

II—KNOWLEDGE
Arming yourself with information

III—THE BEST DECISIONS
Consulting surgeons and making decisions

IV—THE BEST BREAST
Finalizing decisions and preparing for surgery

2

WHAT'S IN THIS FOR YOU?

If you decide to become a breast augmentation patient, you will get what you deserve . . .

What you get depends on how much you know and how well you make decisions.

It's your choice . . . and your responsibility.

3

DOES IT MAKE SENSE TO EVEN THINK ABOUT IT?

First, answer these questions . . .

- Is the procedure medically safe?
- Are there specific issues in my medical history that I should consider before proceeding?
- Am I just being vain?
- Can I achieve the changes I want any other way?

Then, turn this card over and answer the "Am I, Can I" questions . . .

4

CHOICES

Every woman deserves them, choices of . . .

- Surgeon
- Implant pocket location
- Implant type and size
- Incision location

A surgeon can only offer you choices that surgeon knows how to deliver.

3

DOES IT MAKE SENSE TO EVEN THINK ABOUT IT?

The "Am I, Can I" questions . . .

- Am I willing to do my homework and make my own decisions?
- Am I willing to realistically accept the trade-offs and risks?
- Can I handle the costs or the financial burden?
- Am I willing to use common sense when making my decisions?
- Am I willing to remove my implants if necessary?

If you can answer "yes" to all of these questions, proceed . . .

4

ABOUT CHOICES

No choice or combination of choices is perfect.

Every choice has trade-offs — be sure you know them.

The choices you make now, you will live with your entire life.

CHOOSE CAREFULLY.

1

A LOGICAL SEQUENCE OF STEPS TO THE BEST BREAST:

1. Does it make sense to think about it?
2. What you need to know and how to go about it
3. Desires and reality: what my body will allow me to have
4. Breast implants: the devices and the choices
5. Surgical options: Over/under muscle, incisions
6. Trade-offs, problems and risks
7. Learn about recovery before surgery: what it tells you
8. Who do I call? Finding qualified surgeons
9. Information from surgeons: Getting and evaluating it
10. Consulting with plastic surgeons
11. Finalizing your decisions
12. Preparing for surgery
13. Recovery: What to expect
14. Living with your new breasts
15. Visual lessons in augmentation

2

WHAT'S IN THIS FOR YOU?

The more you are willing to learn . . .

The more you will know . . .

And the better chance you'll make good decisions.

5

DEFINING WHAT YOU DON'T LIKE AND WHAT YOU WANT—A LIST

1. List the things you dislike about your breasts.
2. List how those dislikes affect your feeling of being normal, or how those dislikes affect your lifestyle.
3. List the basics of what you would like to have, based on what you know now.
4. Learn about what your body will allow you to have from chapter 4, reconcile desires with reality, then refine your "want" list.
5. Look at your list carefully, and ask yourself if you're willing to live with your choices long term.
6. Finalize your list of "wants" that you'll discuss with surgeons you'll visit.
7. Don't let your window shopping (looking at pictures in magazines and surgeon's "brag books") fool you about reality and the future. Think about your own tissues.

7

GOLDEN RULES FOR GOOD RESULTS— SHORT AND LONG TERM

- For optimal results, the surgeon must adequately fill the existing breast envelope.
- Any more fill than the least amount of fill required for an optimal aesthetic result will detract from the long-term result.
- The size of implant that will be required to fill a larger, stretched envelope will be larger than the size required to fill a smaller, less stretched envelope.
- The smaller and tighter (unstretched by pregnancies) the envelope, the less implant the envelope can accept and give an aesthetically optimal result.
- No implant will produce the same result in two different patients.
- Regardless of your personal choices and choices dictated by your tissue characteristics, you should be informed and aware of the potential long-term implications of those choices before surgery.
- Perfection is not an option. Human surgeons can only produce improvement.

6

WHAT YOU NEED TO KNOW BEFORE CONSULTING A SURGEON

1. What do I want, and what will my body allow me to have?
2. Implant types and options: Shape, smooth or textured shell, type of filler material
3. Possible complications, risks, trade-offs
4. Implant pocket location: over muscle (retromammary) or partially under muscle (partial retropectoral)
5. Incision location options
6. Implant size
7. Options and trade-offs: Sorting them out
8. Complications and trade-offs: Things you and the surgeon can't control
9. Recovery: Ask about it up front, because what you hear can tell you a lot
10. Organizing your information to use it effectively

8

INESCAPABLE TRUTHS ABOUT BREASTS AND BREAST SIZE

1. Cup size is not even a consistent fashion measurement, let alone a medical term that can accurately and consistently define breast size.
2. Cup size is extremely variable and inconsistent from one brand of bra to another.
3. Women buy a bra that they can fill, not necessarily a bra that fits.
4. Women buy bras to push breast tissue where they want it to go to create a specific appearance.
5. Women don't necessarily buy bras that fit their breasts!
6. A certain number of ccs in an implant does not make a certain cup size breast. The final size of the breast depends on the amount of breast tissue the woman had prior to surgery plus the size of the implant that was placed.
7. A surgeon can only work with the tissues that you bring the surgeon.

Turn the card over for more . . .

HOW TO GO ABOUT GETTING THE BEST BREAST

1 List what you need to know (the topics).

2 Review each topic and learn more details.

3 Armed with knowledge, prepare for surgeon consultations

4 Consult surgeons and evaluate what they tell you (using what you have learned).

5 Choose your surgeon.

6 Select from your options and discuss the trade-offs with your surgeon (TEAM DECISIONS).

7 Think about the choices you've made and the trade-offs you've accepted. Be sure you're comfortable.

8 If you have any questions, talk with your surgeon again. The time to clarify every detail is before, not after, your surgery.

9 Have your surgery, and follow your surgeon's instructions for recovery.

INESCAPABLE TRUTHS ABOUT BREASTS AND BREAST SIZE

8. No woman has two breasts that are the same, and no surgeon can create two breasts that are exactly the same.

9. The bigger the breast, the worse it will look over time (augmented or not)! Think about the woman you knew at a younger age with large breasts. How do they look now? Your tissues won't get better as you age; they will get worse! Think about your grandmother's breasts, or any woman's breasts after age 60.

10. Don't let cup size or implant size in cc's be the ONLY way you define what you want— use measurements and descriptions of appearance!

11. The bigger the breast YOU REQUEST, the worse it will look over time.

12. For the best long-term result, you might want to balance what you want with what your tissues will allow you to have and what your tissues can support over time.

Your surgeon should help you understand the characteristics of your individual tissues and which options are realistic for you.

HOW NOT TO DEFINE YOUR EXPECTATIONS OR WHAT YOU WANT

- **Cup size alone** (using cup size as the only description of what you want)

  Try explaining to yourself what a cup size really is . . .

  If you can't explain it to yourself, how do you expect a surgeon to produce it?

- **Implant size in ccs** (cubic centimeters)

  Do you really know what a certain number of ccs produces?

  Will your tissues accommodate that? How will it look?

  How will that many ccs affect your tissues as you age?

WHAT YOU CAN GET DEPENDS ON WHAT YOU'VE GOT

- A surgeon can only work with the tissues you bring.

- A breast implant enhances what you have by giving you a better version of your current breast. It doesn't give you a totally different, new breast.

- Because a surgeon works with the tissues you bring, you can't pick a breast out of a book or magazine and expect that result unless the woman in the picture looked exactly like you look before surgery.

WINDOW SHOPPING 1— PICTURES IN MAGAZINES

- The only picture that represents true breast characteristics is a picture totally without clothing, standing or lying down.

- If a surgeon looks at a picture and says, "Sure, we can make that breast! No problem!" RUN THE OTHER WAY!

- On the other hand, if the surgeon replies, "Let's look at your tissues and compare you as best we can to the person in the picture," BETTER!

- If the surgeon replies, "I'll use the pictures to help me understand what you'd like, and then I'll try to help you understand our best options and trade-offs, given your tissues," GREAT!

THINGS YOU MIGHT NOT WANT TO HEAR ABOUT BREAST IMPLANTS— BUT REMEMBER WE TOLD YOU!

- Breast implants are not perfect.

- Breast implants don't last forever.

- Breast implants may require some maintenance.

- If you can't accept the imperfections of implants or if you're unwilling to have maintenance, don't have a breast augmentation.

WINDOW SHOPPING 3— COMPUTER IMAGING

- Any trained technician can produce changes on a computer that no surgeon can produce with living tissue. Beware of marketing versus substance.

- If the surgeon uses the imager to help you understand some points, fine. If a technician or the surgeon uses the imager to try to sell you something that doesn't make sense or sell you other nonbreast operations, BEWARE.

- If the surgeon morphs (changes the appearance of) your breasts on the computer and prints you a simulated before-and-after picture, don't look at it too much, and try not to fix the image in your mind. Your result definitely won't match the image exactly.

SURGEONS' OPINIONS ABOUT IMPLANTS

1. The best opinion about implants is an opinion based on experience. *If a surgeon has minimal or no experience with a certain type of implant, the surgeon should preface any opinion with, "I've never used that implant, but here's what I think of it."*

2. If your only tool is a hammer, the whole world looks like a nail.

3. If a surgeon has experience with only one type of implant, that's likely the implant the surgeon will recommend—*hopefully. It's scary to think about the alternative.*

4. The more experience a surgeon has with a variety of implant types, the more options the surgeon can offer you, and the better the surgeon can put those options into a realistic perspective for you.

WINDOW SHOPPING 4—
THE INTERNET

- Read the cards for Window Shopping 1, 2, and 3. Apply all the same principles to images on the Internet.

- Almost all images on the Internet are low-resolution images and cannot compare to images you should see in a surgeon's office.

- All images on the Internet could have easily been modified—you have no way of knowing.

- Never select a surgeon, type of implant, or implant size based on images you see on the Internet. You MUST DO ALL YOUR HOMEWORK described in *The Best Breast* if you expect to get the best result.

PREVIOUS PATIENTS' OPINIONS
ABOUT IMPLANTS

1. Most patients who have had an augmentation will tell you that the type of implant they have is best—otherwise, why would they have it?

   When a patient tells you her type of implant is best, ask why.

2. **The more a previous patient knows, the more in-depth information you'll get. But don't be disappointed if you don't get much.**

   Many patients are never offered options. Many patients don't learn about options on their own.

Calling a surgeon's office, using the checklist we give you, and examining the surgeon's written information will always tell you more than a visit to a surgeon's Web site.

WINDOW SHOPPING 2—
BEFORE-AND-AFTER BOOKS

- If you can find a patient in the book that looks very much like you BEFORE her augmentation, it's possible that you MIGHT be able to look SOMEWHAT like her result AFTER your operation.

- If the surgeon doesn't have pictures to show you, consult other surgeons.

- If every result looks good, consult other surgeons.

- If the book does not contain a wide variety of breasts with some results better than others, consult other surgeons.

- A surgeon's habits are reflected in the quality of the pictures as well as the quality of the results. Are the pictures consistent and well lighted or taken with an instant camera?

WHAT YOU CAN'T CHANGE ABOUT
IMPLANTS AND YOUR TISSUES

1. If you are thin and you can feel your breast with your fingertip, you will probably be able to feel the edges or shell of any state-of-the-art implant in the world today, regardless of its shell thickness.

2. If you have thin tissues, you have thin tissues. You can't change that. Your surgeon can't change that.

3. The thinner you are, the more likely you'll feel some portion of your implants after your augmentation.

4. Since you can't change your thin tissues (gaining weight won't change them enough), if feeling your implant is unacceptable to you, don't have an augmentation.

IMPLANT "NATURALNESS" VERSUS DURABILITY

1. The longer an implant lasts, the fewer reoperations you will need during your lifetime. Reoperations increase risks and costs.

2. There are definite trade-offs between naturalness and durability when it comes to breast implants, given today's biomaterials and technology.

3. If you want your implant to last longer, you'll need to accept some trade-offs in naturalness.

4. The only natural breast is a natural breast. Natural breasts don't contain a breast implant. If you want a TOTALLY natural breast, don't have an augmentation.

5. Naturalness is relative. Naturalness depends on what a woman HAS, what a woman WANTS, and what a woman is WILLING TO ACCEPT in trade-offs.

WHAT YOU CAN'T CHANGE ABOUT IMPLANTS AND YOUR TISSUES

1. If you are thin and you can feel your ribs beneath your breast with your fingertip, you will probably be able to feel the edges or shell of any state-of-the-art implant in the world today, regardless of its shell thickness.

2. If you have thin tissues, you have thin tissues. You can't change that. Your surgeon can't change that.

3. The thinner you are, the more likely you'll feel some portion of your implants after your augmentation.

4. Since you can't change your thin tissues (gaining weight won't change them enough), if feeling your implant is unacceptable to you, don't have an augmentation.

IMPORTANT FACTS ABOUT IMPLANT SHAPE AND FILL VOLUME

Round Implants

- All of today's ROUND implants are UNDERFILLED if filled to manufacturer's recommendations. With virtually all of today's ROUND implants, regardless of the filler material or the size of the implant, shell collapse and folding occur if the implant is filled to the manufacturer's recommendations! Watch for new designs with the SafeFill™ designation that we are currently designing to address this problem.

- Manufacturers believe that surgeons won't use (and therefore won't buy) ROUND implants with more fill because the surgeon feels that the implant is too firm. Manufacturers historically respond to the pressures of their market, like most successful companies.

IMPORTANT FACTS ABOUT IMPLANT SHAPE AND FILL VOLUME

Anatomic Implants 1

- ANATOMIC shaped implants are shaped more like a breast, fuller at the bottom, tapering at the top. All anatomic implants are not the same.

- Because of the tapering upper pole, an ANATOMIC implant can be FILLED ADEQUATELY TO PREVENT THE SHELL FOLDING— without producing an unnatural appearing upper breast.

- Allergan has defined the fill volumes of their ANATOMIC implants higher at the outset—so there is no need for the surgeon to overfill the implant to protect the shell!

Continued on back of this card . . .

WHY IS THE AMOUNT OF FILLER IN YOUR IMPLANT IMPORTANT?

1. The more filler you place in the implant, the less risk of shell folding and premature shell failure.

2. Any folding or collapse of an implant shell should worry you if you want the shell to last as long as possible.

3. The more filler you place in the implant, the firmer the implant—slightly firmer is a trade-off for durability.

4. Exceeding the capacity of an implant shell by a larger amount can cause distortions of the shell.

IMPORTANT FACTS ABOUT IMPLANT SHAPE AND FILL VOLUME

Anatomic Implants 2

1. With an anatomically shaped implant, it is possible to adequately fill the implant to prevent shell collapse and folding, and still produce an optimal aesthetic result.

2. For most first-time augmentation patients, anatomics seem SAFER (less risk of shell folding and early rupture) and MORE EFFECTVE (a more natural result with a full but not excessively bulging upper breast).

3. With Allergan Style 468 (saline filled) AND 410 (silicone cohesive, form-stable gel filled) ANATOMIC implants, you get shell protection without filling past manufacturer's recommendations. AND you keep your warranty—no choosing between the two! No Catch-22!

With ROUND saline implants, you must overfill to prevent shell folding, and overfilling voids the warranty.

WHAT AFFECTS HOW NATURAL AN IMPLANT FEELS?

1. **The thickness of the implant shell**
The thicker the shell, the more durable, but the easier to feel.

2. **The thickness of your tissues that cover the implant**
The thinner your tissues, the more you will feel any implant.

3. **The amount of filler material in the implant**
The less filler in the implant, the softer it will feel, but the greater the risk the shell will fold or ripple, causing premature shell failure.

IMPORTANT FACTS ABOUT IMPLANT SHAPE AND FILL VOLUME

Round Implants

• Surgeons feel that firmer implants (even a tiny bit firmer) are unacceptable to patients . . . *Often without ever having used a significant number of the firmer implants or asking patients which they would prefer, slightly more firmness, or a reoperation sooner?*

• When ROUND implants are filled adequately to prevent shell folding, they look very ROUND, and the upper breast can look excessively bulging, even having a sharp and bulging stepoff. *Although some patients request an unnatural, excessively bulging upper breast, most don't.*

• These principles apply to all ROUND implants, regardless of the filler material in the implant.

Continued on next card . . .

17

IMPORTANT FACTS ABOUT IMPLANT SHAPE AND FILL VOLUME

Anatomic Implants 3

4. A major anatomic implant advance is a filler material (cohesive, form-stable gel) that does not migrate following disruption of the implant shell.

5. The Allergan style 410 cohesive-gel anatomic makes three significant advances:
   1) adequate fill to maximally protect the shell,
   2) a filler that doesn't migrate, and
   3) optimal aesthetic results.

6. An ANATOMIC IMPLANT can maintain fill in the upper breast BETTER THAN A ROUND IMPLANT because the upper pole of the anatomic implant doesn't collapse—it maintains its vertical height.

18

ABOUT NEW IMPLANT DESIGNS . . .

- When betting on implant materials and fillers, don't place your bets on a horse until the horse has a track record.

  If you do, you likely won't be collecting money at the winners' window.

- Don't discard SILICONE-and SALINE-filled implants (in that order) until there is an alternative that has at least 5 years of follow-up in a LARGE number of patients.

- Just because a breast implant design or filler is NEW, it's NOT NECESSARILY BETTER—no matter how promising it may seem.

  If it's really good, it will stand the test of time and prove its worth in peer-reviewed scientific studies.

19

FACTS ABOUT SMOOTH AND TEXTURED SHELL IMPLANTS

- Textured silicone shell implants were developed as an alternative to smooth shell implants to reduce the risk of capsular contracture.

- Textured surface implants have a lower risk of capsular contracture than smooth shell implants.

- The difference between smooth and textured implant capsular contracture rates is more pronounced with silicone gel filled implants than with saline filled implants.

  For criteria to choose smooth or textured, see back of this card

---

20

FACTS TO REMEMBER ABOUT ALL SURGICAL OPTIONS

- **No single set of surgical options is best for every patient.** *If you are offered only one set of options, consult other surgeons.*

- **Every patient tends to think that the options she chose are also the best options for someone else.** That isn't true, because no two women are alike in body or soul. Your tissues are definitely different.

- **No surgical option is perfect. No surgical option is without trade-offs.** The question is whether you know the relative benefits and trade-offs, and pick the options that best maximize the benefits and minimize the trade-offs.

- **If you choose surgical options without thinking about your tissues, you'll need to blame something or someone for the consequences.** You'll probably blame the implant or the surgeon, when it's really you who are largely responsible.

CHOOSING A TEXTURED OR SMOOTH IMPLANT

1. If you choose an ANATOMIC implant, it should be filled with form-stable gel. Ideally, it should be textured.

2. If you choose a ROUND implant, and you want the least risk of capsular contracture, choose a TEXTURED surface.

3. Three good reasons to choose a ROUND, SMOOTH IMPLANT:
   You are having a reoperation— not a first time augmentation. Your surgeon has little or no experience with anatomic implants. You are not concerned about the risk of capsular contracture.

4. Two MYTHS that are NOT BASED ON FACTS:
   1) Textured surface implants have thicker shells and are more easily felt in the breast. Not true! The thickness of your tissues over the implant is much more important than the minimal differences in shell thickness. 2) Smooth shell implants have less rippling than textured surface implant Not true! Rippling is the result of underfilling or traction, not the shell surface.

IN FRONT OF, OR BEHIND MUSCLE— THE FACTS

- Partial retropectoral placement means that the upper portion of the implant is partially covered by the pectoralis major muscle.

- A more perfect aesthetic result is usually possible when an implant in the upper and middle breast placed in front of the muscle in the lower breast. But in thin women, behind muscle is preferable because adequate tissue coverage is most important. Dual-plane placement (under muscle in the upper and middle breast, behind breast tissue in the lower breast) provides the best of both worlds.

IMPORTANT FACTS ABOUT IMPLANT SHAPE AND FILL VOLUME

Anatomic Implants 4

7. Some surgeons find the additional demands of anatomic implants too technically challenging or time consuming, and simply don't offer their patients anatomic implants.

8. Anatomic implants may NOT be the best option for REOPERATION cases until a surgeon has gained considerable experience.

9. Anatomic implants may NOT be the best option for THIN patients who request EXCESSIVELY LARGE IMPLANTS, larger than 350 cc.

10. Anatomic, form-stable implants are ideal for the majority of first-time augmentation patients.

ABOUT THE MANUFACTURER OF YOUR IMPLANTS . . .

- The company that manufactures your breast implants doesn't matter until you need to replace their implants. Will they be there?

- It's easier to assure that you'll have a company's guarantee and support when you need it BEFORE you put their product in your body.

- Look into the company that manufactures your implants BEFORE you have an augmentation, or don't complain later.

21

IN FRONT OF MUSCLE (RETROMAMMARY)— THE ADVANTAGES

1. More precise control of cleavage—the distance between your breasts.

2. More precise control of upper breast fill—especially upper fill toward the middle of your chest.

3. Less chance of muscle pressure pushing your implants to the side over time, widening the distance between your breast.

4. Less chance of distorting your breast shape when you tighten (contract) your pectoralis muscle.

5. Dual-plane placement also provides most of the advantages, with fewer trade-offs.

See the back of this card for the trade-offs . . .

22

IN FRONT OF . . . OR BEHIND MUSCLE— HOW DO YOU CHOOSE?

- If you are extremely thin (less than 2 cm pinch thickness above your breast), you should put the implant behind muscle to assure adequate tissue cover over the implant. *If you don't, you run more risks of seeing the edges of your implant, and risk other long-term problems.*

- If you have adequate thickness of tissues (more than 2 cm pinch thickness above your breast tissue), weigh the advantages and trade-offs listed on other cards and choose above, below, or dual-plane based on your preferences and your surgeon's recommendations.

23

BEHIND MUSCLE: REPECTORAL OR DUAL PLANE

1. The major advantage of placing an implant behind muscle is to prevent implant edge visibility.

2. A second stated advantage of subpectoral placement is better reduction of risks of capsular contracture compared to retromammary placement. *This difference is more marked with silicone-gel implants than with saline implants, risks are about the same.*

3. Better mammograms. *Many radiologists feel that mammograms are more accurate with the implant behind muscle.*

4. Dual plane provides muscle coverage advantages without most of the tradeoffs of traditional retropectoral, and recovery is equivalent to submammary placement.

See the back of this card for the trade-offs . . .

24

THE INFRAMAMMARY (UNDER THE BREAST) INCISION

- The greatest advantage of an incision beneath the breast is the degree of control it allows the surgeon in a wide range of breast types. *More augmentation patients have had this incision location than all other incision locations combined!*

- The greatest trade-off of an inframammary incision is the presence of a scar in the fold beneath the breast.

23

BEHIND MUSCLE (RETROPECTORAL)—THE TRADE-OFFS

- Distortion of breast shape when you tighten (contract) your pectoralis muscle; occurs much less with dual plane.

- Shifting of the implants to the side over time, widening the distance between the breasts; occurs much less with dual plane.

- Less control of upper breast fill, especially upper and toward the middle; also less with dual plane.

- More stretch of the lower breast tissues over time. Usually not a big issue, but the muscle puts pressure on the upper implant, transmitting more pressure to the lower envelope; much less risk with dual plane.

- Increased risk of upward displacement of the implant if muscle origins are not adjusted along the fold; almost nonexistent with dual plane.

See the front of this card for the benefits . . .

24

THE PERIAREOLAR (AROUND THE NIPPLE-AREOLA) INCISION

- The greatest advantage of an incision around the areola is that it's located in thinner skin that usually heals well, provided the areola is large enough for access.

- The greatest trade-offs of a periareolar incisions are increased exposure of the implant to bacteria normally found in the breast, and (if you develop a bad scar) a scar located on the most visible location on the breast.

21

IN FRONT OF MUSCLE (RETROMAMMARY)—THE TRADE-OFFS

1. If you are extremely thin, this location may not provide adequate soft tissue cover to prevent your seeing the edges of your implant, especially as you get older and your tissue quality declines and tissues become thinner.

2. This location may make your mammograms more difficult.

See the front of this card for the benefits . . .

22

INCISION LOCATION—IMPORTANT FACTS

1. Most patients worry far more about incision location before the surgery than they care after the surgery (provided they have a good result).

2. If you have a beautiful breast and normal healing, neither you nor anyone else will care where the incision is located.

3. Every patient thinks that the incision location that she has is best.

4. Incision location is a common way that surgeons use to market their augmentation practice. *They may know how to use only one incision.*

5. If a surgeon is experienced with all incision locations, the surgeon will offer you all options.

6. No incision location is always best—each location has advantages and trade-offs.

See additional cards for advantages and trade-offs of each incision location . . .

THE AXILLARY (IN THE ARMPIT) INCISION

- The greatest advantage of an incision in the armpit is that its location makes it the least visible of all scars for augmentation.

- The greatest trade-off of axillary incisions is that a surgeon must be experienced, and the operation time is usually slightly longer (if the surgeon uses state-of-the-art techniques).

- The armpit incision is best for first-time augmentation—if a procedure is necessary later, another approach is better.

BASIC FACTS ABOUT RISKS

- The more you know about what to expect and what is normal, the less confused or frightened you will be when it occurs.

- It's a TEAM JOB to assure that you know what to expect after surgery.

- It's your surgeon's and your surgeon's staff's responsibility to provide information for you. It's your responsibility to use it!

- Every breast augmentation operation carries inherent risks. Medical complications are not totally preventable by you or your surgeon.

- Do not have an augmentation mammaplasty unless you thoroughly understand and accept the potential risks and trade-offs of the procedure.

SURGICAL TECHNIQUES FOR CREATING THE POCKET

BLUNT DISSECTION techniques for creating the implant pocket create *more tissue trauma, tear tissues, create more bleeding, and result in a longer recovery time.* State-of-the-art ELECTROCAUTERY DISSECTION techniques are less traumatic and have a shorter recovery time.

Dissection technique is a major factor that affects your recovery. *The more trauma (blunt dissection), the longer and more difficult the recovery.*

QUESTIONS TO ASK ABOUT RECOVERY BEFORE YOU CHOOSE A SURGEON!

- What will my recovery be like?

- Will I have bruising?

- Will I have drain tubes coming out of my body?

- When can I return to normal activities? Drive my car, lift normal objects, arms above my head?

- When can I bathe?

- Do I need special bandages, bras, or binders?

- When can I return to athletic activities?

- The better the answers to these questions, the better you'll like your recovery . . . and likely your result!

THE UMBILICAL (IN THE BELLY BUTTON) INCISION

- **The main advantage** of an incision in and around the belly button is that the incision is located off the breast.

- **The main disadvantages** of the umbilical incision compared to other incisions are: *It offers the surgeon the LEAST CONTROL of all incisional locations and the LEAST PREDICTABLE RESULTS, and it causes the MOST TISSUE TRAUMA* because more normal tissues are disturbed to get to the breast.

- Access to the breast is created by bluntly pushing a one-inch diameter tube from the umbilicus to each breast, through the tissues of the upper abdomen.

- **The pocket for the implant is developed BLINDLY by inserting an expander and/or tearing tissue to create a pocket.** Most surgeons who use the umbilical approach do not offer implant placement behind muscle. If you are thin, behind muscle is better long term.

TRADE-OFFS AND SURPRISES

TRADE-OFFS always depend on the details of each specific case. The characteristics of your tissues can significantly affect the trade-offs.

The experience of your surgeon with different options can significantly affect the trade-offs.

After a surgeon examines you, be sure to ask about specific trade-offs and how they relate to your specific tissues and the surgeon's experience with different options.

SURPRISES: If it's a surprise, it's a problem.

A surprise can be something you don't know about that confuses or frightens you, OR . . .

A surprise can be a medical complication that causes untoward medical events.

IF PROBLEMS OCCUR, DEAL WITH THEM

- The best way to deal with a problem is to deal with it—now!

- There isn't a surgeon alive who wants an unhappy patient. Keep your lines of communication open!

- No surgeon can solve a problem unless the surgeon is aware that a problem exists!

- Most of the best surgeons will encourage you to seek another opinion—don't hesitate to ask!

RECOVERY: WHAT IS POSSIBLE?

- No bruising, no bandages, no special bras, no drain tubes coming out of your body, no limitation of normal activity from day one.

- Resume full, normal activity the first day after surgery—raise arms above your head, lift normal weight objects, drive your car.

- Shower and wash your hair immediately.

- All of the above true in over 90 percent of our patients even if the implant is behind muscle.

CHOOSING YOUR SURGEON IS YOUR RESPONSIBILITY!

- Many patients spend more time shopping for a car than they spend selecting a plastic surgeon!

- It's your body—you'll be looking at it for the rest of your life.

- It's your job to select your surgeon. Don't complain later if you neglect your responsibilities.

- Selecting your surgeon is the single most important thing you can do to assure an optimal result!

THREE THINGS TO LISTEN FOR WHEN YOU CALL A SURGEON'S OFFICE

Listen for three things in your first call to the office:

COURTESY, KNOWLEDGE, SERVICE

"I want to make this easy for you. Let's get started!"

A CHECKLIST FOR SURGEON CREDENTIALS

Essentials:

- Board certified by the American Board of Plastic Surgery
- Completed an approved residency training program in plastic surgery
- Member of ASPRS and ASAPS (professional societies)
- Has hospital privileges to do breast augmentation at an accredited hospital
- Curriculum vitae documents scientific presentations and publications

Cream on top of the essentials:

- Subspecializes in cosmetic surgery
- Subspecializes in breast augmentation
- Listed in *Who's Who*
- Listed in *Best Doctors in America*
- Recommended by a knowledgeable friend or physician

Not as reliable:

- Advertisements
- Media coverage
- General physician-referral services (most are paid by the surgeon to refer you)
- Recommendations from anyone without in-depth knowledge about augmentation

Red flags:

- Completed residency training in a specialty other than plastic surgery
- Certified in an unrelated specialty
- Not board certified by ABPS
- No hospital privileges
- Any false or misleading information—claims that aren't true
- Unwilling to answer questions about credentials
- Unwilling to provide access to curriculum vitae

WHEN YOU CALL A SURGEON—
A LIST OF BASIC QUESTIONS

When you ask the following questions, stop talking and listen carefully to the answers! Take notes, and keep the answers organized by surgeon. The answers are key to your making good decisions when selecting a surgeon:

1. I'm interested in getting some information about breast augmentation. Does Dr. X do breast augmentation?

2. How does Dr. X do breast augmentation?

3. Could you send me some information about breast augmentation and about Dr. X and your practice?

4. What are the risks involved in having breast augmentation?

5. Do you offer free consultations?

6. Do you have before-and-after photographs that I could see?

7. Would it be possible to speak with other patients of Dr. X who have had augmentations?

8. How long has Dr. X been in practice?

9. How many augmentations does Dr. X do every year?

10. Does Dr. X limit his practice to cosmetic surgery?

11. Where does Dr. X have hospital privileges?

12. Is Dr. X board certified? By which board?

13. How much will my augmentation cost?

HOW TO LOCATE SURGEONS
CERTIFIED BY THE AMERICAN BOARD
OF PLASTIC SURGERY

- The *American Society of Plastic and Reconstructive Surgeons* at

  www.plasticsurgery.org

  or call at **1-888-4-PLASTIC (1-888-475-2784).**

- The *American Society of Aesthetic Plastic Surgery* at

  www.surgery.org

  or call **1-888-ASAPS-11 (1-888-272-7711)**

RED FLAGS WHEN YOU CALL
A SURGEON'S OFFICE

- Not courteous

- No knowledgeable

- Not willing to spend time with you

- Not telling you what you need to know

- Telling you all fluff, no substance

- No offer to send information

- No offer for consultation with patient educator for no charge

ARE YOU READY FOR A CONSULTATION?

If you can check all of the items on the following checklist, you're ready to consult with a plastic surgeon!

☐ I've read Chapters 1 through 10.

☐ I made a list of surgeons and verified credentials.

☐ I called surgeons' offices and requested informational materials.

☐ I evaluated surgeons' staffs on the phone.

☐ I've gathered information from at least three surgeons with solid credentials, good informational materials, and knowledgeable staffs.

☐ I took advantage of visits with patient educators.

☐ I've made a specific list of questions I want to ask the surgeon.

PRICING AND COSTS: KEY TIPS

- If a surgeon offers a "package price," always insist that the price be broken down into the categories listed on the back of this card.

- If you don't, you won't be able to analyze what you're paying for and compare to other surgeons! See Chapter 13.

- Always ask for a written quote for costs, signed by the surgeon or a staff member.

- And ask how long the prices on the quote apply!

HOW TO EVALUATE WRITTEN INFORMATION YOU RECEIVE

A surgeon's habits are reflected in everything a surgeon does—all you need to do is notice!
Informational materials reflect a surgeon's habits and commitment to educating patients.

Is the information generic, or did the surgeon write the information personally?
If it's generic, you can tell—you'll probably see the same thing from other surgeons.

Does it appear and sound distinctively different compared to other surgeons' information?
If it doesn't sound different, it probably isn't much different! What might that say about your result?

What do the informational materials tell you about the surgeon's habits?
Is the surgeon compulsive enough to be different? Better? What might that say about your surgery?

Does the information contain substance, or just fluff?
If you took away the fancy look, what does it SAY? Fluff with little substance? What might that say about the surgeon?

Does the information address most or all of your questions and concerns? How well?
If only 50 percent of the answers are there, what might that say about the percent of knowledge?

Is the information written in language that is easy to understand? At the same time, is it informative?
If not, why not?

PREPARING TO CONSULT A SURGEON

If you have an opportunity to consult a patient educator before consulting the surgeon—DO IT! *The best surgeons will almost always offer this service—they want you to know as much as possible.*

The more PREPARED you are BEFORE meeting with a surgeon, the better you'll understand the surgeon, and the better you can evaluate the surgeon.

COSTS: A CHECKLIST OF QUESTIONS TO ASK

- Surgeon fees
- Laboratory fees (for lab work prior to surgery)
- Electrocardiogram fees (if needed)
- Mammogram fees (if surgeon requires mammogram)
- Surgery facility fees
- Costs of implants
- Anesthesia fees
- Medications fees or costs (for before and after surgery)
- Any other fees

SEEING WHAT THEY DON'T TELL YOU—THINGS TO NOTICE

You're not going to a museum or estate—you're going to see a surgeon. *Statues, art, and expensive furniture don't tell you a thing about the quality of surgery you'll get—but guess who gets to pay for the décor—you!*

A quiet, comfortable atmosphere that reflects good taste is all that's required—anything more, and you're paying extra for the décor. *You want to spend your money on the surgeon, not the decorator.*

If the office looks like it may not belong to a plastic surgeon—there's a message. *An overly "medical" appearing office is not typical of cosmetic surgery offices—do you want someone operating on you that doesn't do those procedures very often?*

The organization, function and flow of every surgeon's office is a reflection of the surgeon's habits. *Ask yourself if you want someone with these habits operating on you!*

Are they trying to inform me or trying to sell me?

Evaluating Surgeons You Consult—Key Questions

You'll recognize a great surgeon without the surgeon's having to tell you!
How much substance is behind what you see and hear?

Caring, thoroughness, and substance definitely contribute to what you'll get in the operating room. *How much of each did the surgeon have?*

Remind yourself: This person will be changing my body forever, and I'll look at it every day! *Are you comfortable?*

Were you offered options? A surgeon can't offer what the surgeon doesn't know how to do! *There is definitely NOT one best way to do an augmentation if you know all the different ways!*

Were you told there was only one best way? *Ask yourself why!*

Did you honestly and frankly discuss complications and what would be done? *If the worst occurred, would you want this person to take care of you?*

QUESTIONS TO ASK EVERY SURGEON DURING A CONSULTATION

☐ In what specialty was your residency training? How many years? Are you board certified? By whom?

☐ How long have you been in practice?

☐ Do you have hospital privileges? Where?

☐ How many breast augmentations have you done, and how many do you perform each year?

☐ What are the three most important things you'd advise me to think about with regard to breast augmentation?

☐ What is your preferred incision location? Why? How many of each location have you done? Can you show me pictures?

☐ Which do you prefer, over or under muscle? Why? Do you do both? How many of each have you done?

☐ What is your preferred implant? Why? Do you offer all different types of implants?

☐ Do you prefer round or anatomic implants? Why? Do you offer both? How many of each have you done?

☐ If you prefer round implants, how do you deal with the fill issue?

☐ Are round implants adequately filled (saline or silicone) to prevent shell folding?

☐ Do you think shell folding can affect the life of the shell?

☐ If we overfill a round implant, are you willing to guarantee the implant if the manufacturer does not?

QUESTIONS TO ASK EVERY SURGEON DURING A CONSULTATION (CONTINUED)

☐ What are the three worst things that can happen following my augmentation? What are the chances they will happen? Exactly what do we do in each case if they happen? What are the costs involved? Time off work, worst possible scenario?

☐ Would you ever recommend implant removal without replacement? If so, why? What affects how my breast will look if we had to remove implants?

☐ Does the size of the implant we choose affect my tissues as I get older? How?

☐ Do you charge me to replace my implant if it ruptures? Is there anything that can occur that you would charge me for in the future, including follow-up visits or surgery?

☐ Will anyone else be performing any part of my surgery? Are they more qualified than you?

☐ When can I lift my arms above my head, drive my car, and lift my children or other objects?

☐ Will I have drains?

☐ Will I have bruising?

☐ Will I wear special bandages, bras, or binders? For how long?

☐ Why should I choose you to do my surgery?

PUTTING IT ALL TOGETHER: FINALIZING YOUR CHOICES

The decisions and the sequence

Who is my surgeon?

- ☐ Dr. X
- ☐ Dr. Y
- ☐ Dr. Z

Which pocket location?

- ☐ Retromammary (behind breast tissue only)
- ☐ Partial retropectoral (behind the pectoralis muscle)
- ☐ Total muscle coverage (behind pectoralis and serratus muscles)

What type and size implant?

- ☐ Smooth
- ☐ Textured
- ☐ Round
- ☐ Anatomic
- ☐ Size

Which incision location?

- ☐ Inframammary
- ☐ Periareolar
- ☐ Axillary
- ☐ Umbilical

SURGICAL ARRANGEMENTS CHECKLIST

- ☐ Select a date for surgery.
- ☐ Review surgeon's financial policies and policies for refunds.
- ☐ Pay scheduling deposit if surgeon requires.
- ☐ Sign informed consent documents and operative consent forms.
- ☐ Review and sign implant manufacturer's documents:
  - ☐ Implant package insert,
  - ☐ Terms of implant guarantee,
  - ☐ Verify that surgeon will register your implants with the national implant registry.
- ☐ Schedule lab tests and mammography.
- ☐ Review medications to avoid and medications to take before surgery.
- ☐ Review instructions for the night before surgery.
- ☐ Review instructions for the day of surgery.

Before Surgery Checklist

- ☐ Read all informed consent documents and operative permits carefully—well in advance of your surgery.
- ☐ Be sure that your surgeon is aware of all medications that you are taking!
- ☐ Avoid all medications that contain aspirin for at least two weeks prior to surgery. *Read the labels carefully for all over-the-counter medications; many contain aspirin.*
- ☐ Be very careful about herbs and herbal medicines. *If you are using any herbal preparations, discuss them with your surgeon.*
- ☐ Never eat or drink ANYTHING after midnight the night before surgery. *If you do, material in your stomach can cause you to regurgitate, aspirate, and possibly die during surgery!*

THE DAY OF SURGERY . . . A CHECKLIST

☐ Wear very comfortable clothing (like a jogging suit) that buttons or zips up the front. *You won't enjoy tugging something on over your head!*

☐ Make arrangements for someone to drive you home from the surgery facility and be with you overnight. *You'll receive medications that make driving yourself unsafe!*

☐ Leave off your eye makeup—otherwise, you'll wake up with it in your eyes! *Protective eye lubricants during surgery make a total mess of makeup.*

☐ Leave your jewelry and valuables at home!

THE ESSENTIALS OF RECOVERY

• Your individual pain tolerance, motivation, and ability to follow instructions will affect your recovery.

• Adopt a positive attitude, follow instructions, and get well sooner!

• The easier your surgeon expects your recovery to be, the shorter the list of postoperative instructions!

• The more the surgeon can do in the operating room, the less you'll be burdened with after surgery!

• Don't try to outthink your surgeon! Follow your surgeon's instructions!

• Don't follow your friend's postoperative instructions if she had a different surgeon.

RECOVERY:
THE MOST IMPORTANT DO'S

☐ Follow your surgeon's instructions—to the letter! Don't try to outthink your surgeon!

☐ Stay hydrated. Drink plenty of fluids for the first few days after surgery.

☐ Eat. And eat well! You need nutrition to heal!

☐ Never take any pain medication on an empty stomach—it'll get even emptier!

☐ Resume normal activity as soon as possible following your surgeon's instructions.

Continued on the back of this card . . .

WHAT'S NOT NORMAL—
CONTACT YOUR SURGEON

If you develop any of the following, you should contact your surgeon:

☐ Fever higher than 102 degrees or fever with chills

☐ One breast that is much, much larger than the other

☐ One breast that appears much more bruised than the other

☐ Noticeable redness and tenderness in any area of the breast

☐ Any drainage from your incision area after three days

☐ Any unusual discomfort

☐ Any other symptoms that your surgeon advises you to call about

RECOVERY:
THE MOST IMPORTANT DON'TS

Your surgeon may give you a longer list of things to avoid, but the following is a basic checklist of don'ts that we use following augmentation:

☐ Avoid any type of aerobic activities (anything that creates a significant increase in your pulse) for two weeks—walking is OK; fast walking is not; sex is OK; olympic sex is not.

☐ Don't lift heavy objects (over 30–40 lbs) or strain hard for two weeks. (And watch those pain pills, they can constipate you.)

• Avoid whatever else your surgeon tells you to avoid.

WHAT TO EXPECT THAT'S NORMAL

If you know what to expect that's normal, you'll be less frightened or concerned!

☐ They don't match! My breasts are different size and shape! And they're different every day!

☐ They're too high! ☐ They're too big! ☐ They're too tight!

☐ They're too swollen! ☐ They're too firm!

☐ I hear sloshing inside my breasts!

☐ They don't move!

☐ They're numb or they're too sensitive or I have weird sensations!

☐ I can't lie on them—they feel like basketballs!

☐ My waist has disappeared!

☐ The magic time when they'll feel like they belong to me is 3 months!

DURABILITY AND IMPLANT RUPTURE . . .

• You don't need to "baby" your implants—they should with stand any type of normal, vigorous activity.

• However, your implants were not designed to withstand closed capsulotomy, the practice of forcefully squeezing your breast to correct capsular contracture.

• If you ever have any type of problem with implant deflation or rupture, insist on a qualified surgeon.

• Implant deflation or rupture is no big deal if your surgeon knows how to deal with it.

RECOVERY:
THE MOST IMPORTANT DO'S (CONT'D.)

☐ Read your postoperative instruction sheets. They'll help you expect what's normal.

☐ Expect to be frustrated that your tissues don't change according to your schedule.

☐ Expect to be too big, too high, and too tight for a few weeks.

☐ Expect differences and constant changes in size and shape of your breasts for 3–6 weeks.

☐ Get out of the house and do something; staring does not reduce swelling and tightness.

☐ If anything seems wrong, check your written instructions and information; then call your surgeon.